AMERICAN DOCTORS
IN
CANTON

AMERICAN DOCTORS
IN
CANTON

MODERNIZATION IN CHINA, 1835-1935

GUANGQIU XU

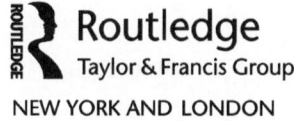

Routledge
Taylor & Francis Group

NEW YORK AND LONDON

First published in paperback 2024

First published 2011 by Transaction Publishers

Published 2017 by Routledge
605 Third Avenue, New York, NY 10158

and by Routledge
4 Park Square, Milton Park, Abingdon, Oxon OX14 4RN

Routledge is an imprint of the Taylor & Francis Group, an informa business

Library of Congress Catalog Number: 2010051386

Library of Congress Cataloging-in-Publication Data
Xu, Guangqiu, 1951-
American doctors in Canton : modernization in China, 1835-1935 / Guangqiu Xu.
    p. ; cm.
Includes bibliographical references.
ISBN 978-1-4128-1829-2
1. Missionaries, Medical—China—Guangzhou—History. 2. Missionaries, Medical—United States—History. I. Title.
[DNLM: 1. Missions and Missionaries—history—China. 2. Missions and Missionaries—history—United States. 3. History, 19th Century—China. 4. History, 19th Century—United States. 5. History, 20th Century—China. 6.
History, 20th Century—United States. 7. Physicians—China. 8. Physicians—United States. W 323]
R722.X84 2011
610.690951'275—dc22
                        2010051386

ISBN: 978-1-4128-1829-2 (hbk)
ISBN: 978-1-03-292126-6 (pbk)
ISBN: 978-1-315-08266-0 (ebk)

DOI: 10.4324/9781315082660

Contents

Note on Transliteration

This book uses pinyin romanization, a system that is applied to Chinese names of persons, places, and terms. However, some popular names have traditional Wade-Giles spellings appealing in parenthesis, and traditional spellings are used for place names and personal names that are long familiar in the West or difficulty to recognize in pinyin. Thus, Canton is retained in preference to Guangzhou, and Sun Yat-sen is used rather than Sun Zhongshan. Names in Taiwan and Hong Kong are not within the pinyin system.

As a convention in this book, total transliteration is employed for Chinese personal names, which means that surnames are in front of given names, exactly as they are in Chinese. For example, in the name of Kang Youwei, Kang is the surname, and Youwei is the given name.

Acknowledgments

I have been interested in medicine for several decades. My father was a physician of Western medicine, who had practiced medicine for more than forty years in China. During the Second World War, he served in the Nationalist army as major physician. After the war, he returned to Guangzhou (Canton) and worked at the Fangbian Hospital in 1946 (Called the First Municipal Hospital of Guangzhou after 1950) until he retired in the 1980s. My father's elder brother and two younger sisters were famous physicians of Chinese medicine or Western medicine. My wife and my younger brother were physicians of Western medicine in China, too.

I had a dream of becoming a doctor, but the Chinese Cultural Revolution destroyed my dream because all schools and universities in China were closed during the period of 1966-68 when I was a middle-school student. Thereafter, I spent four years working in the countryside and seven years working at the railroad station. In 1979, when Deng Xiaoping restored the national entry examination, I passed the examination and was admitted to the Sun Yat-sen University in Guangzhou. I was forced to choose history as my major because it was hard for me to compete with other young students to take medicine as a major. My dream was not realized, but I am very happy that our elder son, Jimmy Xu, will graduate from the Medical College of the University of Arkansas in 2011 and our younger son, Jack Xu, who already took the MCAT, may go to medical school in 2012.

When doing research in Guangzhou, I identified a lot of resource materials relating to American medical missionaries in southern China in the nineteenth and twentieth centuries. As a result, I started doing research in 2005 on American medical missionaries' activities and their medical, social, and political impact on modernization in China generally and in Guangzhou particularly.

I have incurred a number of debts in completing this book. I am appreciative of the suggestions and comments of Professor Tony Clark, Dr. Alex Magoun, Dr. Sibing He, and Antonia Clark, who read and commented on all or part of the manuscript. They criticized style and substance, guided me on points of detail, and helped me reshape my conceptual framework.

I am grateful to the archivists and staff of Guangdong Provincial Archives in Guangzhou, Guangzhou Municipal Archives in Guangzhou, the Special Collection of Sun Yat-sen Library of Guangdong Province, Sun Yat-sen University Library in Guangzhou, the Special Collections of Hong Kong Baptist University Library, the Special Collections of National Library of China in Beijing, the Special Collection of the Library of Hubei Province, and the Special Collections of Shanghai Library. I am also grateful to the archivists and staff of the Presbyterian Historical Society in Philadelphia, the U.S. National Library of Medicine, and the Asian Collections of Library of Congress. Without their support, this book would not have been possible.

I am thankful to Friends University. The faculty research grants of Friends University enabled me to conduct field studies in China. Without such financial support, this project would have been uncompleted. The reference staff of the Edmund Stanley Library of Friends University helped obtain materials through interlibrary loan.

I am also very grateful to Dr. Irving Horowitz, chairman of the board and editorial director of Transaction Publishers, Rutgers University, and the Board. Without their support, this book would have been impossible. In particular, I am very grateful to Andrew McIntosh, senior editor at Transaction Publishers. He did an excellent job and made this book much better.

Finally, I would like to thank my wife, Nanping Wang, and our two sons, Jimmy and Jack Xu, for their support of my project. Unsurprisingly, the opinions in this book are entirely mine and should not be ascribed to the individuals and institutions acknowledge above.

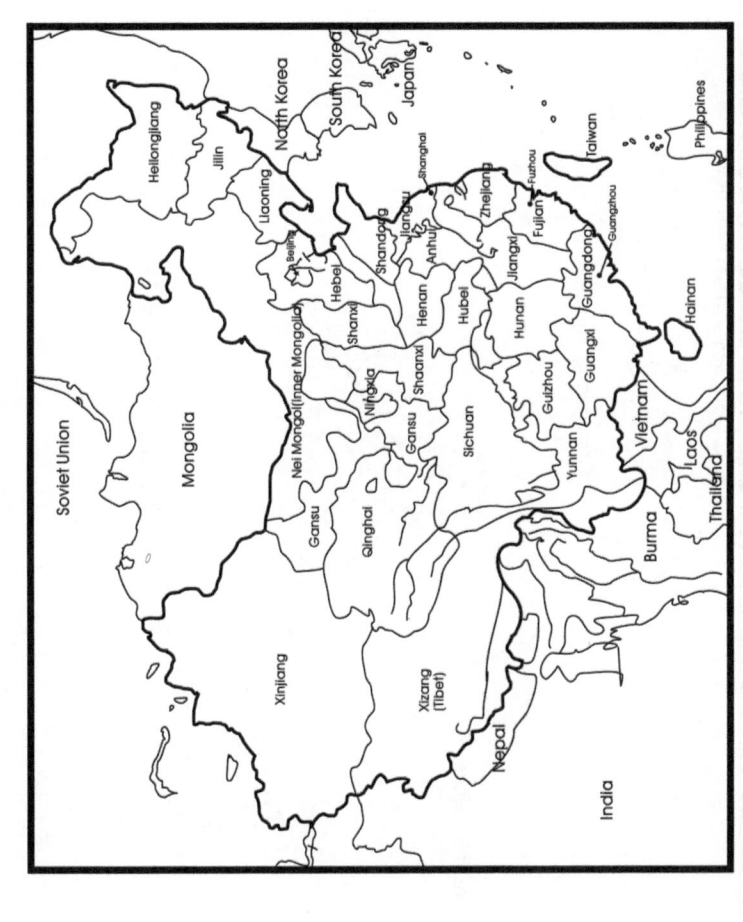

Modern China

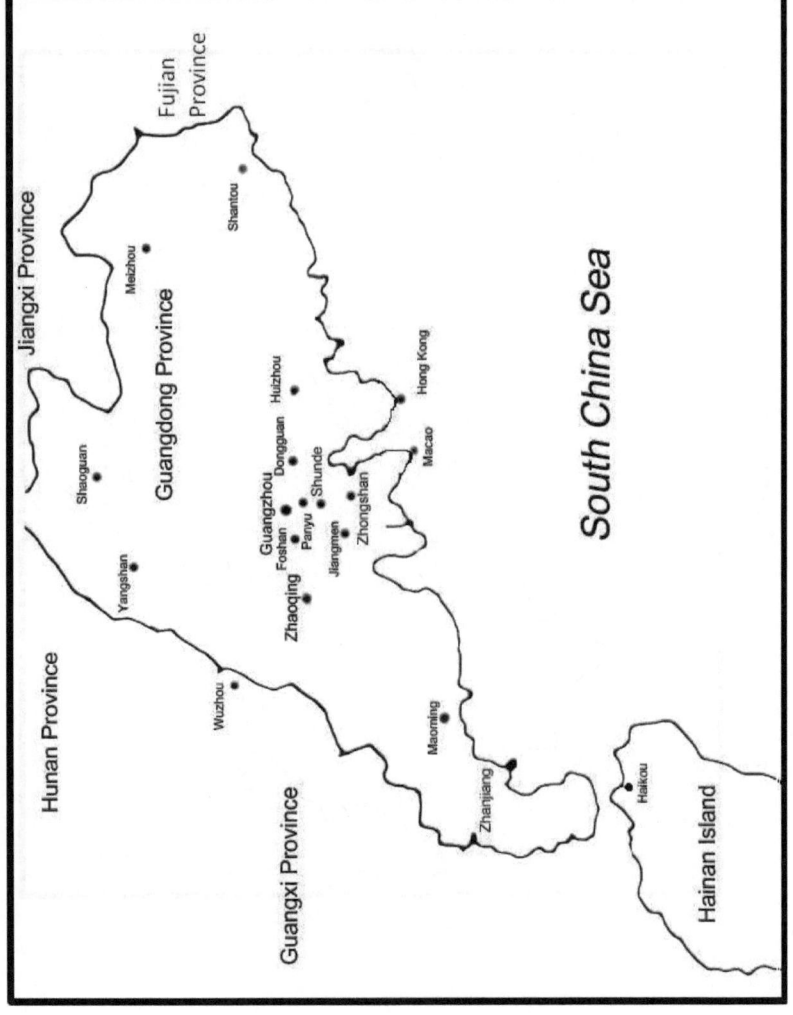

Modern Guangdong

Introduction

Traditional Chinese medicine has a unique theoretical and practical approach to the treatment of disease, which has developed over thousands of years. Traditional treatments include herbal remedies, acupuncture, acupressure and massage, and moxibustion. Chinese physicians had many concepts in large medical writings to clarify the reasons for numerous sicknesses. Chinese medicine is drawn from massive Chinese *materia medica* and native products: medications often contain as many as a dozen ingredients. China's traditional medical education was under the apprenticeship system—often a number of tutors were teaching a student. Until the late Qing Dynasty (1644-1911), most Chinese still had trust in traditional Chinese methods of healing sickness.

According to Western doctors, Chinese medicine was nonscientific because under that system there was little specificity in therapeutics. Since the Chinese believed that the human body, a holy treasure given by their parents, should not be marred in this life and for the spiritual life afterward, dissection was prohibited in traditional China. Thus Westerners believed the Chinese knew little of anatomy because a comprehensive understanding of the construction and function of the human body was impractical to acquire in traditional China.

Western medicine began to expand its scientific base with the first reliable human dissection in 1543 and the discovery of the circulation of the blood later. In the mid-sixteenth century, Western medicine was introduced into the Chinese empire, beginning in 1557 when the Portuguese occupied Macao, which is situated on the coast, less than one hundred miles southwest of Canton (Guangzhou), the capital of Guangdong Province. They set up a hospital and a leprosarium later because Western doctors and dispensaries were allowed in Macao because Christianity was not extinguished as a barbarian faith and Westerners were not considered as uncultured human beings.

Canton's first contact with Western medical practices occurred in 1685 when a surgeon of the British East India Company healed a wounded man in that city. During the eighteenth century, the surgeons of the East India Company continued treating Chinese occasionally. Sent out by the London

1

Missionary Society, Dr. J. Livingston, an East India Company surgeon, and Dr. Robert Morrison, the first Protestant missionary to China, opened a hospital in 1820 at Macao for poor Chinese. Dispatched as an assistant surgeon in 1826 by the East India Company, Dr. Thomas R. Colledge started an ophthalmic dispensary in Macao in 1827 for the therapy of impoverished Chinese, specializing in eye diseases. After taking care of over four thousand patients, he closed the hospital in 1832 and then opened a dispensary at Canton for both foreigners and Cantonese.[1]

American Medical Missionaries in Canton

Assuming that medical doctors would be welcomed when preachers and teachers were hardly accepted in imperial China, the Presbyterian Church in America began to dispatch ordained doctors to China. In accordance with the Presbyterian Church, the practice of medicine by missionaries was considered an evangelistic strategy aimed at securing the confidence of potential converts. Missionaries believed that medicine was a way to lessen physical suffering and to provide the missionaries a chance to talk with their Chinese patients about Christianity; otherwise, the Chinese would stay away from Westerners. Missionary medicine in the Chinese empire thus had a two-fold purpose: to assuage illness and to inform the Chinese of a Christian God who had died for their sins.

American medical missionaries began to establish modern clinics and hospitals and opened medical schools, laying the foundations of modern medicine in China. In Canton, Dr. Peter Parker established China's first Western hospital (The Ophthalmic Hospital) in 1835. Dr. John Kerr founded China's first medical school (The South China Medical School) in 1869 and first mental hospital (Kerr's Refuge for the Insane) in 1898, and Drs. Mary Niles and Mary Fulton opened a dispensary for women and children in 1885 and the Hackett Medical College for Women in 1899, China's first Western medical institution for women. American missionary doctors played a significant role in introducing modern medicine into Canton, which thereafter initiated a transformation of medicine in China.

American doctors were facing many difficulties in Canton. First, the Qing government enforced legal obstacles. Since 1745, the mobility of foreigners in China had been strictly confined by the imperial laws. Canton was the single harbor not closed to international trade in China, and merchants and missionaries were compelled to stay segregated in a limited area—a number of houses about one-fourth mile square with an open space in front. Westerners faced resentment and antagonism, not only from Mandarin administrators, but also from Hong compradors, despite their extensive relations with foreigners. The Qing court banned strictly any relationship between the Chinese and non-Chinese: the Chinese were not allowed to help non-Chinese study Chinese language, and foreigners were forbidden to publish Chinese books. Thus American medical missionaries in Canton worked with great difficulties.

Second, China's traditional rejection of interaction with the Western world was one major obstacle to missionaries' medical practices in China. As the supreme "Middle Kingdom" for many centuries, imperial China scornfully rebuffed every approach made by "Western barbarians." Medical missionaries had to prevail over Chinese mistrust, apprehension, and bias towards what Westerners had done, especially to combat Chinese ignorance of medical practices. The Cantonese later had a positive attitude toward Western medicine, but American doctors, who had to overcome the ancient Chinese superstitions, occasionally heard many nasty rumors regarding their horrifying treatments of the Chinese patients.

Third, official restriction against dissection obstructed Americans' efforts to conduct autopsies and surgeries and to instruct the Chinese in anatomy. Autopsy, partition of the human body, or amputation of any of its parts during life, was still illegal in nineteenth-century China due to both religious and nonreligious cultural attitudes.

Finally, Chinese physicians were not respected by Confucian scholars and the position of Chinese medicine was low in a society dominated by Confucian teachings. The powerful and esteemed system of traditional Chinese medicine remained a principal obstruction for the American medical missionaries in their efforts to introduce Western medicine.[2]

Despite such obstacles and difficulties, American medical missionaries transferred and advanced a broad range of Western medical services and activities to promote the development and popularity of Western medicine in China, including the formation of hospitals, dispensaries and clinics, the opening of medical schools and training of modern doctors, and the promotion of public health education. American medical missions' strategies had several aspects. The first or the most basic one was hospital and dispensary services, the second was medical education, and the third one public health promotion.

The introduction, diffusion, and growth of modern Western medicine, as a technology and a part of Western learning, began to permeate into Canton and cause intense effects on Chinese medical patterns, thoughts, and performances. As the center for interaction between Chinese and Western cultures, Canton became the first noteworthy city for the distribution and practice of Western medicine. By the end of the nineteenth century, Western medicine had secured a firm grip in China. After helping lay the foundation of modern medicine in China, medical missionaries continued carrying out this work devotedly in the twentieth century, and by the 1930s medical schools and hospitals under missionary and other foreign patronage had secured a very important position in the Republic of China.

The Study of Medical Missionaries in China

The role of medical missionaries in China's modernization aroused increasing academic interest, and many books have been published in the past three decades.[3] The study of medical missionaries are found in memoirs of individual medical missionaries, historical articles on Christian missions in China, records of Christian work in rural renovation of China, debate on medical modernization in China, and so on. Ralph Croizier's book points out that medical modernization in China called for institutional and social change, which the Nanjing government was powerless and reluctant to commence, and that the resources of private and religious organizations to sustain the increasing cost of modern medical institutions were limited; the deadly flaw in the missionary effort to start medical modernization was a lack of government involvement.[4] Peter Buck presents the medical missionaries' major efforts as an endeavor to set up the authority of modern medicine, its institutions, and its practitioners in Chinese society, which traditionally assigned a very low position to physicians. Buck argues that, to do this, the medical missionaries generated a typical structure of modern medicine within the mission community, with "the physician as a man of influence," and the "hospitals...as islands of cleanliness and order in an unregenerate society."[5] Some scholarly books on the influence of Western medicine in China also consider the social impact of medical missionaries and their role in the dissemination of ideas and technology in modernization of medicine and health care in China.[6] Some Chinese scholars from mainland China, Hong Kong, and Taiwan have written books and articles on the introduction of Western medicine into China, but medical missionaries in China, especially American medical missionaries, are not studied extensively.[7]

Notwithstanding the voluminous and diverse studies on medical missionaries in China, only a few books in English discuss or study in part American medical missionaries in Canton. Dr. W. W. Cadbury in his book describes how medical missionaries opened the Canton Hospital in 1835 with the great effort of Dr. Peter Parker and later Dr. John Kerr, who became the superintendent of the Canton Hospital before shifting his attention to treating the Cantonese insane in 1899.[8] This work is invaluable for its rigorous details about Drs. Parker and Kerr as well as many medical missionaries. This excellent book contends that the Canton Hospital treated more than two million sick and disabled people and that several hundred doctors and nurses trained by the Canton Hospital were doing valuable work in Chinese society from 1835 to 1935. This book is very useful for the study of this subject, providing a lot of information on the Canton Hospital, but it focuses on the history of the Canton Hospital itself and discusses little of its social and political impact on the Chinese in general and the Cantonese in particular during those 100 years. Edward V. Gulick discusses in his book how Dr. Parker established China's first Western hospital in Canton and how he played an important role in the negotiation of the first U.S-China treaty—the Wanxia Treaty. This book is very important for the study of Dr. Parker and the beginning of the Canton Hospital, but it does not examine the whole development of the Canton Hospital and other missionaries' medical institutions in Canton. In addition, the social and political influence of American medical missionaries, their students, and their patients, is not discussed in this book.[9] Sara Tucker basically reorganizes in her doctoral dissertation the historical documents already provided by Dr. William Cadbury and takes into account the role of the Canton Hospital in the transmission of Western knowledge. She writes, "the history of the Canton Hospital suggests rather that Western technology, at least in the specific form of modern Western medicine, was capable of being both welcomed and constructive within even chaotic nineteenth century traditional China."[10] In this book, the author scrutinizes only a part of the history of the Canton Hospital from 1835 to 1900 and focuses on its medical effect on the Cantonese only. Carolyn McCandliss' monograph, *Of No Small Account: The Life of John Glasgow Kerr*, is a very good biography of Dr. Kerr, including his publications and the statistics of the Canton Hospital from 1854 to 1900.[11] This monograph, however, does not explore what role Dr. Kerr played in early modern transformation in Canton in the nineteenth century. Besides, this monograph was published in small number, and only a few libraries have copies of this book. One of them is located in the Presbyterian Historical Society in Philadelphia, Pennsylvania.

Despite the above works, medical missions in Canton have not yet become the object of adequate scholarly scrutiny. First, some books have assessed in part the work of medical missionaries in relation to the social influence in Canton, but to date, the subject of the social role of American medical missionaries is not well researched. For example, what role did the Americans play in the women's rights movement in Canton in general and in the anti-footbinding crusade in particular? How did the Canton Hospital contribute, directly or indirectly, to the establishment and development of modern charitable institutions in Canton? What part did American doctors play in the modern public sanitation campaigns in Canton, which had an impact on China?

Second, little scholarly work has been done on the effect of the Canton Hospital on the commoners, the elite, and the officials. When the Chinese patients, after being treated successfully by medical missionaries, were restored to health, they might have a new attitude toward Western culture generally and Western medicine particularly. For example, Imperial Commissioners Lin Zexu and Qiying, as well as other prominent officials, received medical treatment at the Canton Hospital. What was the impact of American doctors on them, if any?

Third, the influence of American doctors on their students' nationalism and the role their students played in the transformation of China have not been scrutinized comprehensively. Medical missionaries vigorously attempted to introduce medical technology into China with the specific intention of promoting Western medicine, but they, intentionally or not, imparted Western ideas, in addition to medical arts, to their students. Under such influence, some of them later became revolutionaries or reformers in an attempt to transform their country. Trained by American doctors at the medical colleges, Dr. Sun Yat-sen became the founding father of the Republic of China, Dr. Zhang Zhujun turned out to be one of the pioneers of the modern women's rights movement in China, and Dr. Kang Guangren turned into one of the leaders of the 1898 Reform movement. What role did the American-trained Cantonese medical students play in the revolutionary and reform movement? Why did Chinese nationalism gain its strength in Western medical institutions in Canton in the 1920s and 1930s?

Finally, the impact of Western medicine on the Cantonese progressive reformers is not investigated thoroughly. Few historians examine Western medicine to assess its consequences for political and social development and pay attention to its role in political and social transformation in China, although some scholars assert that the introduction of Western technology was a factor contributing to political and social changes in the country.[12] After Western medicine was first introduced by medical missionaries into Canton, hundreds of thousands of Cantonese patients, including progressive Cantonese elites, benefited considerably from its positive effect, although they were not treated at missionaries' hospitals. Western medicine had an impact on the Cantonese, including the Cantonese reformers, in late imperial and early republic China. What role did Western medicine play in nurturing the reforming ideology of the Cantonese reformers—Kang Youwei, Liang Qichao, and Zheng Guanying—when they were involved in shaping Chinese modernity?

Structure and Arguments

This book will try to answer all the above questions. First, this study will discuss the role American doctors played in promoting modern medical transformation in Canton and medical modernization in China. Canton was the cradle of modern medicine in China, from where Western medicine spread to the rest of the country. By 1935, the Canton Hospital and the Hackett Medical College for Women had been taken over by the Lingnan University (the Canton Christian College originally founded by Americans) and the administration of Kerr's Refuge for Insane had been shifted to the Canton government. From 1835 to 1935, approximately thirty American medical missionaries participated in the development of hospitals, medical schools and public health programs in Canton. The strategy of medical missionary work was defined into three areas: principal medical work (hospitals and dispensaries), medical teaching (medical schools and colleges), and minor medical work (public health).

With regard to Americans' medical influence, the book focuses on medical missionaries' ideas, the methods with which they diffused their medical technology to the Cantonese, and the outcomes of their approaches to medical modernization in Canton. In contradiction of the assessment that medical missions focused their medical work on erecting large city hospitals in China that persisted for only a limited time, the book argues that American missions instituted a model of differentiated levels in medical work that is preserved in Guangdong Province today, with rural dispensaries, smaller hospitals in local cities, and the largest and well-resourced hospitals in Canton with a population of ten million.

On medical education, American doctors' ambition was to train Cantonese medical elites who would become the pioneers of China's medical modernization. They made an effort to standardize the training of Chinese physicians and hospital technicians and translate medical texts into Chinese. To promote medical modernization in Canton, the modernizing Cantonese elite, in part encouraged by American doctors, started to train native medical doctors, construct the medical infrastructure to provide medical care, and rally local social forces and governmental officials to maintain the institution of a modern health care system in Canton, which had an effect on China.

Second, the book will investigate what role American doctors and Western medicine played in social and political changes in Canton. Undergoing a tumultuous transition from a dynastic kingdom to an independent republic, China endured the Opium War of 1839-1842, the Sino-France War of 1883-1884, the 1898 Reform Movement, the 1900 Boxer Rebellion, the 1911 Revolution, the rise of the Chinese Communism movement in the 1920s, and the growth of strong Chinese nationalism in the 1930s. Modern medical institutions served several purposes: health care, charity, research, education, and business, but they were a mirror of many central events, forces, and changes, affecting traditional Canton. The Qing high-ranking officers had different attitudes toward Western culture or Americans after they received effective treatments from American doctors at the Canton Hospital. The growth of the varied and increasingly well-trained Cantonese medical staff reflected parallel changes within the Cantonese society. It is not surprising that several Cantonese medical students trained by American doctors became the leaders of the 1898 Reform Movement and the 1911 Revolution. This study also analyzes the relationship between Western medicine and the well-known Cantonese reformers who first started the modern reform movement in China in the late nineteenth century. When realizing that Western medicine, a part of Western learning, was more efficient and practical than Chinese medicine, the elite Cantonese changed their attitude toward Western learning. Thus Western medicine became one of the inspirations of those enlightened Cantonese reformers, who had to resort to Western medical treatment to restore their health.

Finally, this book will concentrate on three major movements in the process of the modern transformation of Canton. The first one was the women's rights movement, an important part of the modern transformation of Canton.[13] China's nation-building program contained the causes of women's rights. Since the Cantonese modernizers regarded the poor physical condition of the Chinese population to be a major obstruction to modernization in China, the health of Chinese women became the nucleus of a range of endeavors of both Cantonese reformers and American medical missionaries to renew or transform China. To both sides, Western standards of health should be imposed upon the Chinese women, and Western medicine was considered to be an instrument with which Chinese women's lives would be saved. American doctors' care of female patients and the introduction of modern midwifery not only improved the health of Cantonese women at its most basic level, but also decreased the high infant mortality rate. More importantly, American doctors contributed to the development of the modern women's rights movement in Canton through their work at the hospitals and medical schools. They challenged traditional Chinese attitudes toward women, participated in the anti-footbinding movement, caused the women to become interested in maternal and child health, and trained China's first female professional midwives, nurses, and obstetricians/gynecologists. In this movement, there was a link between the new class of Cantonese women medical professionals (doctors, nurses, and midwives) who were instituted into Canton by Americans on one side and nation building, modern transformation, and changing gender ideologies on the other.

The second one was the modern charitable movement in Canton, another key part of the modern transformation of Cantonese society.[14] Charity and welfare in traditional Chinese society were strictly the responsibility of families and lineages. In the late Qing and early Republic periods, the Cantonese charitable institutions and local philanthropies were commonly run virtually alongside charities operated by the medical missionaries. American medical missionaries arrogantly believed that only Christian charity could stimulate genuine compassion in China and that Christian morals and, unreservedly, Western values, helped direct the Cantonese to inaugurate a modern philanthropic movement in Canton. This book examines how medical missionaries were adept in attaining the endorsement of the Cantonese officials and merchants, whose philanthropy was crucial to the formation of mission medicine in Canton, and how the growth of the municipal elite interested in generosity adequately accounted for the adaptation of the Kerr Refuge for the mental patients, as well as other American benevolent institutes in Canton.

The third one was modern hygiene campaigns in Canton, a significant component of modernization.[15] Modern practices of sanitation emerged in the complicated environment of Canton in the late nineteenth century. American doctors not only criticized the Chinese for lacking modern concepts of bodily cleanliness and fitness, but also participated in campaigns against contagious disease. Both American doctors and the Cantonese government took part in the health management of Cantonese residents. When the Health Department of Canton took charge of health-related work in the city, health care became a part of the modern municipal administration in the 1920s. The implications of hygiene began to develop in Canton: hygiene meant not only personal health, but also civic order and national strength. This relationship of hygiene, civic order, and the nation was revealed in modern sanitary campaigns, in which sanitation became a political motto and a theme of mass mobilization activities. Placing meanings of health and disease at the center of modern Cantonese consciousness, the book discloses how, partially under American doctors' influence, modern hygiene became an essential element in the formulation of Cantonese modernity and how hygienic modernity not only transformed Canton but also manipulated Cantonese perception of hygiene requirements for national survival in a modern world.

Briefly, from 1835 to 1935 American missionary doctors in Canton successfully trained more than two hundred Chinese medical doctors, men and women, and effectively healed more than three million Chinese patients in southern China, which had an impressively positive impact on the Chinese. Challenging published literature in this field, the book argues that American doctors not only introduced Western medicine into Chinese society but also facilitated political and social reforms in China to a certain extent, although their role cannot be exaggerated in this regard. The Cantonese elite, in part inspired by Western medicine and influenced by American medical missionaries, promoted social and political reforms to modernize Cantonese society and the country. They contributed to the vision of a new political and social order, helped arouse modern consciousness and nationalism among the Chinese, and held a disproportionately large role in movements for social and political reforms in China, such as the 1898 reform movement, the 1911 Revolution, the campaigns for women's rights, the modern charitable movement, and the public hygienic campaigns.

The Canton Hospital's social and political role was significant, as American doctor Dr. J. Oscar Thomson commented in 1935:

> Our institution [the Canton Hospital] has helped to produce, directly or indirectly, many of the constructive movements in the modernization of China. It has been an important factor in opening the doors of China.[16]

This book explores Western medicine as a broad enterprise in two spheres: American medical institutions and China's modernization with a focus on Canton. The major theme threading through and emerging from this study is American doctors' medical and social influence in Canton as well as in China. Mission sources are important in this book, but the chief focus of the study is not on missionaries themselves or the missions as institutions, but on how both American doctors and the Cantonese promoted modern transformation in China generally and in Canton particularly.

This book is divided into five chapters. Chapter 1, "The Canton Hospital and Its Impact on Chinese Society, 1835-1935" studies the origins, development, and expansion of the Canton Hospital and its dispensaries and its medical achievements from 1835 to 1935. This chapter also examines how the Canton Hospital contributed to modern hospitalization in Canton as well as in China. Special attention is paid in this chapter to the new attitude the Chinese high-ranking officials Lin Zexu and Qiying took, both of whom were Dr. Peter Parker's patients, toward Western medicine in general and Western culture in particular during that time. This chapter also studies how Western medicine affected such Cantonese reformers as Kang Youwei, Liang Qichao, and Zheng Guanying.

Chapter 2, "Western Medical Education in Canton and Its Influence in China, 1835-1935" discusses the development from medical assistantship to medical schools at the Canton Hospital, as well as the development of the modern medical education in Canton, and examines the impact of Canton's modern medical education on China. This chapter also investigates what social and political role Sun Yat-sen, Kang Guangren, Zheng Shiliang, and other Chinese medical students of the Canton Hospital played during the revolutionary and social reform movements from 1835 to 1935.

Chapter 3, "The Hackett Medical College and the Women's Rights Movement, 1899-1935" studies how American women medical missionaries Dr. Mary Niles and Dr. Mary Fulton established China's first medical college for women and the impact of the Hackett Medical College for Women on China. This chapter also explores the Cantonese women doctors' medical contributions to Cantonese women's health and their role in women's rights movement in Canton.

Chapter 4, "American Doctors and the Modern Philanthropic Movement in Canton, 1835-1935" investigates how American doctors promoted modern charitable movements in Canton, opening China's first mental hospital and China's first school for blind girls in Canton. This chapter also looks into how the Cantonese reformers, under American influences, initiated a modern philanthropic movement in Canton.

Chapter 5, "American Doctors and the Modern Health and Hygiene Movement in Canton, 1835-1935" focuses on how American doctors promoted public hygienic movement in Canton, made great efforts to control the 1894 bubonic plague, and helped establish public health system in Canton from 1835 to 1935. This chapter also studies the enlightened Cantonese elites who, in part under American doctors' influence, established China's first municipal health administration, launched epidemic prevention campaigns, initiated food hygiene drives, and promoted street sanitation works in Canton.

Significances

This study, offering an in-depth look at the role American medical missionaries played in modern transformation in China during an unprecedented period of socio-political upheaval, is significant. First and foremost, this book engages with debates in the ever-growing body of studies on Western missionaries in China, addressing a broader issue in the history of the relationship between the West and China. Historians are fascinated by the work of missionaries in the age of high imperialism.[17] The work of Protestant missionaries has been recognized as one of the most important points of contact between China and the West in late Qing and early Republic China, a transition from imperial China to Republic of China and from a traditional society to a modern society. Many factors were responsible for such great transformation. What was the place of Western missionaries, and, in particular, what was the place of medical missions in China's early modernization? Some historians have admitted that the missionary enterprise in China failed in its ambition to Christianize that nation, but its secular contributions were momentous in such transformation. John King Fairbank and his students were doubtful of missionary evangelism, but they had an affirmative attitude toward other achievements of missionary work, such as the anti-opium campaign, anti-footbinding crusade, educational work, medical work, and others, while pointing out the cultural arrogance of missionaries.[18]

In recent years, much of the debate on missionary work in China concentrates on whether missionaries and their institutions were instruments of cultural imperialism (the practice of promoting or artificially injecting the culture of one society into another) or compassionate distributors of outstandingly Western contributions to the world—Christianity, medicine, science, technology, law, democracy, and so on. Students of American missionary work raise the hypothesis and dispute whether missionary experiences met the criteria of cultural imperialism with all its negative definitions. Arthur M. Schlesinger, Jr. was unwilling to regard the missionary movement as a tool of Western imperialism, but he portrayed it as "cultural aggression, or the communication of ideas and values across national borders ... accompanied by political, economic, or military pressure." He did not consider the missionaries in China as agents of typically defined Western economic or political imperialism, but he built the concept of cultural imperialism.[19]

Cultural imperialism is a dominant notion in the contemporary account of the modern Christian missionary movements. Current scholarship witnesses the shift in attitude toward mission work from a laudable undertaking of putting forward Western, or more explicit Christian, values and culture to cultural imperialism. Some historians even suggest the concept of "cultural transfer," or "cultural transmission," to some extent, to keep away from the involuntary denunciation of "cultural imperialism," and, to some degree, to focus on the genuine course of transmission. They point out that cultural transmission is a mutual connection in which two parties are engaged and that cultural messages are repeatedly arbitrated, collaborated, compromised, and deformed by the requirements, wishes, and objectives of the receivers.[20] In the case of China, Gael Graham wrote in her book published in 1995 that Protestant missionary education work in China was a story of "cultural exchange and interaction, borrowing back and forth across a selectively permeable cultural border."[21]

In the case of medical missionaries in China, a number of historians have regarded medical missions in China as agents of change. After using the archival records of two Canadian Protestant missions in China from the late 1880s to 1937 to examine medical missionaries' commitments, administrative procedure, and performance, Yuet-wah Cheung recounts a charming story of communication between them and the Chinese society where they practiced medicine. The theoretical models that the author uses are very helpful in exploring the social role of medical missionaries as agents of change and the connection between agents of change and Chinese society is complicated.[22] Edward Bliss, Jr. offers a lovely account of Dr. Emily Bliss's enduring commitment to China and the Chinese, completely balancing an impartial account of Dr. Bliss's contributions as a doctor and Christian missionary with a sincere affection and admiration for him. It is accepted practice at the present time to regard missionaries as agents of Western imperialism, but in this book Bliss is regarded as benevolent instead of being paternalistic and helpful rather than being dictatorial.[23] Karen Minden helps understand the role of Canadian medical missionaries who built a medical and dental education program in Chengdu, the capital of Sichuan Province in China. The author lays emphasis on the role of Canadian medical missionaries as agents of change in China and explicates the cross-cultural transmission of technological information.[24] Michelle Campbell Renshaw's recent book, *Accommodating the Chinese: The American Hospital in China, 1880-1920*, is an exhaustively comparative analysis. This study maintains that the hospital established by Americans in China was different from its counterpart in the United States and these dissimilarities were a result of a complicated development involving accommodation, comprehension, compromise, opportunism, and practicality. She argues that American doctors were trying to balance the pressures of the political, cultural, economic, and physical realities in China while upholding their own professional criteria.[25]

This book would not like the argument that medical missionary activities were covert cultural invasion because the cultural imperialism method has a number of weaknesses. For example, this theory does not hold true in all situations of the phenomenon that it attempts to explain, and the cultural component is much more difficult to measure. Since this method is inadequate to comprehend American medical missionary institutions in Canton, this book would not like to use the cultural imperialism structure to examine the medical missionary movements in Canton.

This book, like other books, contends that American medical missions in Canton positioned themselves as negotiators of progress, bringing medical science and rationality to China, and that they were more effective distributors of non-religious than of particularly religious characteristics, making an important and admirable contribution to Canton's modernization and China's national development. The praise for arousing the Cantonese and refreshing their creative vigor has to be given, to some extent, to American doctors in their ability as transmitters of the secular elements of Western learning. In proportion to the standard of efficiency and the scope of transformation, their scientific contributions and success in Canton were calculated as agents of transformation and their role was determined as agents of modernization.

This book, however, not only regards medical missionaries as agents of modernization, but also furthermore argues that the medical missionary movement in Canton, insightfully placed within the context of global modernity, has to be regarded as one campaign in the development of modern globalization, one element in a globalizing modernity that had altered Western countries as well as non-Western countries in the nineteenth and twentieth centuries.

When American doctors introduced Western science and culture to the Cantonese society, they also tried to learn Chinese knowledge so as to help them promote their work in China. When the Cantonese were absorbing Western science and culture, they tried to maintain the merits of their own culture, too. Thus China's modernization or modernity was a process of making of a hybrid culture. American medical missionaries in Canton can be defined as a part of globalization that breaks social and technological barriers across the world toward the creation of a one-world network of increasing connection, interdependency, and homogeneity.[26] The study of American medical mission in Canton will help shed light on the process of China's modernity and modern cultural globalization.

Second, the study of this subject helps comprehend modern history of Canton. Canton was chosen for the center of attention of this study because of its unique place in the history of Sino-Western relations. Canton, the business doorway of China, was the main point of entry into China for the West and the primary area for East-West contact: the largest metropolitan area in south China and China's first city open to the West. Canton grew to become one of the largest, most prominent and affluent cities of the empire. It was the only port officially open to foreign trade before the mid-eighteenth century and then as one of the five earliest treaty ports created by the Treaty of Nanjing of 1842. For its position in the early twentieth century history of China, Canton was the stormy setting for the revolutionaries, variously labeled "the cradle of revolution" or described as "a case of seemingly local development affecting the revolutionary transformation of the entire nation."[27] Canton was also the location of the first modernist municipality in the Republic of China. Canton held a significant position in modern Chinese history, especially in China's modernization. Thus, the study of modern Canton provides students of Chinese history with a fuller and more comprehensive picture of Chinese political, economic, and social life and popular way of thinking.

Yet despite Canton's role in the political and social drama of the period, surprisingly little has been written in English from the perspective of the city and its inhabitants; the study of Canton is not comprehensive.[28] Why did Canton become the cradle of the revolutionary and reform movements? What role did Western medicine play in the shaping of the cradle of revolution? Why were the common Cantonese more receptive to a pro-Western mentality? Why did the Cantonese establish China's first modern municipality? American missionary hospitals provided a unique window into the political, cultural, and social conditions of life in Canton at that time.

This book asserts that Western medicine helped in part to make the Cantonese more open-minded, more receptive to a pro-Western way of thinking, and more reformed. The purpose of medicine is to help patients to restore their bodies to health. Critically ill patients ask for help urgently when having a sense of pain in their bodies. When having indisposition or ailment, patients would try anything when in a desperate situation and turn to any doctors they could find. Since Guangdong's prevailing humid climate with the intense heat, semitropical in nature, resulted in wider prevalence of epidemic diseases than many other provinces in China in the nineteenth century, many Cantonese patients were in more urgent need of efficient and practical medication than other people in China.

During that time, Canton and the surrounding areas were productive grounds for missionary activities, especially medical missionaries. While eye surgery had already been identified as a valuable propaganda weapon for Western medicine before Parker's arrival, it formed the bulk of his workload there. As a specialty in which Western practice was clearly superior to local efforts, and with its results seemingly miraculous to those unfamiliar with surgical intervention, it was to be a mainstay of both Cantonese and mission practitioners of Western medicine in competition with local systems. American medical institutions were then becoming a society where ordinary Americans met ordinary Chinese in the friendliest circumstances on the whole. As time went on, more and more Cantonese found that Western medicine, part of Western learning, was more efficient and practical than Chinese medicine, and they adopted Western medicine. Thus the ordinary

Cantonese adopted Western medicine earlier and more comfortably than other people in China, which had an effect on their attitude toward Western learning. Western medicine not only had an impact on the commoners, but also on the elite. The Cantonese modernist elites, in part under American doctors' influence and their efforts, began to cry for medical modernization and subsequently cried for political and social reforms in China. Therefore, the introduction of Western medicine constituted the early period of the transformation of Canton into a modern city, and the growth of Western medicine in Canton contributed to intercultural transfer of medical technology and social institutions. This book, broadening understanding of the culture and society of Canton, argues that Canton became the cradle of revolution and reform, and played a significant part in the early modernization of China because both American medical mission and Western medicine, to some degree, played a role.

Third, the study of American doctors in Canton facilitates comprehension of the current medical system of the People's Republic of China (PRC). China's current health institutions can be traced to many of the medicines, methods, and systems introduced by medical missionaries in Canton. In the 1930s, the Chinese Nationalists took over American medical institutions in Canton, and the Chinese Communists controlled them after taking over mainland China in 1949. Since then, those hospitals and colleges have become an important part of the medical system in Canton until today; medical missionary institutions remain as the major source of modern health care in Canton. Existing literature discusses how the Chinese Communists promoted Western medicine after the establishment of the PRC, but few scholarly books study why the PRC adopted Western medicine while maintaining Chinese traditional medicine. Since China is the only country in the world where Western medicine and traditional medicine are practiced alongside each other at every level of the healthcare system, the study of American medical institutions in Canton will contribute extensively to a deep perception of this subject.

Finally, this book fills a real gap in the literature, especially important at this time in which there is a developing relationship between China and the United States. This research on American-Chinese contact within the medical sector provides important data and analysis of how Americans affected China that can be applied to strengthen the positive aspect of U.S. China policy today. What made Western medical practices transformative for China? What does the microcosm tell about this example of American medical missions that promoted hygiene, women's rights, and philanthropic activity within a nation that was very suspicious of things Western? The study of these positive transformational impacts of Western medicine on China has spillover applications to U.S. foreign policy on the whole and to the U.S.-China relationship above all today.

Sources

In this book, the author tries to make conceptual sense of facts from numerous sources—archives, documents, interviews, observations, books, articles, and so on. This book tackles more on an empirical than on a theoretical level, assembling data and evidence. This book fully utilizes the available resources in the United States, including the Archives of Presbyterian Church Board of Foreign Missionaries, Presbyterian Historical Society, Philadelphia, Pennsylvania; Dispatches from Consuls at Canton (1790-1906) of U.S. Department of State, the National Archives in Washington, D.C., the U.S. National Library of Medicine, and the Asian Collections of Library of Congress.

This book uses the Chinese resources at Guangdong Provincial Archives in Guangzhou, Guangzhou Municipal Archives in Guangzhou, the Special Collection of Sun Yat-sen Library of Guangdong Province, Sun Yat-sen University Library in Guangzhou, the Special Collections of Hong Kong Baptist University Library, Special Collections of National Library of China in Beijing, the Special Collections of Shanghai Library, and the Special Collection of the Library of Hubei Province, which have a large number of books, monographs, newspapers, journals, and archives with regard to the Canton Hospital, the Refuge for the Insane, and Hackett Medical College for Women. The author also conducted research at the Archives of the Medical School of Sun Yat-sen University, the Archives of the First Municipal Hospital of Guangzhou, and the Archives of the Mental Hospital of Guangzhou in Canton. In addition to archives, the author interviewed several Chinese medical doctors in Guangzhou and in other cities in China. Using extensive multi-archival research, the author, moving his study away from the usual one-sided approach, looks at both sides with a more balanced view. This distinctive analytic framework, a new research method using multiple perspectives, will sharpen readers' interest in this book.

Notes

1. For a study of Elijah Coleman Bridgman of the American Board of Commissioners for Foreign Missions, see Eliza J. Gillett Bridgman, ed., *The Pioneer of American Missions in China: The Life and Labors of Elijah Coleman Bridgman* (New York: Anson D. F. Randolph, 1864), 20-27.
2. For a study of Canton in the early nineteenth century, see W. Hunter, *The "Fan Kwae" at Canton, Before Treaty Days 1825-1844* (London: Kean Paul, Trench, 1855), 27-29.
3. With regard to contextualization of the mission effort in Canton in relation to medical missions elsewhere in China or in the colonies, or of China's modernizing reforms and Western influence in other periods or regions, there is considerable scholarship on these subjects. A very brief list includes David Arnold, *Colonizing the Body: State Medicine and Epidemic Disease in 19th-Century India* (Berkeley: University of California Press, 1993); Teresa Meade and Mark Walker, eds., *Science, Medicine and Cultural Imperialism* (New York: St. Martin's Press, 1991); Philip D. Curtin,

Disease and Empire: The Health of European Troops in the Conquest of Africa (New York: Cambridge University Press, 1998); and Sheldon Watts, *Epidemics and History: Disease, Power, and Imperialism* (New Haven and London: Yale University Press, 1997).

4. Ralph Croizier, *Traditional Medicine in Modern China: Science, Nationalism, and the Tensions of Cultural Changes* (Cambridge: Harvard University Press, 1968).

5. Peter Buck, *American Science and Modern China* (Cambridge: Cambridge University Press, 1980), chapter 2.

6. See, for examples, G. H. Choa, *"Heal the Sick" Was Their Motto: The Protestant Medical Missionaries in China* (Hong Kong: Chinese University Press, 1990); M. Cristina Zaccarini, *The Sino-American Friendship as Tradition and Challenge: Dr. Ailie Gale in China, 1908-1950* (Bethlehem: Lehigh University Press, 2001); John Bowers, *Science and Medicine in Twentieth-Century China* (Ann Arbor: The University of Michigan Press, 1988); John Z. Bowers and Elizabeth F. Purcell, eds., *Medicine and Society in China* (New York: Josiah Macy, Jr., Foundation, 1974); Paul Starr, *The Social Transformation of American Medicine* (New York: Basic Books, 1982); AnElissa Lucas, *Chinese Medical Modernization: Comparative Police Continuities, 1930-1980s* (New York: Praeger, 1982); and R. Holden, *Yale in China: The Mainland, 1901-1951* (New Haven, Conn.: Yale in China Association, 1964).

7. See, for example, He Xiaolian, *Xi yi dong jian yu wen hua tiao shi* (Introduction of Western medicine to China and cultural accommodation) (Shanghai: Shanghai guji chubanshe, 2006); Li Jingwei and Yan Liang bian, *Xi xue dong jian yu Zhongguo jin dai yi xue si chao* (The introduction of Western learning and modern medical ideology in China) (Wuhan: Hubei ke xue ji shu chubanshe, 1990); Wang Meixiu, *Jidu jiao shi* (The history of the Protestant movement) (Nanjing: Jiangsu renmin chubanshe, 2006); Cao Zengyou, *Jidu jiao yu Ming Qing ji Zhongguo she hui: Zhong xi wen hua de tiao shi yu chong zhuang* (The Protestant movement in China between the Ming and Qing dynasties: Sino-Western Cultural exchanges) (Beijing: Zuojia chubanshe, 2006); Wu Ziming ed., *Zhongguo jiao hui da xue li shi wen xian yan tao hui lun wen ji* (Essays on historical archives of Christian higher education in China) (Hong Kong: Chinese University Press, 1995); and *Zi xi cu dong: Malixun mu shi lai Hua er bai zhou nian ji nian* (Meeting of East-West culture: celebrating the 200th anniversary of Rev. Robert Morrison's arrival in China) (Xianggang: Xianggang zhongwen daxue chong ji xue yuan zong jiao yu zhongguo she hui yan jiu zhong xin, 2007).

8. W. W. Cadbury, *At the Point of a Lancet; One Hundred Years of the Canton Hospital, 1835-1935* (Shanghai: Kelly & Walsh, 1935).

9. Edward V. Gulick, *Peter Parker and the Opening of China* (Cambridge: Harvard University, 1973).

10. Sara Tucker, "The Canton Hospital and Medicine in Nineteenth-Century China, 1835-1900" (Ph.D. dissertation, Indiana University, 1982), vi.

11. Carolyn McCandliss, *Of No Small Account: The Life of John Glasgow Kerr* (The Washang Press, 1996).

12. See, for example, Christina Gilmartin, *Engendering China: Women, Culture, and the State* (Cambridge: Harvard University Press, 1994), Denis Goulet,

The Uncertain Promise: Value Conflicts in Technology Transfer (New York: IDOC, 1977); J. Ramesh and C. C. Weiss, eds., *Mobilizing Technology for World Development* (New York: Praeger, 1979); R. Braibanti and J. Spengler, *Tradition, Values, and Socio-Economic Development* (Durham, NC: Duke University, 1961); and D. M. Apter, *The Politics of Modernization* (Chicago: University of Chicago, 1965).

13. For a study of the women's rights movement in modern China, see Claudie Broyelle, *Women's Liberation in China* (Atlantic Highlands, NJ: Humanities Press International, Incorporated, 1977); Rey Chow, *Woman and Chinese Modernity: The Politics of Reading between West and East* (Theory and History of Literature, vol. 75. Minneapolis, MN: University of Minnesota Press, 1991); Gail Hershatter, *Women in China's Long Twentieth Century* (Berkeley: University of California Press, 2007); Ono Kazuko, *Chinese Women in a Century of Revolution, 1850-1950* (Stanford, CA: Stanford University Press, 1989); Caroline Beth Reeves, "The Power of Mercy: The Chinese Red Cross Society, 1900-1937" (Ph. D. Dissertation, Harvard University, 1998); Janet Yi-chun Chen, "Guilty of Indigence: The Urban Poor in China, 1900 1949 (Ph D. Dissertation, Yale University, 2005); Jane Hunter, *The Gospel of Gentility: American Women Missionaries in Turn-of-the Century China* (New Haven: Yale University Press, 1984); Jessie Gregory Lutz, ed., *Pioneer Chinese Christian Women: Gender, Christianity, and Social Mobility* (Bethlehem: Lehigh University Press, 2010); and Hu Ying, *Tales of Translation: Composing the New Woman in China, 1898-1918* (Stanford: Stanford University Press, 2000). For a study of the footbinding movement, see Hong Fan, *Footbinding, Feminism, and Freedom: The Liberation of Women's Bodies in Modern China* (Ilford, Essex: Frank Cass Publishers, 1997) and Ping Wang, *Aching for Beauty: Footbinding in China* (Minneapolis: University of Minnesota Press, 2000).

14. For a study of the modern charitable movement, see Vivien W. Ng, *Madness in Late Imperial China: From Illness to Deviance* (University of Oklahoma Press, 1990), which focuses on the legal status of the insane, particularly the criminally insane, as revealed in 105 case studies ranging in date from 1697 to 1892. Ng argues that the state was in no position to enforce new registration and confinement procedures and that the authorities continued to afford special consideration to the insane as not responsible for their actions. Veronica Pearson analyzes the history of China's psychiatric services from an explicitly Western social welfare perspective. She concludes that the grafting of "modern" Western psychiatric services onto Chinese practice is problematic due to the culture-bound nature of psychiatric knowledge and practice. Pearson argues for cultural and historical sensitivity when interpreting cross-culturally, as was the case with the Kerr Refuge. See V. Pearson, "The Development of Modern Psychiatric Services in China 1891-1949," *History of Psychiatry* 2 (1991) 133-47. Neil Diamant analyzes the Kerr Refuge from a political science perspective and claims "mass confinement" in China was not the result of state building initiative but rather the product of local activism. He states that "in the absence of a national health policy, municipal elites initiated the expansion of mental institutions founded by Protestant and Catholic medical missionaries. Diamant recognizes the shift role of household and state policy

that encouraged social innovation at the local level. His insights support claims made explicit by the theory of a shifting welfare mix. This research builds upon Diamant's insights by recognizing local activism within the marketplaces as well. See Neil Diamant, "China's Great Confinement? Missionaries, Municipal Elites and Police in the Establishment of Chinese Mental Hospitals," *Republican China* 19 (1): 3-50.

15. For a study of the modern hygienic movement in China, see Kerrie Macpherson, *A Wilderness of Marshes: The Origins of Public Health in Shanghai, 1843-1893* (Oxford University Press, 1987). This book explores the origins of communal health in the city and the measures deemed essential for its protection as well the efforts directed toward the implementation of the preventive medicine. The author maintains that the institutionalization of public health claimed a central place in both the private and public sectors of foreign settlements. Ruth Rogaski, *Hygienic Modernity: Meanings of Health and Disease in Treaty-Port China* (Berkeley, California: University of California Press, 2004), describes the intersection of significant military and political events in Tianjin and the transformation of practice related to health—the arrangement of space, the provisioning of water, the care of the body, and the management of human excreta. The book demonstrates how the debates about hygiene alternately united and fragmented the imperial powers in the city, at the same time creating an important link between the goals of imperialist and the goals of modernizing elites. This book is one of the best books in English on the modern hygiene movement in China in the nineteenth and twentieth centuries.

16. J. Oscar Thomson, "A Century of Medical Work in China," *The Missionary Review of the World* 2 (February 1935), 55.

17. There is an extensive literature on Western missionaries in China. G. Thompson Brown, *Earthen Vessels and Transcendent Power: American Presbyterians in China, 1837-1952* (Maryknoll, N.Y.: Orbis Books, 1997); Kathleen L. Lodwick, *Crusades against Opium: Protestant Missionaries in China, 1874-1917* (Lexington: University Press of Kentucky, 1996); Michael C. Lazich, *E.C. Bridgman (1801-1861): America's First Missionary to China* (Lewiston: The Edwin Mellen Press, 2000); Daniel H. Bays, ed., *Christianity in China: From the Eighteenth Century to the Present* (Stanford, CA, 1996), and Murray A. Rubinstein, *The Origins of the Anglo-American Missionary Enterprise in China, 1807-1840* (Lanham, Md: Scarecrow Press, 1996). Xi Lian's *The Conversion of Missionaries: Liberalism in American Protestant Missions in China* (University Park: Pennsylvania State University Press, 1997) is an account of one of the often neglected aspects of the Christian mission enterprise in China, namely, what impact did it have on the missionaries and their home churches. The author tells American Protestant missionaries' stories in China, showing how their priorities changed from predominantly evangelical to humanitarian ones and making it clear that missionaries, like thoughtful Christians everywhere, had to make their peace treaties with the modern one by one, each in their own way.

18. John King Fairbank, ed., *The Missionary Enterprise in China and America* (Harvard University Press, 1974); Suzanne Wilson Barnet and John King Fairbank, eds., *Christianity in China: Early Protestant Missionary Writings* (Cambridge, MA, 1985).

19. Arthur M. Schlesinger, Jr., "The Missionary Impulse and Theories of Impe-
    rialism," in *The Missionary Enterprise in China and America*, ed. Fairbank,
    363-64, in which he compares missionary activity to classical economic,
    sociological, and political theories of imperialism.

20. For a thoughtful historiographic survey of the cultural-imperialism debate
    and the concept of cultural transfer, see Jessica Gienow-Hecht, "Cultural
    Transfer," in *Explaining the History of American Foreign Relations*, 2d ed.,
    ed. Michael J. Hogan and Thomas J. Paterson (New York, 2004), Reinhold
    Wagnleiter, *Coca-Colonization and the Cold War: The Cultural Mission
    of the United States in Austria after the Second World War*, trans., Diana
    M. Wolf (Chapel Hill, N.C.: University of North Carolina Press, 1994), and
    Richard F. Kuisel, *Seducing the French: The Dilemma of Americanization*
    (Berkeley, CA, 1993).

21. Gael Graham, *Gender, Culture, and Christianity: American Protestant
    Mission Schools in China, 1880-1930* (New York: Peter Lang Publishing,
    1995), 1. Some scholars of mission studies consider that Graham's work
    is riddled with errors, and some statements of the book are open to
    discussion.

22. Yuet-wah Cheung, *Missionary Medicine in China: A Study of Two Canadian
    Protestant Missions in China before 1937* (Lanham, Md.: University Press
    of America, 1988).

23. Edward Bliss, Jr., *Beyond the Stone Arches: An American Missionary Doctor
    in China, 1892-1932* (New York: John Wiley, 2001).

24. Karen Minden, *Bamboo Stone: The Evolution of a Chinese Medical Elite*
    (Toronto: University of Toronto Press, 1994).

25. Michelle Campbell Renshaw, *Accommodating the Chinese: The American
    Hospital in China, 1880-1920* (New York: Routledge, 2005).

26. For a discussion of the issue of modernity, see Warwick Anderson, "In-
    troduction: Postcolonial Technoscience," *Social Studies of Science* 32,
    5(2002): 648-50 and Ibrahim Kaya, "Modernity, Openness, Interpretation:
    A Perspective on Multiple Maternities," *Social Science Information* 43,
    1 (2004): 49-50. With regard to China's modernity, see Benjamin Elman,
    On Their Own Terms: Science in China, 1550-1900 (Cambridge: Harvard
    University Press, 2005).

27. C. Martin Wibur, *The Nationalist Revolution in China, 1923-1928* (Cam-
    bridge: Cambridge University Press, 1983), 1; Chan Ming K., "A Turning
    Point in the Modern Chinese Revolution: The Historical Significance of
    the Canton Decade, 1917-27," in *Remapping China: Fissures in Historical
    Terrain* (Stanford: Stanford University Press, 1996), eds. Gail Hershatter,
    Emily Honig, and others, 224-41.

28. See, for example, Virgil K. Y. Ho, *Understanding Canton: Rethinking
    Popular Culture in the Republican Period* (New York: Oxford University
    Press, 2005), which studies six different aspects of culture in Canton in the
    period between the two world wars, examining the matters of patriotism
    and anti-foreignism, gambling, prostitution, and opium in Canton as well
    as a widely accepted form of commercialized mass entertainment—Canton
    opera. See also, Michael, T. W. Tsin, *Nation, Governance, and Modernity
    in China, Canton, 1900-1927* (Stanford, California: Stanford University
    Press, 1999), which is a study in English of the city of Canton (Guangzhou)

in the first quarter of the twentieth century, using a social history of early twentieth-century Canton to explore the meaning and mechanisms of the political culture of modernity. Ezra F. Vogel, *Canton under Communism: Program and Politics in a Provincial Capital, 1949-1968* (Harvard University Press, 1969), is a study of Canton under the Chinese Communism, an excellent book on the history of Canton.

1

The Canton Hospital and Its Impact on Chinese Society, 1835-1935

This chapter examines the origin, development, and expansion of the Canton Hospital and its dispensaries from 1835 when Dr. Peter Parker opened China's first Western hospital in Canton, until 1935 when the Canton Hospital was formally taken over by the Lingnan University. This chapter also studies how American doctors in Canton made contributions to the introduction of Western medicine into China and analyzes Western medicine's impact on the Qing officials, Lin Zexu and Qiying, who received medical treatments from American doctors. Finally, this chapter examines the relationship between Western medicine and the progressive Cantonese reformers, Kang Youwei, Liang Qichao, and Zheng Guanying, whose illnesses were cured with Western medicine.

The Canton Hospital, 1835-1935

The Ophthalmic Hospital, 1835-39

The institution of the American Board of Commissioners for Foreign Missions (ABCFM) in 1810 was the starting point of the ABCFM movement because no Protestant missionaries had been dispatched outside the United States prior to this time. On October 14, 1829, two young American missionaries, Elizah C. Bridgman and David Abeel, departed from New York for Canton (Guangzhou), China. Their arrival in February 1830 was the beginning of the ABCFM mission in China.[1] The Qing government banned the introduction of any new religion into imperial China and expelled any persons caught proselytizing from the empire, and the policies of the Canton system prevented any types of close communication with the Chinese. Thus it was very hard for missionaries to have a sure tactic for spreading the Gospel in China. The earlier missionaries to China were compelled to present the Chinese something, in addition to Christianity.[2] As a result, Bridgman and his colleagues in Canton became more and more persuaded of the remarkable possibility of a missionary hospital for preaching to the Chinese the tenets of Christianity, believing that a dispensary in Canton would be a perfect example of Christian philanthropy.[3] In the subsequent years, five other ABCFM missionaries were dispatched to Canton, and Peter Parker (1804-1888) was one of them.[4]

Peter Parker started his journey on the ship *Morrison* on June 4, 1834, together with Mr. D. W. C. Olyphant, the ship's owner and a well-to-do New York businessman famous for his support for American missionaries in China. They arrived in Canton on September 8, 1835.[5] Luckily, Dr. Parker won support in his ground-breaking enterprise from the chief Hong merchant Howqua (Wu Chongyao), who was respected by the Cantonese and Westerners alike, and who enthusiastically accepted Parker's scheme for the creation of a hospital.[6]

Eye trouble was very common in Canton at that time, possibly because of the strong heat and dryness of the air. Additionally, the physical characteristics of the Chinese people might be responsible for this commonness of eye diseases because the curve of the eyelid universal to all Chinese made the eyelashes turn in upon the eye, resulting in inflamed corneas and, in many instances, loss of sight. Finally, Western medicine in treating cataracts with surgery to help patients to restore their sight was more efficient than Chinese medicine. As a result, Parker decided to focus on one specific type of disease—eye disease; if not, he would be overcome by too many patients by reason of the extraordinarily large population of Canton. In November 1835, Peter Parker, the first medical missionary to China, opened his Ophthalmic Hospital in a street not frequently visited by foreigners.[7] The intention of the Hospital was to demonstrate Christian compassion to the Chinese by healing their sick, and to create an opportunity for preaching and teaching the canons of Christianity to the patients who gathered there.[8] As its name suggests, the hospital was anticipated to serve predominantly for the treatment of eye diseases. This hospital was the first of its kind in China and the first mission hospital in East Asia, after that recognized as the celebrated Canton Hospital.

Eye diseases established the majority of the cases at the Hospital, but other ailments were treated by the American doctor.[9] In the first three months of the hospital's operation, 1,020 cases of eye disease were treated, while the total number of other cases (mostly ear diseases and large tumors) was forty-one. During the first nineteen months following the founding of the hospital, Parker dedicated almost all his time to healing his patients. The hospital was doing well from the start. Basically, all patients treated successfully by Parker had proved to get better, and a large number of patients were entirely restored to health. There were several reasons for such success: the American doctor's skill as a surgeon, the courage and strong constitutions of his patients, and possibly, the most imperative, the advantage of Western medicine over Chinese medication.[10]

The success of the hospital was so great that news of the American doctor spread speedily, appealing to an increasing number of patients, even from remote provinces. Some of the local patients left their homes at midnight to be the earliest in line at the hospital door; others came the previous evening and waited all night. During the spring of 1837, the number of patients was occasionally 200 or 300 in one day. One day as many as 600, in the company of their friends or relatives, arrived in the hospital. In the early days, new patients were accepted day by day, but patients turned up in so large a number that the hospital later had to arrange admission days. Parker also started to build up quite a large private practice so that patients could seek him out for medical treatments, and he was then given numerous opportunities to visit the homes of his patients.[11]

At the commencement of the Canton Hospital, the Canton Mission of the ABCFM was responsible for the initial expense of the hospital and financed Dr. Parker. Parker was pressed to concentrate his efforts on the circulation of Scripture and other religious books and on the direct preaching of the Gospel.[12] The American Board repeated that the leading duty of their missionaries was to sermonize the Gospel to the Cantonese in Cantonese dialect.[13]

Parker, however, argued that "pious men who are physicians ... have a peculiar advantage in imparting instruction to the heathen," and recognized that it was crucial to first heal the wounds of the body before treating infections of the spirit.[14] In the meantime, Peter Parker and E.C. Bridge were discussing the establishment of a medical missionary organization.[15]

In the end the Canton Mission claimed in 1837 that its budget would not support the Canton Hospital in the future because it was not among its aims as a missionary society. It was quickly obvious that if the hospital was to continue its work, a society had to be created to oversee and make plans for the collection of funds to support it, and to get hold of additional doctors for medical work in China. For this reason, Dr. Parker, together with Dr. Colledge and Dr. Bridgman, made a proposal to set up a society. In February 1838, they held a public meeting at the Canton Chamber of Commerce, during which a medical missionary society was established. By then American medical missionaries in Canton were represented by the Medical Missionary Society, an evangelical association of Protestants.[16]

The creation of a bi-national institution helped make known a new profession and secure new recruits for it. More importantly, the formation of the Medical Missionary Society indicated that American medical missionaries had to adjust themselves to Chinese society when implanting a Western institution in China—they had to put the medical work before the religious work because most Cantonese were more interested in Americans' medical arts than their sermons at the hospital. Since then, the Canton Hospital, as well as other missionary hospitals in China in the following decades, became a mainly medical center rather than a religious center, although it was performing two functions.

The General Hospital, 1839–59

Dr. Parker aimed initially to treat eye diseases only, but actually he was dealing with so many different kinds of diseases that the Ophthalmic Hospital decided to become a more general one. In August 1839, Dr. Parker moved into the Canton Dispensary, which had recently been evacuated by British doctors, and turned it into a general hospital, no longer limiting himself predominantly to ophthalmic diseases.[17]

When the Opium War of 1839-1842 erupted in November, Parker left Canton for the United States. After the war, Dr. Parker arrived in Canton on November 5, 1842 and reopened the Canton Hospital on November 21, a general rather than an ophthalmic institution. More and more patients came to visit this general hospital. According to the Medical Missionary Society's report in December 1847, "The aggregate number of patients admitted at the close of 1847 was 26,504, of which 8,247 have been received since the period of the last report."[18]

Dr. Parker continued his medical work during the first few months of 1855. In April he suffered a complete physical breakdown, seemingly from overwork. As the work proved eventually to be too much for his physical condition, he spent several weeks recovering at Macao, but his health improved only a little. Since he became conscious that he had to return to America to gain a full recovery, he asked Dr. John Kerr (1824-1901) to assume responsibility of the Canton Hospital during his absence. Parker left for the United States in the summer of 1855 after handing over the Canton Hospital to Kerr who agreed to the doctor's call.[19]

Dispatched by the American Presbyterian Board in 1853, Dr. Kerr and his wife sailed for China on November 28 and arrived in May 1854. Soon after his arrival in Canton, Dr. Kerr took over Dr. A. P. Harper's medical work at the Huiji Dispensary of the Presbyterian Mission in the southern suburb of Canton. After the Canton Hospital was shifted to his care in May 1855, Kerr managed both the hospital and dispensary. The number of patients visiting the dispensary during the twenty-two months of its existence was greater than that of those visiting the Canton Hospital. After the Second Opium War between China and England-France broke out in 1856, hostilities between the Chinese and the Westerners became so great that the Canton Hospital was forcibly closed in October. At the end of the month the Huiji Dispensary, which held most of the tablets, was on fire. The Hospital itself, the old factory building, was burned to the ground on December 14, too, thus destroying the place of Parker's previous work and Howqua's charity. During that time, Dr. Kerr was forced to return to the United States. There he married Miss Isabella Jane Mosely in 1858, and in the later part of that year, they returned to Canton.[20]

The Boji Hospital, 1859–99

When returning to Canton in November 1858, Dr. Kerr found a fairly satisfactory building facing the river in Zhengsha Street in the southern suburb of Canton. To return to his medical work for the sick, Kerr purchased a piece of land near the building and opened in mid-January 1859 a new hospital, called by the name of Boji (Spreading benevolence).[21] By 1860, the Boji Hospital had treated 17,631 patients.[22]

Dr. Joseph Clarke Thomson was chosen to take up the responsibility of the Hospital during Kerr's absence at the annual meeting of the Medical Missionary Society in January 1884 when Dr. Kerr asked to be allowed to return to America as a result of ill health. It was the Franco-Chinese War of 1883-84 that fanned the flames of the anti-foreign ferment, and a gang went so far as to assault the Boji Hospital. Fierce anti-foreign outbreaks took place in 1885, forcing the missionaries to close their dispensaries and withdraw. Placards expressing disapproval of foreigners were put in the most well-known places throughout the city. As a result of Dr. Thomson's bravery and manner of dealing with the angry mob, the gang was disbanded, and the Boji Hospital continued its work, although the number of patients was reduced. As a promising doctor, Dr. Thomson's years at the Canton Hospital during exceedingly troubled times proved that he was a man of extraordinary ability and character.[23] This young man from Ohio came out the previous year under the American Presbyterian Board and proved himself to be a worthy successor by directing the hospital for many years, leading it through turbulent times and augmenting its competence and size.[24]

Dr. Swan's Hospital, 1899-1914

Dr. Kerr quit both the Hospital and the Canton Medial Missionary Society in 1899 because he had entered into many disputes with his mission colleagues. Dr. John Myers Swan came after Dr. Kerr as the medical superintendent of the Boji Hospital in 1899. Swan arrived in Canton in December 1885 and spent his first year studying the Cantonese dialect, but quickly he was summoned to be responsible for various duties of the Canton Hospital. In 1887, he was assigned Dr. Kerr's assistant in the Hospital, and from then on he was associated with the celebrated surgeon, Dr. Kerr.[25]

John Swan was an energetic, vigorous man. Building upon the excellent work of Dr. Kerr and his colleagues and forerunners, Dr. Swan carried the institute progressively ahead and all alone transformed the hospital into a new, efficient one. He cut all translation and dispensary tasks associated with the Hospital in order to concentrate the money on improving the Hospital.[26]

In 1906, new rules were added to the constitution of the Canton Medical Missionary Society, and, in consequence, a defined scheme for specializing the work was commenced.[27] Andrew H. Woods for some years was a physician of the Canton Christian College (later Lingnan University) and linked himself with the work of the Boji Hospital as early as 1900, both in medical and surgical work. He approached Dr. William W. Cadbury and Harvey J. Howard of the University Medical School in Pennsylvania and persuaded them to come to Canton as visiting physicians. In 1912, Drs. Andrew H. Woods, William W. Cadbury, and Harvey J. Howard of the Canton Christian College were employed as visiting members of the Missionary Society Hospital staff. With their initiation, the proficient work of the Canton Hospital was specialized, the first doctors taking total responsibility for the medical, pathological, ophthalmological, neurological, and dermatological services. Dr. Swan, the recognized surgeon, performed most of the operations from 1891 to 1910. After leaving the Hospital and quitting the service of the Medical Missionary Society in May 1914, Swan built a private hospital in an eastern suburb of Canton and engaged in private practice, making with noticeable accomplishment. Unfortunately, while on a visit to America in 1919, he was knocked down and killed by a vehicle. During the fifteen years of superintendence, Dr. Swan increased the facilities and equipment of the hospital in many ways. The Canton Hospital had 300 beds, received roughly 30,000 patients, and performed surgery on 2,000 cases yearly, the largest hospital in East Asia and commonly known as "Dr. Swan's hospital" during that time.[28]

From Missionary Hospital to University Hospital, 1914–35

Dr. William W. Cadbury went to the Canton Hospital and became its superintendent in June 1914. Dr. Cadbury graduated from Haverford College in 1898 and the Medical School of the University of Pennsylvania in 1902. He practiced and taught medicine in Philadelphia for several years. As a member of the University of Pennsylvania Christian Association, he was employed to serve in the new medical school in Canton. He left his home, not as a Quaker or a missionary, but as a physician and teacher, and arrived in Canton in 1909 as a member of the staff of the University Medical School in connection with the Canton Christian College, winning the support of members of the Society of Friends in Philadelphia.[29]

In 1914, the departmentalization of the professional work was initiated. Hence, for the first time in the history of the Canton Hospital, the work was divided among proficient specialists, a system of interns was introduced, a clinical and pathological laboratory was founded, a training school for nurses was started, a system of records was established, and a complete system of registration of patients with history sheets for both inpatients and outpatients was organized.[30]

In 1916, the Canton Hospital passed through perhaps the gravest period in its long history. It was faced with a serious financial deficit, and was obliged to borrow on the security of the Medical Missionary Society's assets so as to continue functioning. Maybe the most crucial lesson learned from the 1916 crisis was the requirement of a better and more stable organization. A new strategy was designed, and the Canton Medical Missionary Union was established that year. The Canton Hospital handed over to the Union the assets owned by the Board of Trustees of the Medical Missionary Society.[31] The Canton Medical Missionary Society continued to be present as owner and trustee of the Hospital and its assets, but it was to operate by means of the Canton Medical Missionary Union, of which it was a member and was entitled to supply three people to the Board of Directors.[32]

The Canton Hospital became more popular than before. In 1919, 2,493 inpatients and 11,654 outpatients were treated at the Hospital.[33] In the 1920s, more than 3,500 inpatients and more than 20,000 dispensary patients were treated annually.[34] The Canton Medical Missionary Society, threatened by an ultimatum from the Miscellaneous Workers Union, resolved to shut down the Hospital, and from then on patients and employees were forced to leave on March 11, 1926.[35]

The Hospital remained closed until September 5, 1929 when medical work was recommenced, in the beginning on a restricted scale.[36] The Hospital, however, with the new arrangement, was shifted to the directors of Lingnan University on July 23, 1930, provided that they would carry on the objectives of the Medical Missionary Society as articulated in its constitution—healing patients, teaching medicine, and preaching Christianity—and use all funds received from the Society and its properties for these objectives. A definite plan of affiliation was passed in 1933 whereby the Hackett Medical College for Women, Lingnan University, and Canton Hospital were united with an agreement that Lingnan University would take full responsibility for a new medical school in 1935.[37]

The Dispensary Movement: Canton Hospital Extensions

China had become the largest operation of the Board of Foreign Missions of the Presbyterian Church in the United States. The Canton (South China) Mission, which was created in 1845 and one of eight missions in China, was restructured as a separate mission because of its distance from other stations in south China. In the late nineteenth century, new mission stations—Lianzhou, Yangjiang, Hainan, Shilong, and Gaozhou—were opened at other south China locations. Hainan station, originally an outpost of the Canton Mission, was formally recognized as a separate mission in 1893. Missionaries from other Presbyterian denominations were also active in Canton during that period. In this way, American medical missionaries were not only working in Canton but also in south China.

The Canton Hospital was located in the city of Canton, but it had branches in many places, numbering in all more than thirty at the beginning of the twentieth century. Many other dispensaries or medical services were attached or related to the Canton Hospital and were sponsored by the Canton Mission. The hospital and dispensary work of the Canton Medical Missionary Society was assiduously carried out both in the city and in a varying number of out-stations. Branch hospitals and dispensaries in the countryside interested doctors of the Canton Hospital irrespective of mission or denomination. The Canton Hospital assisted new physicians in buying drugs and helping select and pack drugs from the hospital storeroom, and medical missionaries in south China had to go to Canton at least once a year on hospital business. The American medical missionary movement had started not only in Canton, but also in south China.[38]

Foshan

The Canton Mission decided to establish a second mission station in the city of Foshan, located about fifteen miles west of Canton on the connecting Xi River system, thus beginning its expansion outside the city of Canton through a system of outstations. The Canton Mission hoped that this new station would eventually reach a population of more than seventeen million in that area. Dr. Kerr then opened a dispensary in Foshan in February 1860; patients came in so large a number that it became unworkable to take care of them all. Dr. Kerr reported that "the gratuitous healing of the sick will be a tangible demonstration to the people that the foreigner comes not just to destroy, but that he also brings a message of peace and good will."[39] Dr. Kerr, visiting the clinic twice a week until 1864, was welcomed by the people, and had opportunities to pass on some knowledge of Western medicine. The clinic was closed later by Dr. Kerr, and in 1881, the London medical missionaries took it over and turned it into a hospital. Today it is the largest hospital in the city of Foshan.[40]

Zhaoqing

Reverend R. H. Graves of the Southern Baptist Convention of America opened a dispensary in Canton in 1856 after arriving in China in 1855. Dr. Graves, the son of a physician, received medical education before becoming a missionary.[41] In February 1861, Dr. Graves made great progress when launching another outpatient station at Zhaoqing, the old capital of Guangdong Province, situated on the West River, 60 miles upriver from Canton. This dispensary maintained relations with the Canton bases both through its Medical Missionary Society funding and its round of visits, consultations, and medical supplies from Dr. Kerr. Dr. Graves, for example, sent a letter in 1860 to the twenty-second annual meeting of the Medical Missionary Society in Canton, requesting an appropriation of $60 for medical missionary purposes in Zhaoqing and some adjacent locations.[42]

Dr. Graves reported that he started normal medical work at Zhaoqing, first in the back of a shop, then in better premises, and that three days of each month were arranged for taking care of outpatients while vaccinations were performed every Monday. According to Dr. Graves, a total of 3,060 visits were paid to the dispensary in 1861, about half of the patients suffering from eye diseases. Those small surgeries were performed at the dispensary, and severe cases were sent to the Canton Hospital.[43] In 1862-3, the work at the two dispensaries continued; the attendance at Zhaoqing was somewhat less because Dr. Graves had to spend much time at Canton, leaving the work in the hands of his assistant. Dr. Graves, for instance, was not present during the latter half of 1863, but his competent assistant was keeping on the work. In May 1873, Dr. Graves opened a new station at a town of Xinan, thirty miles from west of Canton and at the junction of the North and West rivers. Dr. Graves later reported the opening of another dispensary at the city of Wuzhou in Guangxi province, 200 miles from northwest of Canton. The work there was mainly in the hands of his helper, too, who had been with him since the opening of the Zhaoqing station and who gained the patients' full confidence.[44] In 1882, Dr. Graves' work at the dispensary in Xinan was closed, but his work at the out-station at Zhaoqing was continued in 1897.[45]

Lianzhou

In 1883, the Reverend Joseph C. Thomson and Mrs. Thomson, with their infant son, made a pioneering trip to Lianzhou, 120 miles north of Canton, living for six months in a boat anchored close to the city. Dr. Thomson established a dispensary for the sick and a small school for boys, but it was very challenging because the Chinese were doubtful that the foreigners had come to help them. Due to the anti-foreign antagonism, American medical missionaries left and did not come back until the circumstances in Lianzhou were getting better in 1887. Dr. Edward C. Machle of the American Presbyterian Church arrived in 1889 and commenced permanent medical work at the station in Lianzhou. Dr. Machle opened a dispensary in 1891 and treated 6,720 patients in just one year.[46] In 1894, Dr. Eleanor Chesnut took over the medical work for women in Lianzhou. Dr. Chesnut, born in Waterloo, Iowa, took full courses at the Women's Medical College. She left America for China in the fall of 1894. Once in China, she studied Mandarin, Cantonese, and Lianzhou dialect and made several useful translations into Chinese. Chesnut, in charge of a hospital and dispensary, every week traveled ten miles on horseback to hold a clinic in other counties. At that time, she was the only foreigner in Lianzhou and treated 5,479 patients at the Women's Hospital in one year. Throughout her life, she was self-sacrificing to the last degree, by no means looking out herself, but only considering others. On one occasion, because a patient's survival depended upon surgically receiving a skin graft, she did not hesitate to give from her own body what was necessary to make the surgery successful.[47] In 1905, the men's hospital under Dr. Edward Machle and the women's hospital under Dr. Eleanor Chesnut treated 13,056 patients with 195 operations. Three lepers who had been expelled from their village came to stay at the hospital, and American doctors built a hut for them just outside the Hospital. Dr. Eleanor Chesnut also began the principles and practice of nursing, but she was killed in an anti-foreign riot at Lianzhou in 1905 when she caused an incident by destroying idols, infuriating the local people. The hospitals were destroyed, too.[48] In 1908, American missionaries reestablished two hospitals and started medical work again after the Qing government paid a huge amount of indemnity. The 1911 Revolution brought a number of inpatients to the Hospitals. Most of them were injured by bomb explosions. The hospital treated 1,340 patients in just one month.[49] This American missionary hospital helped treat about 200 soldiers of Mao Zedong's Communist Red Army during the Long March of 1934-35 when they were marching on Lianzhou. At present this hospital is the largest hospital in the city of Lianzhou.[50]

Yangjiang

In 1886, Dr. Thomson made Macao his headquarters but practiced medicine as much as he could, setting up a clinic at Yangjiang, a seaport on the western coast and a city 200 miles southwest of Canton. In the beginning, posters were put up against the missionaries and some hostility was revealed, but no fighting occurred. Having endured many problems and much unfriendliness, he had secured a grip and won the confidence of the Chinese by his compassionate effort. The medical assistance that Dr. Thomson was adept in providing during a cholera epidemic made him more welcome among the Confucian scholars and well-to-do families. Sir Robert Hart, the inspector general of the Customs Service in China, while visiting in south China, was so impressed by the Americans' medical achievements that he made a donation of five hundred dollars to Dr. and Mrs. Thomson for their work in 1886.[51] Dr. Thomson treated 6,050 patients in 1886, and the number of outpatients treated was 16,548 in 1890.[52] In 1893, the Thompsons were united with two brothers, the Reverend Andrew Beattie and David Beattie, M.D., their two wives and two Chinese pastors. This mission station south of Canton near the south China coast had a chaotic year when a fatal bubonic plague spread from one side of the province to the other in 1894, leaving tens of thousands lifeless. As the presence of foreigners was held accountable for this tragedy, a riot occurred and a violent mob broke into the Beattie residence and destroyed their two homes. The two families with their children took shelter at the government compound where they were saved from harm. They departed when their property was demolished by rioters. The station was closed in 1894 for a short time and again during the Boxer Rebellion in 1900.[53]

Dr. William H. Dobson (1870-1965) on behalf of the Northern Presbyterian Church opened the Fumin Hospital (Foreman Memorial Hospital) in 1902 at Yangjiang. Dobson, born in 1870 in New Jersey, went to Yangjiang in 1897 after receiving his medical degree. Tan Yunchang, a native Chinese, became Dr. Dobson's assistant after graduating from the Guanghua Medical School in Canton. Dobson often traveled to the countryside to take care of patients and to promote knowledge of hygiene.[54] The hospital, the only one within a radius of 150 miles, won the support of local officials, who participated in the hospital's opening ceremony. During the first year, Dr. Dobson treated 6,178 patients and performed 216 operations, and the hospital reported a variety of unusual medical cases. The hospital received 7,000 calls, had 300 patients in the wards, and performed 300 operations every year before 1914.[55] By 1915, 60,000 patients had passed through the dispensary, 3,000 had averaged twenty days in the wards, and 1,000 major and 2,000 minor operations had been carried out.[56] The outlook for the station took a turn for the better, and by 1932, the Hospital owned twenty-two buildings.[57] Today Dr. Dobson's Hospital is the foremost hospital in the city of Yangjiang.[58]

Hainan

American missionaries became interested in the Hainan Island in south China in the late 1880s. Carl C. Jeremiassen was a sea captain from Denmark. In 1868, he went to China and was employed later by the Canton Customs Service, making the acquaintance of Dr. Kerr. He served an apprenticeship for two years at the Canton Hospital where he acquired enough knowledge of medical practice to enable him to commence medical work in the following years. Then single-handedly Jeremiassen went to Hainan in 1881, the tropical island divided from the extreme point of southern Guangdong Province by a narrow twelve-mile strait. He started mission work there as an independent self-supporting missionary and opened a dispensary, where he was able to cure many of the patients who came.[59]

In 1885, the Presbyterian Board decided to appoint Dr. H. M. McCandliss and Rev. Frank P. Gilman as missionaries to Hainan. Dr. McCandliss, the son of a physician in Philadelphia and John Kerr's grandson, left America for Canton in May 1885. He pursued his course at the Jefferson Medical College in Philadelphia. On reaching Canton, he spent some months working at the Canton Hospital before he went to Hainan. In November 1885, Dr. McCandliss and Mr. Jeremiassen established a hospital in the city of Haikou, the first Western hospital in Hainan Island. In 1886, Dr C. S. Terrill and his wife came to serve in the hospital. Dr. Terrill had already had many opportunities to exercise his surgical skill, and a number of patients were anxiously awaiting his arrival. About seventy outpatients were treated at the hospital daily.[60]

During the hot summer months of 1887, an epidemic of malaria broke out and many troops died. Jeremiassen began to treat the ill soldiers with quinine; all patients under his care were restored to health. So the grateful general gave land to him, and a thatched-roof building was erected, becoming the site for the mission compound with its dispensary, manse, and chapel. Mr. and Mrs. Jeremiassen became something of a legend on the island as they traveled on long trips into the mountains. In 1892, 15,681 patients came to visit the hospital and dispensary, and Mr. Jeremiassen treated 3,500 patients.[61] Their annual report of 1894 recounted their experiences, "We stayed among the Tahan hills for about a fortnight, having daily service and healing the sick."[62] By 1919, the hospital established by Dr. McCandliss had 100 beds and had an average of 150 patients all the time.[63] Today this hospital is the largest hospital in Hainan Province.[64]

In brief, the dispensary movement of the medical missionaries helped found hospitals and dispensaries in the rural areas in south China to provide medical services to the sick. They played a role in promoting modern medical work in the countryside. Those hospitals and dispensaries became admired among the poor peasants, gentries, and merchants, and some of them even won the support of the local governments. American medical missionaries were welcomed in those communities basically because of their successful treatments, although they were in trouble and sometimes killed during the anti-foreign campaigns. More importantly, American medical missionaries paved the way, in some measure, for the spread of modern medicine in south China in the following decades, and many hospitals they established during that time are still serving the Chinese today after the People's Republic of China was established in 1949.[65]

American Doctors' Medical Achievements and Influences

Modern Hospitals

The rising of the Canton Hospital and the dispensary movement in south China contributed to the founding of more private and public modern hospitals in Canton; by 1935, a total of nearly twenty existed. American physicians were hardworking in those private hospitals in Canton in the 1930s. The Two Guang Baptist Hospital and Paul Todd's Hospital were two examples. A dispensary was established in Canton in 1901 to promote Christianity, but it was closed half a year later due to the low number of patients. Later, Dr. Zhang Xinji, Dr. Kerr's student, was determined to organize medical work under the Two Guang Baptist Association. He took over and successfully expanded the dispensary in 1916 so as to provide free medical care and medicine to poor patients and to use medicine to spread God's blessing to the Cantonese. In 1917, Dr. Zhang handed the hospital over to Liangguang Jinxinhui (Two Guang Baptist Association). The Board of Trustees of the

Two Guang Baptist Association was created to take care of the hospital, and they named it Liangguang Jinxinhui Hospital and appointed Dr. Zhang Xinji as its supervisor in 1919. In the 1920s, the Hospital was expanded when a fine, new building was erected in eastern Canton, modernized equipment was purchased, and the number of patients was greater than before.[66]

Dr. Charles A. Hayes played a role in the expansion of the Two Guang Baptist Hospital. Dr. Hayes and his wife came to China in 1902 under the auspices of the Mission Board of the Southern Baptist Church. As a medical missionary, he started working at a hospital in northern Guangdong Province, and later at a hospital in the city of Wuzhou, Guangxi Province, approximately 250 miles northwest of Canton. Many years were spent in Wuzhou where Dr. Hayes developed a zealous interest in diseases of the eye, ear, nose, and throat. After special study in these areas, he was invited by the Canton Hospital to join its staff, becoming the chair of the Department of Eye, Ear, Nose, and Throat at the Canton Hospital and professor of eyes at Gongyi Medical College. He began work at the Liangguang Jinxinhui Hospital in October 1918, and was appointed in 1919 as chairman of the staff, during which period Dr. Calvin C. Rush was working together with him in this department. The Hospital treated 688 outpatients in 1919 and 328 inpatients 1922. Later, Dr. Hayes became a doctor-in-chief of the Two Guang Baptist Hospital due to the closure of the Canton Hospital as a result of its workers' strikes in 1923. In early 1926 he was assigned to the Department of the Eye, Ear, Nose and Throat in the newly finished Two Guang Baptist Hospital where he still continued working in a dedicated manner. The Hospital was expanded during that time and treated 22,000 outpatients and 1,700 inpatients in 1933. Dr. Hayes contributed significantly to the expansion and works of the Hospital until he retired and returned to the United States in 1937.[67]

Dr. Paul Todd also played a role in the development of modern hospital services in Canton. After resigning from the Canton Hospital, Dr. Todd helped establish the Gongyi Medical School and its hospital. Later, he returned to the Canton Hospital in 1929 as superintendent but resigned again and went into private practice. In 1929, Todd's hospital was established, having fourteen ward beds, four doctors, and six nurses. By 1934, it had forty beds, four doctors, and six nurses. Every year about 1,500 patients visited and 1,064 stayed at his hospital for treatment. Dr. Todd became one of the best-known and most beloved physicians in Canton.[68]

Medical Associations

The beginning of the Medical Missionary Society, the first of its kind in the world, was an eminent achievement of American missionary doctors in Canton. The society had its birth in Parker's medical work in 1838 and remained the government body of the institution until 1930 when the Canton Hospital's administration was transferred to the directors of Lingnan University. When Peter Parker realized the Ophthalmic Hospital could not be run by only one man, it was instantly put under the Society's control. The first draft of the propositions pertaining to the organization was issued in 1836, and the first manifesto published by the Medical Missionary Society made an articulate statement about the statesmanlike nature of the founders and their broad vision of the undertakings of medical missions. The goal of the Society was to push the medical professionals to be present and work among the Chinese, introduce the Gospel, instruct Chinese youths in Western medicine, expand general medical knowledge through practice which would be secured in China, present an opportunity for Christian kindness and service, and offer to the Chinese people some of those advantages which modern sciences and technology had bestowed upon the West world. The medical missionaries anticipated that the Chinese would enjoy the advantages of modern medicine and their confidence and companionship would be gained by the Westerners.[69] As Dr. Thomas Richardson Colledge stated, "The great object of this Society is to aid the Missionary of the Gospel and the philanthropist, in the execution of their good works, by opening avenues for the introduction of those sciences and that religion."[70]

Dr. Colledge was elected the president of the Society, but he left China in 1838 and never returned, continuing to hold the position of honorary president of the Society. Elected as one of the vice presidents of the Society, Dr. Parker always took the chair at annual meetings while still retaining his office of senior vice president. After the Opium War, the Nanjing Treaty of 1842 forced the Qing government to open a total of five Chinese seaports to Westerners. As a result, the Medical Missionary Society was, in some measure, prepared to take advantage of these new openings, announcing its statement at the annual meeting of the Society held on September 1842.[71] The Medical Missionary Society made great efforts to establish new hospitals in the treaty ports in the following decades.

On February 21, 1857, the meeting presided over by Dr. Parker was his last appearance as a medical missionary in China. On the word of the twenty-second annual meeting report of 1861, Dr. Kerr was a correspondent and recording secretary. Parker did not become the president of the Medical Missionary Society in China until 1879 when Colledge died in that year.[72]

Since the number of Protestant missionaries had augmented quickly after the opening of the Chinese hinterland to foreigners in 1860, thirty-four medical missionaries decided to coordinate the medical work of the roughly sixty different Protestant societies that were separately backing medical missionary work in China. Thus Dr. H. W. Boone in Shanghai proposed in 1885 the creation of the China Medical Missionary Association (CMMA).[73] When the medical missionaries in various parts of China had a conference in 1886 in

Shanghai, Dr. Kerr was unanimously chosen by ballot the first president of the CMMA because he was much more famous than any of the other surgeons in China. The first medical organization was formally established in China. During the conference, President Kerr's speech and several papers dealing with the problem of medical education in China were in favor of promoting medical education for the Chinese. The goals of the new Association were summarized in the first number of the *China Medial Missionary Journal,* of which Dr. Kerr was the editor. The CMMA's objectives were to promote medical science amongst the Chinese and mutual assistance derived from the varied experiences of the medical missionaries in China, cultivate and advance mission work and medical science in general, and preserve the nature, curiosity, and reputation of the fraternity by upholding a coalition and accord of the ordinary professionals in China. A list of the original thirty-four members included: John Swan, John C. McPhun, Mary H. Fulton. In 1890, CMMA established a Medical Terms Committee to standardize the translation of medical terms into Chinese.[74]

In Canton, when the fiftieth anniversary of the founding of the Medical Missionary Society was commemorated in 1888, Dr. Parker died, and Dr. Kerr succeeded him as the president of the Canton Medical Missionary Society, an office Kerr held until his resignation in 1899.[75] At a meeting called by Dr. John Kirk on February 26, 1909 at his home in Canton to discuss the formation of a Canton branch of the China Medial Missionary Association, new officers were elected: Dr. John Kirk, president; Dr. Josiah C. McCracken, vice president; and Dr. J. Allen Hofmann, secretary and treasurer. Other branches of the CMMA were opened in Shanghai, Wuhan, Fujian, Taiwan, and others thereafter.[76]

In the spring of 1912, all members of the Canton branch of the CMMA were privileged with a visit from Sun Yat-sen, the founding father of the Republic of China, for whom a party was organized at the hospital. Dr. Sun was honored to become a life member of this society and was elected as a director for life. The British and American consuls in Canton as well as prominent British and American merchants were elected vice presidents.[77]

The China Medical Missionary Association partially inspired the Chinese physicians of Western medicine to organize a national association. In May 1915, the idea of creating a National Medical Association was again being discussed. A good chance to make good progress came when the doctors got together in Shanghai during the 1915 biennial conference of the China Medical Missionary Association. The National Medical Association of China, a professional organization mainly composed of modern Chinese physicians, was founded, and the first issue of the *National Medical Journal of China* (English and Chinese editions) appeared in October 1915. Next year the first conference of the National Medical Association was held in Shanghai at the Y.M.C.A. building on February 7-12, 1916, and about eighty members participated in this meeting. Its original membership of seventy-seven soon increased to ninety-two, including twenty-six medical women. The Guangdong branch of the National Medical Association was formed during the Canton Conference in 1917.[78]

The Canton Medical Missionary Society had its meetings every year. On January 17, 1924, thirty-six members attended the eighty-fifth annual meeting.[79] The South China Branch of the China Medical Missionary Association in 1926 elected President J. Allen Hofmann and Secretary A. Clair Siddall. The last and most compelling evidence of the merit and eminence of the medical missions was the merger of the China Medical Missionary Association and the National Medical Association of China in 1932; this new national organization also established a Council on Medical Missions, of which the Chinese president of the Association was a member.[80]

In a word, the Medical Missionary Society played a part in the founding of a national medical association in China, which is still operational. The doctors at the Canton medical mission were no longer isolated from their colleagues who were then scattered in all parts of China: Fuzhou, Xiamen, Shanghai, Ningbo, Hangzhou, and Beijing. Inspired by the Medical Missionary Society, the Chinese founded their own national medical association for the first time in modern China. The establishment of the Chinese Medical Association was a wonderful example of a union between the missionary and the Chinese medical organizations and a fine instance of friendly internationalism in medical science, a tremendous step forward in the introduction of Western medicine in China. After the establishment of the China Medical Missionary Association, American medical missionaries worked together with it to promote Western medicine in the new Republic.

Medical Journals

As early as 1868, Dr. Kerr had started the publishing of a newspaper *Guangzhou Xinbao* (Canton's New Newspaper), the first newspaper in Chinese language to introduce Western medicine. It was a weekly sheet, one foot square in size, printed on one side and sold for one case on the street. In 1880, Dr. Kerr published a small Chinese medical journal called *Xiyi xinbao* (Western Healing News) in quarterly installments, which continued for two years only.[81] It was the first journal on Western medicine in the Chinese language in China, although it had a very short existence because it was stopped with the eighth issue. The purpose of the journal, according to Kerr, was to help Chinese practitioners of Western medicine exchange their medical experiences, and to provide latest medical achievements to the public, because no medical journal in Chinese was available in China at that time.[82] Dr. Kerr contributed an article in each issue during his editorship. The publication of *Xiyi xinbao* was so popular in Canton that *The China Review* published in Hong Kong praised it for being a Western medical journal for the Chinese public that provided them with an opportunity to compare and contrast Chinese and Western medicines.[83] Dr. Kerr published many articles in the periodical on popular diseases, their symptoms and their treatments in Western medicine, which attracted so many Chinese that these articles were republished in other magazines. *Wanguo gongbao* (Global News), for example, published Kerr's "Lun Neizhi" (On internal piles) first published in *Xiyi xinbao.*[84]

Yixue bao (The Medical Journal) was first published monthly in Canton in 1886, the first journal on Western medicine run by the Chinese in China. Dr. Yin Duanmo published several articles in the journal on how to prevent the spread of plague, to quit opium, and to protect eyes in an attempt to promote the spread of knowledge of hygiene. Kerr was an editor for two years of the *China Medical Missionary Journal,* which brought out its first issue in March 1887. This journal, produced in quarterly installments, was the periodical of the China Medical Mission Association. Beginning on January 1, 1905, it was published every two months, and in May 1907, its title was changed to the *China Medical Journal.*[85]

In May 1912, a Chinese bi-monthly, called the *Zhonghua yi bao* (The Chinese Medical Journal) was published in Canton under Dr. William W. Cadbury. Among the scientific papers, reports, and other items published before July 1913, thirty-five articles were written by modern-trained Chinese physicians and thirty-four by foreigners. Two of the most notable articles were on the administration of sanitation and on government sanitary regulations of Guangdong Province. Dr. Todd reported at the 1913 conference that the journal had 221 subscribers and was self-financing, and the publication committee suggested that the China Medical Missionary Association should take over its financial tasks and make it an official periodical of the Association, though it was still prepared for publication in Canton at that time. Dr. Cadbury remained editor of the journal until the later part of 1915 when he went on leave of absence and was succeeded by Dr. J. A. Hofmann. The Journal remained in publication until 1917 (a total of thirty-two numbers were published). When it became obvious that the National Medical Association of China was competent to issue a magazine in Chinese, the medical missionaries were delighted to surrender the responsibility and transfer it to the Chinese. As a result, the *China Medical Journal* integrated with the *National Medical Journal* to form the *Chinese Medical Journal* in January 1932, which is still operating today in China.[86]

In summary, American medical journals enabled the Chinese physicians of Western medicine to have an organ for the first time, in which they would express themselves and report upon their medical works. Those academic journals also helped the Chinese to gather the continuously mounting collection of observations and experience for the good of their own organization and the world in general. By means of the medium of the journals, the Chinese were able to read medical achievements, which were of imperative interest, and medical problems of the different parts of China were brought together. In the establishment of the medical journals, American doctors took a step ahead and played a role in promoting Western medicine in China.

Surgical Treatment

Surgery is a branch of medicine, and modern surgery developed rapidly in the Western countries in the nineteenth century. All through the hundred years of its history, the Canton Hospital was well known for its surgical treatment. When Parker first began his work, surgery of the eyes and, slowly but surely, the amputation of unusual growths of the body occupied the greater part of his time. When sufficient sterilizing apparatus was introduced, the greatest amount of key operations in the city was performed at the Canton Hospital. The surgery consisted of three main lines, operations on eyes, lithotomies (removals of stones), and removal of tumors (including ovarian cysts).

Dr. Parker carried out a large number of operations for the removal of cataracts on children and adult patients, including a case of double cataract in a child of five years old. In these cataract operations, as in most of his other surgical procedures, Parker was, by and large, successful, and few of his patients grumbled about post-operative nuisances.[87]

The Canton Hospital was also in a way popularized by its lithotomies and lithotritries (stone crushings). Augmenting the reputation of the hospital, on July 17, 1844 Dr. Parker performed the first successful lithotomy operation in China at the Canton Hospital to remove a kidney stone, a common disease in China. American doctors had just started to perform such an operation in the United States. The Chinese and government officials were very impressed by the first case so treated in China. Thirty-one lithotomy cases, when lithotrity was replaced with lithotomy, were treated in the year 1845.[88] Dr. Kerr performed a crushing operation in 1856 with the use of the lithotritor of charrière, the first successful case of lithotrity in China. Operations for stones in the bladder continued to play an outstanding part in the surgical work. The largest stone, nearly half a pound, was removed in 1870, and the operation took one hour and a half. The rise in the number of such cases was so amazing that Dr. Kerr published an article in 1894, focusing on his personal practices in many cases.[89]

Vesical calculi (bladder stones) were "found pretty much all over China," but were particularly widespread in Guangdong, according to Dr. Hamilton Jeffreys' 1910 report. The Canton Hospital, which was made famous by Peter Parker for the number of bladder stone operations, continued to enjoy its eminence under Kerr, who, it was said, had performed more "stone operations [than any] other known surgeon, barring one."[90] Since the first operation was performed by Peter Parker, the Canton Hospital held the record for the highest number of surgical treatments for vesical calculus in China.

Finally, American doctors took care of countless patients badly affected with tumors of numerous types. The removal of tumors posed the most difficult task to Dr. Parker.[91] The first attempt in China to remove an ovarian tumor was made by Dr. Kerr in 1875, but because of adhesions, the surgical work was not finished. The patient in this case recovered from the incision, which was made in the abdomen. Dr. J. F. Carrow in his report mentioned two operations for ovarian tumor in 1876 and four in 1877. A successful ovariotomy (ovarian operation) was completed by Dr. Kerr in 1880. In 1902, two ovariotomies were performed. In 1903, an ovarian tumor was removed, weighing forty-eight pounds. By 1905, there were eighteen operations for ovarian tumor, five for appendicitis and one for strangulated hernia. In 1875, the first laparotomy (surgical opening of the abdomen) was performed in the Hospital, again the first case of such surgery in China. It was not until the 1890s that much was done in abdominal surgery, and the period between 1902 and 1907 was considered the beginning of abdominal surgery.[92] An amputation of the arm for a male patient in a life-threatening situation was carried out at the Canton Hospital when Dr. J. Jardine offered fifty dollars to the man. The patient allowed the operation, and his life was saved. In 1900, Dr. Andrew H. Woods removed a thyroid gland, the first time such an operation was done in the Hospital. Therefore, operations occupied a great percentage of the cases, as many as 10 percent of the total admissions, or more than 200,000 out of the two million patients.[93] The Canton Hospital took the lead in the development of modern surgery in China when Western medicine was introduced into Chinese society at that time.

Autopsy and Dissection

In the history of Chinese medicine, dissection and most surgery were forbidden as mutilations of the human body. Even in late nineteenth century China, it appeared that most students' interest in anatomy had to make their studies at sites of the execution or on the bodies of animals. After obtaining the permission of the patient's relatives to extract the stone, Dr. Parker, for the first time, was allowed to perform a partial autopsy on a man who had been suffering from a bladder stone and had died at the hospital on May 18, 1849. The doctor considered this a great breakthrough because, as he wrote, the Chinese were very intolerant of autopsy. Another medical leap forward was made when a second autopsy was performed at the Canton Hospital in November 1850.[94] In 1867, Dr. Huang Kuan started teaching an anatomy course at the Canton Hospital and next year carried out a postmortem examination, the first case in China. The Canton government did not approve postmortem examinations until 1912, the first local government to legalize postmortem examination in China.[95]

Medical Technology

The introduction of ether and chloroform as anesthetics was another pioneering achievement by the Canton Hospital. The use of ether or chloroform as anesthetic was unknown during the early years of Western hospitals. Only a few instruments and drugs were obtainable; patients were given an opiate just before an operation, but it did not always sufficiently lessen pain. Dr. Charles Thomas Jackson, a renowned Boston chemist and geologist, was the inventor of ether as anesthetic, dispatching Parker his breathing equipment along with a supply of ether and a description of the practice. Parker used the new innovation in a tumor surgery on October 4, 1847. The patient stayed awake but did not suffer any pain, a triumphant surgery. According to Dr. Parker, "I selected for its first trial a Chinese, a robust farmer.... He was then directed to inhale deliberately with full inspirations the ether from Dr. Jackson's apparatus."[96] This was the first time ether was employed as an anesthetic for surgical procedure in China. Parker began to use ether frequently in his operations after that. Quickly adopting a new anesthesia, Dr. Parker performed a successful operation on November 24, 1849 for calculus under the influence of chloroform as an anesthetic, the first time used in China.[97]

The year 1861 witnessed first example of medical photography in China.[98] A case was illustrated at some length of a man whose body was covered with countless tumors, and the number had been evidently mounting over the years. This was not the first case at the Canton Hospital, which concentrated on such problems, but a photograph of this was taken that year.[99]

Modern management measures were introduced into the Canton Hospital when rules of the hospital were established by Dr. Parker. Patients were required to queue up to register at the register office before seeing doctors and were admitted by a porter who gave them a numbered slip. They then progressed to the receiving room where they were treated in order of coming. Patient records were also established to trace patients' history, and thorough records were maintained with the patient's number, disease, time of admission, and medicine. A copy of this record was given to the patient to be used as identification by the porter on subsequent visits.[100] The Canton Hospital was leading the way in medical science in China in terms of medical technology and management.

The Impact of Western Medicine on the Commoners

American doctors found esteem in the eyes of the Chinese patients. The patients of the Canton Hospital were from different classes, from the homeless persons in the street to gentlemen and merchants. Most patients were satisfied with the medical treatment at the Canton Hospital and grateful to American doctors. An old Cantonese gentleman, for instance, requested to be permitted to send a native artist to paint Parker's portrait with the intention that he might be able to kowtow (ritual bow usually held in reserve for the imperial rulers and the city gods) before it every morning because Dr. Parker was successful in restoring his sight. In keeping with Chinese tradition, Dr. Parker usually returned gifts in an effort to demonstrate his fair-mindedness, but offerings of food were held in reserve and used to supplement the hospital supplies. To demonstrate their thankfulness, some patients compiled verses of gratitude, which were forwarded to the Canton Hospital on decorated rolls, and some wished to present kowtow to Dr. Parker.

Dr. Parker became popular not only in Canton but also in China. Many patients traveled more than one thousand miles from "Fujian, Jiangxi Zhejiang, Anhui, Jiangsu provinces to Canton to see Dr. Parker. Some patients even came from Shanxi Province in North China."[101] A 48-year-old gentleman of Zhejiang Province, for instance, had a tumor of nearly one foot circumference positioned upon his left cheek. He learnt of the Canton Hospital through his friends and traveled sixty-two days to Canton. He seemed quite affected when informed that it could be safely removed. The surgery was, without delay, performed, and the tumor was extirpated. The patient awoke from the sleep with minor sickness, but it soon abated. He suffered relatively little, either during or after the surgical procedure, and on July 4, 1849 was ready to commence his long journey home.[102] The Canton Hospital under the direction of Dr. Parker was admired greatly, with as many as 1,000 patients requesting to be admitted on the receiving days. Dr. Parker's medical contributions were abundant and extraordinary: the treatment of 50,000 patients and implementation of the most advance operations of that time.

Dr. John Kerr was hospital superintendent, medical educator, and medicinal philanthropist as well as medical missionary. Dr. Kerr had been an administrator of the Canton Hospital for forty-five years, during which time, the number of patients under his treatment totaled 39,440 inpatients and 740,324 outpatients. His patients came from about 4,000 villages and towns in south China.[103] Kerr was a competent surgeon, mainly proficient in lithotomy and lithotrity. He performed some 48,918 surgeries, of which 1,284 were for urinary calculus.[104] Kerr's celebrity as a surgeon became widely known, and he was recognized not only in China, but also in Europe and America. It was said that only one surgeon in the world exceeded him in the number of operations performed for bladder stones in his time. Dr. Kerr attained this most remarkable accomplishment and earned the highest reputation, despite the fact that his surgery was in no way restricted to this area of expertise alone. Dr. Kerr was so appreciated by the community he served that thousands of people took part in his funeral. The stone that marked his resting place was a block of gray granite bearing these words: "John Kerr, M.D. LL.D., 1824-1901. Missionary of the American Presbyterian Board came to China in 1854 for forty-five years in charge of Medical Missionary Society's Hospital, Canton. Afterwards, he founded the first Refuge for the Insane in China."[105]

Dr. John Swan spent thirty-four years in China, of which twenty-nine years were in missionary service. He was a superintendent, business manager, surgeon of the Canton Hospital and a medical doctor to the Chinese Maritime Customs at Canton for the foreign community and port surgeon for the American consulate. As a meticulous and professional family physician, he inspired confidence and won the admiration and thanks of his patients from hundreds of villages and towns in south China; stories of his competence as a surgeon spread everywhere. The most unprivileged people eagerly got hold of his help, and he was never too tired to answer the call to attend. Apart from city or country calls or petitions for endowments, he hardly ever left the Hospital; he had no other ambition than his hospital work. It was indisputable that no other name was more commonly known to the Cantonese patients than "Guan Yisheng" (Doctor Swan), uttered with friendliness in nearly every part of Canton in the 1910s.[106]

The Canton Hospital was so popular in the Cantonese society that it helped, to some extent, not only the patients but also ordinary Cantonese take a new attitude towards American doctors. In 1847, for example, in a placard denouncing the British and paying tribute to Parker, the Cantonese wrote that Parker practiced the therapeutic arts and commonly alleviated the poor Chinese, whose high merit had been praised by all the Chinese.[107]

The Boji Hospital's survival during the anti-foreign missionary campaign of 1870-1871 in China was another example. When the Tianjin Massacre occurred in that city in June 1870, a rumor was widespread that the French Catholic Sisters abducted or purchased children for their orphanage with the aim of taking away their hearts and eyes for medicine. Such gossip was intended to provide the Chinese with pretexts as a grievance against the reviled foreigners. Tianjin suffered more than any other cities, but anti-foreign sentiments were rising throughout the empire so that Canton could not be avoided. The Boji Hospital's medical work was able to persist without any disruption, but in 1871 its buildings and Dr. Kerr's residence scarcely evaded destruction by fire because some shops in the vicinity were ablaze. Anti-foreign emotion was powerful during that year. The number of patients at the hospital was exceedingly reduced the moment the rumor about poisoning was prevalent. In all the accusations made against foreigners in Canton, none were targeted against the Boji Hospital. This was because the caring nature of the institute towards the Cantonese people was known, and nobody accepted as true the tales that some of the inpatients at Boji had been poisoned by the powders or capsules which were given by the doctors.[108]

Arriving in China in 1834, Parker found a people very unfriendly to all foreigners and particularly suspicious of Westerners. After putting up with many problems and much unfriendliness, American doctors secured a foothold and won the confidence of the Chinese by their compassionate efforts. The medical assistance that American doctors were adept in providing gave rise to a more welcoming reaction from the commoners as well as Confucian scholars and well-to-do families. By the end of the nineteenth century, much of the opposition and mistrust had disappeared; many Cantonese had accepted and esteemed Western medicine in general and Western medical doctors in particular. This change in attitude resulted, to some extent, from American medical doctors' successful medical treatment of hundreds of thousands of Chinese patients.

The Impact of Western Medicine on the Officials

The Canton government originally gave unspoken recognition to the Canton Hospital and remained silent and suspicious when it was founded. Later, some Qing officials occasionally visited the Canton Hospital for medical attention and consultation. Since Dr. Parker occupied a key position as one of the few successful doctors in the Chinese empire and the prestige of the hospital remained high, more eminent Chinese officials often went to seek Dr. Parker's services. A district magistrate, who had become blind due to much reading of official papers late at night with insufficient light, was treated for four months. An operation was performed finally, but it produced no results. As a result, he was discharged, weeping. Later, he sent a testimonial back to Dr. Parker, expressing his gratitude. He wrote that Dr. Parker daily treated several hundred with kindness for a long time without weariness and that "Although my sight is not yet restored, nevertheless I have received the doctor's diligent attention and become inseparably attached to him."[109] When the provincial judge came to Parker to have his ears treated, a malformation of the ear was discovered. After his condition was improved, the judge was very pleased with Parker's treatment.[110]

A crucial event occurred at the Canton Hospital in January 1838 when a woman patient died, the first death recorded in the history of the hospital. The Hong merchants asked for interment, the customary Chinese practice. The magistrate, a former patient of Parker, conducted an investigation of this case and suspended inquest. After the examination, the government did not make an objection, and the dead body was buried, an important step in the history of both medical missions and Sino-Western relations because for the first time in Chinese history, a local government gave unspoken recognition to missionaries' practice of medicine in the empire.[111]

When Western medicine appealed abundantly to the Chinese officials in Canton, more officials often eagerly sought American doctors' medical treatments. In 1839, Parker treated a number of influential patients. The prefect of the province suffered from a bad case of neuralgia; Parker explained the real character of his disease and assuaged his grief. A district magistrate with a painful peptic ulcer was treated successfully by Dr. Parker, too.[112] According to Dr. Park's annual report of 1840, in 1839, "among the more distinguished personages who have, directly or indirectly, availed themselves of the benefits that the institution affords, were a commissioner" of "circuit in Kwangse [Guangxi], heads of the judicial and the financial and territorial affairs of this province, and, not least, the high imperial commissioner, of which all have heard so much."[113]

Dr. Parker was also invited to attend to the wives or children of government officials. He removed a tumor from the son of a local official; he successfully treated the wife of another official for skin poisoning, caused by a native doctor's "medicine." Maybe the most fascinating of these instances was that the wife of an army officer from Nanjing refused to visit the hospital, so Parker had to treat her on a boat on the river, just outside the foreign factories. The therapy went well, and the American doctor later learned that she was associated with the emperor himself.[114]

During the Taiping Rebellion in the early 1850s, the city of Guilin in Guangxi Province was defended by a Tartar general, Ou lan-tai, who was one of the best generals in the Qing army. While fighting on the fortifications, where they were attacked relentlessly by the insurgents, a small iron ball penetrated into his knee. As the injury was regarded exceptionally hazardous and Chinese medicine was judged inadequate in so critical and urgent situation, a prompt letter was dispatched to Canton, inquiring Dr. Parker's instruction. The American doctor himself was entirely prepared to pay a quick visit to the wounded general to pull out the ball, but his suggestion was not allowed because foreigners could not enter the inland of the empire, as indicated by the Qing laws. For that reason, Ou-lan-tai set out on the journey to Canton so as to receive Dr. Parker's surgery there, but the deficient medical attentions of the Chinese physicians, which he had received earlier, caused the wound to deteriorate, and he died en route.[115]

Many high-ranking officials of Guangdong Province were impressed by Western medicine because American doctors successfully treated their illness in the 1880s.[116] On October 17, 1884, Dr. J. C. Thomson received a letter from Viceroy Zhang Zhidong of both Guangdong and Guangxi provinces, who asked Thomson to pay a visit to him.[117] Dr. Thomson had prescribed for him in the past, and afterwards his son informed Dr. Thomson that his father had been restored to health. While calling on him this time, Dr. Thomson found him extremely friendly.[118] In 1885, Dr. Kerr went to see Governor Zhang Shusheng of Guangdong Province, and Zhang returned to health after Kerr's careful treatment. In 1889, Dr. Kerr was called to attend a Tartar general, who was a military commander and held the highest rank of any official in the province. After his recovery, he came personally with a large number of followers to show gratitude to Dr. Kerr.[119]

American doctors not only took care of the Qing officials' health but also treated the sick in the Qing armies. On April 29, 1885, for example, Viceroy Zhang Zhidong sent a request through U.S. Consul Paul Seymour to the Canton Hospital for a military surgeon to serve in the Taiwan Army.

American doctor L. W. Luscher, together with two native assistants from the hospital, left for Taiwan on May 10. The hospital of the North Taiwan Army near Jilong was closed in September 1886 when Dr. Luscher returned to Canton, after serving there for a year and a half.[120]

American doctors' successful treatment of the Qing officials helped the Canton Hospital not only win official recognition but also protection. During the Sino-French War of 1883-1884, for example, mobs that did not distinguish Americans from the French attempted to attack the Canton Hospital—although after the Opium War Western hospitals and schools were protected by the Qing government, in accordance with the Treaty of Nanjing. As a result, the American consulate in Canton sought official protection of American medical missionaries' lives and property, and the Canton government quickly published an announcement on June 27, 1884 that all foreigners' churches and hospitals were legal under the treaties and that those who hurt and attacked the Westerners would be punished. On July 19, the Canton government published another official declaration that all American churches and hospitals were protected by the Chinese government because the United States was in good relations with Imperial China and that those people who occupied Americans' property would be punished severely, according to Dr. Kerr's report.[121]

The American doctor's treatment of the Qing officials had an effect, even if small, on their attitude toward the Westerners and Western culture. The medical treatments of both Lin Zexu and Qiying were two good examples.[122]

Lin Zexu

Lin, a Fujian scholar-official and a *Jinshi* degree holder of 1811, worked at the Hanlin Academy, the esteemed official center for Confucian learning in the imperial capital.[123] Lin's father was a good friend of a famous Chinese physician, Chen Nianzu, both often discussing Chinese medicine and ways to maintain long life. While they were discussing, young Lin always stood by and listened carefully to their conversations. Later, Lin became interested in Chinese medicine and began to link medicine with the Chinese empire's might. In February 1830, he was asked to write an introduction for a medical book, *Jinkui yaolue qianzhu* (Annotation on Medicine) written by Chen Nianzu. Lin wrote in the introduction that good medicine was important not only for people's health but also for a strong state and that both physicians and officials had the same important duties in terms of people's lives.[124]

Since Lin was good on Chinese medicine and realized the harmful consequence of opium smoking, he tried to use Chinese medicine to cure opium addiction at that time. With the help of a famous physician of Chinese medicine, He Qiwei (1774-1837), Lin effectively created treatments for opium addicts of Chinese herbs. His treatments to cure addicts were successfully in Hupei

Province, and many addicts got rid of the opium evil. Lin thus submitted his treatments to the imperial court in 1838.[125]

Since more and more Chinese became opium addicts due to the opium traffic, Emperor Daoguang made his decision firmly to stop the opium trade. To enforce his decree, the emperor chose and ordered Lin in November 1838 to proceed to Canton as a specially appointed imperial commissioner to end the practice of the opium trade. Lin left Beijing on January 23 and arrived in Canton on March 10, 1839. To put an end to opium, Commissioner Lin tried to muster all the traditional powers. As regards the foreigners, Lin employed a comparable mixture of rationale, proper advice, and intimidation, so as to compel the Westerners to abide by their legal business in tea, silk, and porcelain, and so on and to restrain them from hurting the Chinese people and violating the international laws. Considering opium as less destructive than alcohol, the English traders refused to abandon the opium trade during the anti-opium crusade in Canton in the summer of 1839, and Lin first forced them out of Canton and Macao thereafter. After Lin seized the opium of the British merchants in June, the British merchants mobilized all their traditional forces to urge Parliament to declare war on China in order to punish the Chinese.[126]

Lin was not in good health while in Canton. By that time Lin had realized that Western medicine was more scientific and practical than Chinese medicine. In a letter of May 1, 1839 to his friend, Lin wrote: "Western medicine had advantages over Chinese medicine because Western doctors dissected the dead person's body to identify the reasons for the death."[127] Thus it was not surprising that Lin decided to consult Dr. Parker about his own health, using Howqua as an intermediary. At that time, the commissioner was suffering from a hernia and desired to have Dr. Parker treat his illness but refused to come to see the doctor personally. Parker finally agreed to send him medicine and bandages, recommending a truss. Since Lin declined to come in person to be fitted, Parker passed along six he had in stock. Later he learned that one of the six suited Lin tolerably, although "when he coughs, the contents of the abdomen are liable to descend."[128]

Dr. Parker's treatment apparently was fairly successful, and Lin remarked positively upon Parker's medical ability. Parker later wrote, "Many of the chief officers of the empire (including Imperial Commissioner Lin,) had sought and obtained relief, and their expressions of gratitude were unbounded."[129] Lin also praised highly the Canton Hospital. In the tenth report of the Ophthalmic Hospital for the year 1839, Parker wrote, Lin "has inquired particularly regarding the ophthalmic institution, and has been correctly informed with respect to this, as well as like institutions in other counties, he has expressed himself favorably with reference to it."[130]

Western medicine helped, in some measure, establish good relations between Lin and Parker, who was becoming an advisor to Lin. In a letter of

May 1839 to Lin, Parker advised him to reach a deal with the British treaty and to persuade him to use normal diplomatic channels to solve the disputes between China and Western nations. Keen on acquiring more advantages for Western traders and missionaries, Parker was looking forward to meeting Lin in consequence of his letter. This did not take place, but Lin did seek advice from Parker about opium addicts. Lin wanted to have a formula from Dr. Parker, which would help treat those opium patients and speculated whether Dr. Parker could blend some twenty or thirty ingredients and identify the quantity of the mix necessary to heal each addict. Parker provided the treatments on opium, but informed Lin that there was no particular remedy that would heal opium patients, each patient having to be cured in proportion to his symptoms.[131]

In the meantime, Imperial Commissioner Lin also asked Dr. Parker's help for translating Western laws into Chinese. In July, Dr. Parker was visited by two of the commissioner's deputies who made various inquiries. A few weeks later, the commissioner asked Parker to translate a part of E. de Vattel's book, *Law of Nations,* into Chinese. Dr. Parker translated a long paper into Chinese, with respect to the laws of nations, particularly national wars and national relations.[132]

During the crisis, Lin believed that there were conflicts between the English and Americans who had the power to challenge the English and that it was possible to carry out different trade policies toward different powers so as to establish an alliance between China and the United States against Great Britain. In his memorial of July 1839 to the emperor, Lin suggested the establishment of the Sino-U.S. alliance against the British for three reasons.[133] First, Lin wrote that since trade was both bait and weapon, every power was willing to carry out trade with China and that the Chinese should trade with those nations observing the Chinese laws and stop doing business with those nations violating Qing laws. If Chinese trade with England was closed, in Lin's opinion, Americans would benefit significantly from Chinese trade at the cost of the British, and Americans would be willing to cooperate with China against Britain.[134] Second, Lin wrote that Americans were observing the Chinese trade laws and were friendlier with the Chinese than the English.[135] Finally, Lin asserted that since England was the most powerful nation in the world and only America and France would be able to challenge it, the Sino-U.S. alliance would be a means to resist British aggression. As a result, Lin suggested establishing an alliance with Americans against the English. Lin's suggestion, however, was not adopted by the emperor.

Lin then submitted a memorial to Emperor Daoguang on August 3, 1839, a letter to send to the queen of the United Kingdom, encouraging the British government to stop the illegal opium trade. After the emperor approved it on August 27, Lin asked his senior interpreter to translate it into English. Lin was not entirely sure of the interpreter's competence in English; therefore he had another man translate the English version back into Chinese to check its accuracy. Apparently, Lin was not satisfied with the translation. In October 1839, Lin had Howqua request Peter Parker to translate the emperor's correspondence into English. Parker did study the letter and pointed out that it contained convincing arguments along with "nonsense and insult" which would worsen Lin's diplomacy.[136] Lin's diplomatic efforts failed, and war finally broke out on November 3, 1839.

In short, Lin was at that time one of the most enlightened, progressive, and open-minded officials in the Qing empire when most Qing officials were uninformed and arrogant. Most Qing officials' views of Westerners remained totally negative when they emphasized how ignorant and uncultured Westerners were. It is very interesting that an American doctor had become a high-ranking Chinese official's friend and adviser when Lin asked Parker to use Western medicine to treat the opium addicts, especially to translate Western laws into Chinese and the emperor's correspondence into English. Lin advocated an alliance with the United States against Britain, a strategy on the basis of China's traditional statecraft of playing barbarians off against barbarians, but his view of Americans was not totally negative. There were several reasons for Lin's better attitude towards Americans than towards the English. Western medicine was one of the forces, if not the sole one, to inspire Lin to take different attitude towards Westerners in general and Americans in particular because he considerably appreciated an American doctor's medical treatment and an American hospital's medical achievements when his illness had been cured by Dr. Parker with Western medicine.

Qiying

Qiying was another eminent official having closing relations with an American doctor. Imperial Commissioner Qiying was the chief negotiator during the negotiation of the Treaty of Nanjing in 1842. After signing the Treaty, Commissioner Qiying was promoted to the governor-general of Guangxi and Guangdong, and sent to Canton on June 10, 1843 to negotiate with Americans.[137]

While in Canton, Qiying consulted Dr. Parker for medical advice. Qiying, not in good health, had been afflicted for more than twenty years with a troublesome skin problem, so painful that it delayed his work from time to time and forced him several times a day to seek momentary relief by showering. It was through the Hon. J. R. Morrison that Qiying first sought medical aid. After the American consul presented Dr. Parker's records on October 2 to Qiying, the Manchu official had a chance to talk directly with the American doctor. Qiying stated that his ailment originated some twenty years before, stemming from long contact to rain on horseback and that since the pain struck almost in all seasons and weather, he had up till then refused to go along with any therapies. The treatment of his illness was successful at the

Canton Hospital.[138] As a result, during an open event, Qiying, expressing how much he had benefited by the treatment of his case, happily alluded to the Canton Hospital in excellent terms of praise before the provincial judge and many other bureaucrats and employees. He subsequently requested a supply of medicine to take with him and made some small presents, accompanied by two autography tablets, enclosing such sentences as: under your skillful hand, from the winter of disease the spring of fitness returns; with long life, you sanctify mankind.[139] Clearly, the imperial commissioner was very grateful to the American doctor who had effectively healed his sickness.

Dr. Parker was engaged not only in medical work but also in the field of diplomacy after the Opium War. When the Nanjing Treaty between China and Britain was signed in 1842, American President John Tyler dispatched Caleb Cushing to China as minister plenipotentiary in an attempt to negotiate a treaty with the Chinese empire, similar to the clauses of the Treaty of Nanjing and its supplements. Arriving at Macao on February 24, 1844, Cushing, in need of a secretary and Chinese interpreter, discovered that Peter Parker was the only American capable of filling both offices. In the summer that year, Parker joined the American delegation at Wangxia, a village suburb of Macao. In the negotiations of June 17–July 3, Parker noted that he already knew almost the whole Chinese mission: Qiying and his several subordinates. Two of them were of great importance in the following negotiation: Huang Entong, the provincial treasurer and an old hand of the Nanjing compromise in 1842, and Pan Shichen, assistant in naval building to Qiying, an expert, a collector, and a pioneer of Westernization. Both had a pleasant and personal relationship with Dr. Parker. Pan's father (a former Hong businessman) and mother were Parker's patients, and Parker successfully took out a large nasal polyp from each nostril of Pan's father. Parker felt confident because these relationships would be extremely importance in the Sino-U.S. negotiation.[140]

At the commencement of the negotiation, Pan, knowing what Americans wanted from the Chinese empire, suggested the additional and most important provision, "Temples of Worship," having an article in the treaty specifically providing for the free toleration of Christianity throughout the empire. As a result, during the negotiation, Peter Parker required the insertion of "Temples of Worship" into Article 17, which provided for leasing of land for businesses and dwellings, burial grounds, and hospitals at the treaty ports. With regard to this important issue, Imperial Commissioner Qiying declared that he did not have any authority to make a conclusion until the emperor's final approval and that he would send a memorial to the monarch seriously and truthfully.[141]

The Treaty of Wangxia, which Caleb Cushing negotiated, was signed by both parties in 1844 in four copies, a milestone in the history of U.S.-China relations. Parker was delighted over the outcomes of the cooperation of both sides, stating on August 1, 1844, "Nearly everything that America could ask, or China consistently concedes, has been secured."[142] All the imperative goals of Americans were realized, especially one of the objectives—the article, which Parker had helped write, providing for the foundation of hospitals and Christian churches at five treaty ports, Canton, Xiamen, Fuzhou, Ningbo, and Shanghai. This additional article was considered as remarkably momentous because it served as a springboard for Théodose de Lagrené, the French envoy, to ask afterward for toleration of Christianity throughout the empire and helped prepare the way for the imperial edict of 1845 extending toleration to Protestants.[143]

In October 1844, the French envoys arrived in Canton to urge the Qing government to lift sanction on Christianity in China. Qiying, in his October memorials to the emperor, was in favor of lifting the embargo on Roman Catholics. He claimed that the Qing emperors had never prohibited Roman Catholics in China and that the Catholic missionaries, unlike such secret Chinese organizations as Society of Lotus, which had plotted to overthrow the Qing government, had never made any trouble in China in the past 200 years. Understanding that the French were determined to force the Qing court to lift the ban on Catholic missionaries, Qiying implied to the emperor that if the Qing court rejected the French demand, the consequence would be severe. On December 28, 1844, Qiying obtained an imperial rescript granting full toleration to the Catholics in China, a provision inserted into the Sino-French treaty of 1845.[144] This provision paved the way for extending Catholic influence throughout the empire. In a complementary proclamation of 1845, Qiying extended the same rights to Protestants. This provision, which was first conceded by the imperial rescript, was several years later included in the treaties of the Western nations—England, Russia, and the United States, a real inauguration of Christian toleration in China.[145]

Like Lin Zexu, Qiying was considering the establishment of a China-U.S.-France alliance against Britain at that time. In a memorial of January 1846 to Emperor Daoguang, Qiying suggested that since the English had conflicts with both the Americans and the French, both of whom maintained good relations with imperial China, China needed to win the support of both the Americans and the French so as to resist the English barbarians' aggressions in China.[146] The Qing court, however, did not adopt Qiying's suggestion, which remained a strategy of playing barbarians off against barbarians.

Qiying left Canton for Beijing in the spring 1848, but the commissioner still sent all the way to Canton for medical advice. His successor, despite his prejudice against foreigners on public occasions, made honorable and complimentary allusion to the Canton Hospital, according to the missionary reports for the years 1848 and 1849.[147]

Qiying started to develop a new attitude toward Christianity in a couple of years, showing his sympathy to Christians in China. In 1851, Qiying's article,

"A Form of Prayer to the God of Heaven with Preface," was translated and published in the *North China Herald*, an English journal in Shanghai. This article claimed that Jesus was the founder of Christianity and God incarnate, who came to provide salvation and reconciliation with God and that Man was created to have fellowship with God but, because of his stubborn self-will, he chose to go his own independent way, and fellowship with God was broken. Qiying wrote in his article:

> Formerly, I was commissioned to the Two Kwang Provinces, having also received the Emperor's commands to take control of the affairs of the foreigners and having closely examined the Religion practiced by the said foreigners, whether true or false, depriving or correcting and, from first to last, having watched and examined. I was brought to know that that which they preached, was true and entirely good; and that it was my duty to memorialize his Imperial Majesty, that this (Religion) might not be interfered with, and that [a] Proclamation might be issued accordingly, in order to manifest kindness toward men from afar.[148]

Qiying further claimed in his article that one of his colleagues was severely sick last winter, asking for help from the Buddhist monks and fortunetellers, but they would not cure his disease. Qiying continued that after learning that the Westerners prayed in the name of God of Heaven, his colleague prayed in the name of Jesus toward the Heaven, and the next day "he found relief in his illness. After this, whatever he prayed for his request was granted." Therefore, Qiying concluded that God existed in the universe and took care of mankind, but that many people were not grateful to Him and that people needed to pray and ask God for forgiveness of their sins.[149] Apparently, Qiying's article indicated that he had adopted more liberal attitudes toward Christianity than before and had realized the existence of God.

Qiying was one of the most conservative, intolerant officials in the Qing government before the Opium War. He was condemned later by other eminent Qing officials because he had made too many concessions to the Western powers when granting full toleration to the Catholics in China and extending toleration to Protestants under the Treaty of Wangxia of 1844 and the Sino-French Treaty of 1845 as well as other treaties thereafter. In addition, Qiying showed his sympathy to Christians in China in his article of 1851, a great leap forward in his attitude toward Western culture. It is not very clear why Qiying changed his attitude toward the West, but several reasons may help interpret Qiying's concessions and new perspective on Christianity. The pressure of the Western powers was one of the major reasons that forced Qiying to comprise with the Westerners in order to avoid a war. Second, during the negations with the Western countries, Qiying was in direct contact with the

Westerners, which helped him gradually identify the advantages of Western culture and therefore develop a new attitude toward Western religion, an important part of Western culture. Finally, Western medicine was one of the inspirations, if not the only one. Western medicine helped cure the disease that had bothered him for more than twenty years. The successful treatment helped him realize the advantage of Western medicine from his personal experience and helped him have new perception on Western culture in general and Western religion in particular. Western medicine to some extent helped make Qiying to become more tolerant and open-minded.

The Impact of Western Medicine on the Cantonese Reformers

Western medicine had an effect on not only the commoners and the officials but also the Cantonese Confucian elite, especially the progressive reformers. Western medicine helped them realize not only the disadvantages of Chinese medicine but also the shortcomings of the Chinese cultures. For this reason and others, they pushed for medical modernization and promoted social and political reform in China.

Kang Youwei

Kang Youwei (1858-1927), a great Cantonese reformer, was born into a scholarly family near Canton, where a famous educator inspired his passion for classical learning.[150] Kang successfully passed the civil service examination and thereafter earned *Juren* degree. In 1879, at the age of twenty-two, he was admitted to a private academy near Canton, therefore traveling often to Canton and Hong Kong. During the Sino-French War, the French troops threatened Canton in 1884, forcing Kang to leave Canton for his hometown and to start writing his book, *Renlei gongli* (Universal Principles of Mankind). He was working so hard that he felt sick with severe headaches. He thought he was going to die. While waiting for death, he read many books, including books on Western medicine, which encouraged him to take Western medication.[151] After taking Western medicine, Kang began to recover, as he wrote,

> On the April 7, 1885, I had such a violent headache that I thought I would die. I read medical books till my eyes hurt and the words I was reading became blurred. The doctors were unable to cure me. With my head swathed in bandages, I remained in my room for several months, checking over my notes and papers, and calmly awaited death.
>
> Later, after reading Western medical works, I came to believe in Western medical science. I followed their prescriptions and tried Western medicine, and gradually I felt better. Every day I rested under a tree back at the back of our village. By the seventh month, I was fully recovered.[152]

Western medicine cured Kang of a serious sickness in his youth and saved his life. Kang's experience of illness helped him realize the advantage of Western medicine over Chinese medicine—Chinese medicine could not cure his disease while a Western remedy was effective in saving his life. Kang began to develop his medical thought in the following years.[153]

First, Kang increased in value the role of medicine in the society to the highest degree. Kang began working on his book, *Renlei gongli*, in 1884, and parts of it were completed in 1885, later titled *Datong shu* (Great Harmony). He had exceedingly elevated ideas of the role medicine should play in a perfect society. As indicated by Kang, human history was divided into three phases: the first phase would be an anarchic world, where warlords had the uppermost part in the world because of frequent wars; the second phase would be a peaceful world where intellectuals played a fundamental part in societies because people sought to be knowledgeable; and the third would be an ideal world, where many general practitioners had foremost ethical judgment, first-rate medical talents, and unlimited authority, because people needed to preserve their excellent physical condition.[154] In his imagination of the ideal world, Kang put physicians at the top of society to take charge of everything after society was put in natural, effective order. They would have a lot of power and be responsible not only for everyone's health monitoring and medical treatment, but also for peace, order, and social justice, as Kang wrote:

> And so, in the Age of One World, physicians will be the most numerous, medical capabilities will be the most highly developed, medical responsibilities will be the heaviest, and medical [personnel] will be selected from the finest [talents], and medical authority will be the greatest.[155]

The power of the doctors was so great that it was necessary to pass new bylaws so as to prevent the doctors from abusing their supreme power because of "the rise of some medical Napoleon, who might gather together a great following and become a world ruler," according to Kang.[156] Otherwise, the perfect society would return to an anarchic world again due to power struggles among the doctors and civil rebellions arising from doctors' oppression, as Kang claimed. This book clearly disclosed Kang Youwei's intense admiration of the social function of medicine. Kang did not mention Western medicine, but the source of stimulation was evidently Western medicine.[157]

In another of his books, Kang also showed his great interest in the highest status of Western medicine in a society. Since Kang realized that the strength of Western countries lay in their specialization in studies and it was difficult to learn Western languages, a book, based on the numerous Japanese works, would be useful for the Chinese in acquiring Western learning through the Japanese translations available in large numbers at that time. As a result, Kang collected many Japanese books and completed his 1897 edition of the bibliography of Japanese books, *Riben shumu zhi* (Bibliography of Japanese Books), the first one of such a kind in China.

Kang's book listed 7,725 books in fifteen volumes with his comments of 109 paragraphs. The first volume is on physiology, the second natural science, the third religion, then politics, and others. Explaining why the volume of physiology was put at the beginning of the book, Kang claimed that in a peaceful and harmonious society, punishment by law was not necessary to be carried out and that the people would be very happy in their peaceful existence and their lifespan would be increased. Consequently, people would need more medical and hygienic knowledge to maintain their health, and physiology was the source of philosophy, psychology, and others, according to Kang. Kang might exaggerate the social role of Western medicine, but he already realized the significance of Western learning in a society.[158]

Second, Kang encouraged the Chinese, like the Japanese, to adopt Western medicine. Japan adopted Western medicine while abandoning Chinese medicine in early Meiji Restoration. Kang believed that Japan's modernization started first with the adoption of Western science and technology, including Western medicine, then carried out social and economic reforms, and finally embraced Western political institutions. In his 1897 edition of the bibliography of Japanese books, *Riben shumu zhi* (Bibliography of Japanese Books), the volume of physiology listed 366 titles of the books in Japanese with Kang's annotations of about 1,500 words and included several books on modern hygiene and anatomy in Japanese, such as *Dongwu bijiao jiepo tu* (Diagrams of the Dissection of Animas), *Xusi zuzhi xin lun* (New Comments on the Human Tissues), and *Renti zuzhi lanyao* (An Outline of Human Body), which Kang regarded as excellent. This volume indicated that Kang was in favor of dissection of the human body and that Kang had understood the significances and meaning of modern medicine and sanitation because those new medical and hygienic terms in Chinese translated by Kang were adopted by Chinese doctors of Western medicine in the following years.[159]

Kang believed that medical modernization was an important part of modern transformation in Japan and that the health of the Japanese was improved significantly after they adopted modern medicine and hygiene. Kang considered that a revolution in medical science in the West introduced a lot of modern medical terms into Japan, such as tissues, arteries, clinical manifestations, anti-epidemic measures, pathology, agential, and others. He asserted that after learning from the Westerners who were experts in modern sanitary technique, the Japanese were keen on cleanness, drinking clean water, breathing fresh air, and adopting preventive measure to safeguard health.

Kang compared and contrasted Japan with China, praising Japan's prompt acceptance of Western medical science and hygienic measures and criticizing China's slow acceptance of modern medicine and hygiene. Kang believed that since Western medicine and hygiene played a role in modern transformation of Japan, the Chinese had to embrace Western medicine and sanitation in an attempt to promote not only a modern medical revolution in China but also modern transformation of China.[160]

Third, Kang encouraged the Chinese to apply medical principles to the Chinese society. To encourage more Chinese to participate in the reform movement, Kang applied the principle of *Duizheng xiayao* (suit the medicine to the illness) to Chinese society, as he wrote:

> If a doctor prescribes wrong medication to a sick person, the patient's health will deteriorate; only the right medicine will restore the patient's health. In the case of China, in the past fifty years many Chinese attempted to revive China, but they used wrong means, sometimes emphasizing fighting their enemies and sometimes negotiating with their enemies. Consequently, China, after being defeated by other powers, was forced to surrender a lot of territories and to pay huge amount of reparations. This giant—China—is very unwell and dying, and if no new means are immediately used to diagnose the causes of its infirmity and if no new medications are instantly prescribed, this empire will collapse in next to no time.[161]

Applying the law of suiting the remedy to the Chinese case, Kang, as other reformers, comprehended clearly that without adoption of efficient and practical Western medicine, many people's lives would not be saved, and that without any reform, imperial China, like a very sick man, would not be rescued. He believed that the Chinese had to find new means to save the Chinese race, an important message to the Chinese in a national crisis, encouraging the Chinese to participate in social and political reform in China.

Finally, Kang, a strong Confucianism advocate, obviously admired Western medicine but undoubtedly defended the fundamental essentials of Chinese culture, including Chinese medicine. Kang believed that the ancient philosophers, both Confucius and Mencius, had started China in the right direction for good physical shape by laying emphasis on both natural, individual mental and physical maintenance of the bodies their parents bestowed, and claimed that the ancient philosophers had never opposed dissection of deceased bodies. Kang admitted, however, later both Confucianism scholars, who had complicated and abandoned those principles, and Buddhist monks, who had disrespected life and ignored the body, had directed the Chinese in a wrong path and were in opposition to the ancient essence of Chinese civilization. To Kang, Confucius stressed sanitation and hygiene 2000 years earlier than the Westerners did in the nineteenth century.[162]

Kang became more vigorous in advocating medical as well as social and political reforms in China in the 1890s. Kang set up a private school at Canton in 1890 and began to formulate a new synergetic interpretation of Confucianism for his students while promoting reforms. Immediately after the Sino-Japanese War of 1894-95, Kang Youwei stressed the necessity of state medicine and public health institutions. In 1895, he advocated the continued vitality of the Chinese people in his "Ten Thousand Word Memorial." By that time, Kang's political reform contained reference to the need for a modern medical and public health system in China.[163]

In summary, Kang Youwei was a Confucian scholar but read Chinese translations of Western works, which were accessible to him in Canton. His knowledge of the West remained fragmentary and superficial, but Western medicine had an impact upon Kang's mind because it had saved his life. To Kang, Western medicine would play a significant role in Chinese society, making the Chinese healthy, especially in his utopian society as he claimed in his book. Medical reform became a part of his great social reform program.

More importantly, Kang realized that Western medicine was more successful and more efficient than Chinese medicine because of its practical and scientific features. From the study of Western culture generally and Western medicine particularly, Kang reconsidered *ren* (humaneness), a fundamental virtue of Confucius, which had pervaded all the activities of Chinese society for more than two thousand years and started to identify the concept of wisdom, an elementary virtue of Western culture, and the rational thinking pattern of the Westerners. As Chinese historian Jiang Yihua wrote, "Kang began to abolish the traditional, irrational thinking pattern of Chinese culture while adopting the rational thinking way of Western culture in the late 1880s."[164]

Western medicine was only one of the many factors for Kang's reform ideology formation and in part encouraged Kang to take a new attitude to Western learning generally and Western medicine particularly. Kang's reform ideas began to take shape in the late 1880s. He first turned to Western learning, including Western medicine, because of its efficient, practical, and scientific features, and then referred to the Western political system—constitutional monarchy—because it was working in the Western world and could be able to save a deteriorating nation in a critical condition.[165]

Liang Qichao

Liang Qichao (1873-1936) was another influential Cantonese reformer, on whom Western medicine had an impact.[166] Liang was born into a family at a village in Xinhui country, southwest of Canton. At the age of four, he studied Confucianism under his grandfather and his mother, and when he was eight years old, he was intelligent enough to write lengthy theses, obtaining a standing as a child genius. He succeeded in the county level of examinations and became a *Shengyuan* (junior scholar) in 1884. In 1885, Liang studied at a private school in Canton and passed the provincial examinations in 1889, attaining the title *Juren* (senior scholar) and becoming a provincial official candidate.[167] In 1891, Kang Youwei opened Wanmu caotang, a private school in Canton, where Liang studied sporadically at Kang's guidance for four years as a superior student. As Liang recollected later, these were years of serious study and questioning, which laid the scholarly groundwork for his entire life.[168]

Liang became interested in political affairs in 1895. When the news of the humiliating Treaty of Shimonoseki came in April after the Chinese were defeated in the Sino-Japanese War, Liang hastened to organize a petition, and obtained the support of 190 senior gentries from his home province, Guangdong. When Kang went north to launch a campaign for reform in 1895, Liang left Canton and joined his teacher as a young political activist. In next to no time, he helped Kang lead a national appeal to demand reforms and a strong stand against Japan. In August, Kang established in Beijing, Qiangxue hui (Society of the Propagation of Learning), the first political organization in China, and opened a translation house of the reformers so as to spread Western learning and put forward reform. As the chief secretary of the Society, political thinker Liang was becoming energetic in the political reform movement and the transmission of Western learning.[169]

Liang became interested in Western medicine when promoting the study of Western learning. To carry out the reform movement, Liang edited a book, titled *Xixue tiyao* (An Outline of Western Books of Knowledge), in August 1896, introducing books on Western sciences and social sciences to the Chinese. In October, Liang wrote an article, "Xixue shumu biao," (A List of Western Books) and published it in the journal *Shiwu biao*, of which he was the editor. In this article, thirty-nine books on Western medicine were included.[170] Liang attached to this article his another article, "Du xixueshu fa," (On Reading Books of Western Learning) in 1897. By that time, Liang had read more than twelve books on Western medicine.[171] Laing became engrossed in Western medicine and began to develop his medical thought.[172]

Liang also became more enthusiastic in promoting modern medicine in China. In 1897, Liang and other reformers founded Yixue shanhui (Medical Philanthropic Society) in Shanghai, and the purpose of this Society went far beyond familiar philanthropic motives. Liang published an introduction to the Society's objective in a journal, declaring that the goal of the Medical Philanthropic Society was to improve or reform medicine in China as an essential step in strengthening the race and, through it, the nation.[173]

Liang, like Kang Youwei, was not in good health during that time. In early 1898 when Liang was teaching at his Shiwu School in Changsha, the capital of Hunan Province, he contracted a near-fatal illness. As a result, Liang left Changsha for Shanghai for Western medical treatment in February.

Meanwhile, Kang Youwei asked Liang to come to Beijing to take the official, national examination while launching a reform campaign there. Liang was recovering but decided to go to Beijing. Since Liang was still ill, Kang Youwei asked his younger brother Kang Guangren to accompany Liang. Kang Guangren, who studied medicine at the Canton Hospital for three years under Dr. John Kerr, treated Liang's illness with Western medicine during the trip in March.[174] Liang thereafter adopted Western medicine and saw only doctors of Western medicine for the rest of his life.

Since then, Liang advocated Western medicine until he died in 1936. Before his death, Liang published an article, titled "The Union Hospital and I." He wrote that the X-ray identified the failure of the kidney on the left side of his body, but during the surgery performed by the famous doctors of Western medicine, they accidentally cut out his good kidney on the right side. He claimed that many people had used his case to express disapproval of Western medicine while justifying the advantages of Chinese medicine and that the criticism was completely wrong because this incident was not a fault of modern medicine. He argued that the doctors of Western medicine were able to use up-to-date scientific means—X-rays—to single out his kidney as the major cause of his illness while the physicians of Chinese medicine were using a mysterious principle—Yin and Yang—to diagnose his sickness and did not pinpoint the cause. He finally appealed to the Chinese not to use his case to erect obstacles to block the progress of medical science in China.[175]

Liang's medical thought had taken shape in the late 1890s. First, Liang was concerned about the poor features of Chinese medicine and its harmful effect on the health of the Chinese. Liang condemned strongly doctors of Chinese medicine because they could not understand the nature of the human body, identify different herbs and plants, and find the causes of the illnesses. Liang claimed that a bad physician restored to health only 20 percent of his patients but continued to practice medicine, and that Chinese medicine had declined and the medical system was becoming inefficient in recent centuries because it focused its attention only on the classic theory without any new theories. Liang also denounced the Chinese medical system because it did not have any formal training programs, any regulations for punishment and reward, and any official hygienic administration, which resulted in the practice of many quacks, an unclean environment in the cities and countries, and transmission of disease everywhere in China. Liang also condemned the Qing government for ignoring medicine, neglecting public health, and disregarding the parlous state of medical practice in the country. Liang castigated this indifference, not only on humanitarian grounds for the countless number of unnecessary deaths each year, but also for its long-range effects in debilitating the Chinese race and even reducing its numbers. Liang encouraged the Chinese to abandon their attitude toward physicians, which traditionally regarded medical callings as beneath a scholar's notice, while calling for raising the social status of physicians of Chinese medicine.[176]

Second, Liang strongly advocated the study of Western medicine to reform Chinese medicine so as to improve the health of the Chinese. In discussion of the advantages and disadvantages of both Western and Chinese medicines, Liang, believing that Western medicine had advantages over Chinese medicine in terms of knowledge, institutions, and others, urged the Chinese to open Western medical schools, recruit good students for the study of Western medicine, publish medical newspapers and journals, and create medical associations. Liang also believed that the Chinese had to adopt Western medicine because it had helped make Western society better and Western states stronger. He even claimed that the reform in England was an example of the significance of modern medicine. He alleged that the goal of the British revolution was to seek means of maintaining good health. He asserted that the English had to limit the power of their monarchy because they needed more freedom to study sciences, technology, social problem, and the human body so that they would produce good babies, raise good children, eat healthy food, do physical exercises, and improve their living environment, all important for good health. Looking to Western countries, Liang advanced medical science to promote people's health as a foundation stone for national prosperity and power because modern medicine would produce strong bodies, which would create a strong race, and the consequence would be a powerful and prosperous state.[177]

Finally, Liang, like Kang, applied the medical principle to Chinese society that only political and social reforms would rescue China. The progressive reformers launched a second campaign of reforms in 1898, a year witnessing Liang's strong determination to carry out reforms immediately. On April 22, Liang delivered a very emotional speech at the second meeting of Baoguo hui (Safeguard China Association), China's first political party established by Kang Youwei and other reformers in Beijing in March 1898. In his speech, Liang stated that today China was severely sick and could not be saved if it did not take any medicine and that many Chinese people had identified the illness of China, but they were only watching China dying instead of helping it recover. He appealed to 400 million Chinese people during the meeting that this nation was dying and the Chinese had to use their wisdom and to take all measures to safeguard China.[178] Liang did not mention Western medicine in his speech, but it was clear that the medicine he mentioned meant Western medicine because he was taking Western medicine to restore his health when traveling from Shanghai to Beijing in March. By then Liang was determined to call for immediate social and political reforms in China; otherwise, this giant empire would soon die of social disease.

In short, Liang's study of Western medicine helped him understand much better its efficient role in the treatment of illness and its advantages over Chinese medicine. His concern about Chinese medicine was due to his concern about China's fate. He believed that Western medicine, critical to preserving the Western race, was exceedingly practical and would play a critical part in safeguarding the health of the Chinese people.

Liang not only identified the advantages of Western medicine, but also realized the advantages of Western culture and sciences over those of the Chinese. He advocated not only reforming Chinese medicine, but also abandoning the old knowledge. Liang envisaged a faulty China that was stalled in false thinking and ailments while imagining a perfect Western world that placed emphasis on scientific standards in all aspects of life in Western society. To Liang, the study and practice of modern medicine, as well as other sciences in the Western world, was the most respectable of studies and careers in the modern world of life-threatening battles for endurance among rival powers, while Chinese intellectuals were still studying the old learning, which constructed the core for the eight-legged essays (*bogu wen*) (a style of essay writing which was divided into eight sections and had to be mastered to pass the imperial examinations) and seemed impractical. Focusing on the race as the unit of endurance and paying tribute to medicine as critical to a race, Liang had done away with the old knowledge, culture, and values.

Liang's medical thought, a part of his reform ideology, was similar to Kang Youwei's, but there still one major difference. When Kang Youwei still paid respect to Confucianism and unquestionably preserved the essential elements and values of Chinese culture, Liang's concern about the state's existence and racial survival noticeably took him far away from the Confucian sphere. Liang had entered a completely new sphere of values, not just a new medical sphere.

Zheng Guanying

Zheng Guanying (1842-1922) is best known for his participation in the *yangwu* (overseas affairs) movement of the late nineteenth century. Born in Zhongshan county in 1842, Guangdong, not far from Canton. Zheng left for Shanghai in 1858 to study at Shanghai's Anglo-Chinese school and served as a comprador at the British shipping firm of Battlefield and Swire before he went on to create his own business empire. Zheng was a principal person in several Qing government—supported commercial ventures, such as the China Merchants Shipping Company and Kaiping Mines. He was in favor of governmental control of steamships, telegraphs, and railroads, and gave suggestions to the Qing government on diplomatic and military affairs.

Zheng was one of the pioneers of the reform movement in the late Qing dynasty. Between the 1870s and 1880s, Zheng wrote many articles on his reform ideas. In 1873, Zheng published his first book, *Jiushi jieyao* (Essentials to solve the crisis), advocating that China should learn from the West and carry out political and social reforms, which would help make China strong. In 1880, Zheng completed another book, *Yiyan* (Words of change). This book advocated reforming traditional and old systems and customs of the Qing dynasty and emphasized understanding, learning, and adopting Western sciences and technology, with the aim of resisting and defeating foreign invasions. Most Chinese books on Western leaning at that time focused on only Western sciences and technology. Zheng's book divided Western leanings into four parts: medical science, religions, laws, and intelligence, and the first part was Western medicine, which suggested that Zheng had realized that Western medicine was the first and foremost part of Western leanings.[179]

Since Zheng was not in good health when he was young, he paid attention to the study of health and the way to lengthen life. After being ill and deteriorating physically during his numerous tours to Southeast Asia in support of his businesses, he resorted to Daoism to find the solution to his physical problem and to hunt for a therapy for spiritual impoverishment in years chasing money. Zheng studied long life methods with Cantonese Daoists in the 1880s and continued until his death in 1922. During that time, he caught pulmonary tuberculosis and asthma so severely that he had to cease working in the second half of 1885. While building up his strength at home in Macao in 1886, Zheng was writing two books, *Zhongwai weisheng yaozi* (Chinese and foreign essentials to hygiene) and *Shengshi weiyan* (Words of warnings to an affluent Age).[180]

During that time, Zheng was putting up with inexpert doctors of Chinese medicine, who took an extensive amount of time to treat his disease. The quack doctors of Chinese medicine forced Zheng to read many books on Western medicine and sciences, and he began to pay attention to medical science and social problems regarding people's health. When cholera occurred in both Macao and Canton in 1887, Zheng hired one man to collect and compile previous good prescriptions for cholera into a book, titled, *Huoluan yanfang* (Prescription for cholera), and many copies of this book thereafter were distributed to the public. In 1890, he returned to Canton to take rest and nourishment to regain his health.[181]

In view of the fact that both Zheng and Sun Yat-sen, a physician of Western medicine and the founding father of the Republic of China, were born in Zhongshan County in Guangdong Province, they soon became good friends. Zheng, a successful merchant twenty-four years older than Sun, often provided financial support to Sun for the reform and revolutionary movement. While in Macao, they frequently discussed Chinese and Western medicines as well as how to reform Chinese society. There is no doubt that both Dr Sun's perspective on Western medicine and the Western hospitals in Canton had an impact on Zheng when he was writing books and articles on medicine.[182]

While in Canton, Zheng's books, *Zhongwai weisheng yaozi* and *Beiji yan-fang* (Prescription for emergency), were completed on December 22, 1890, and his five-volume book, *Shengshi weiyan*, was completed in 1892.[183] The major theme of his last book was how to rescue China. It advocated political and social reforms, such as establishment of the constitutional monarch system and promotion of education for both men and women, abolishment of the social evils—footbinding and opium, creation of modern charitable institutions, and formation of a welfare system. The book was widely read at the end of the nineteenth century for its truthful information on the functions of Western capitalism and its imperative request for the Qing court to embark on feasible economic reform and economic expansion in a global commercial war so as to make China rich and strong.

In this famous multiple volume book, several articles on medicines were put into a chapter, *Yidao* (Medical essences), introducing Western medicine.[184] Zheng's medical thinking began to develop at that time, and his distinctiveness as a businessman and Daoist worked together in this remarkable anthology on Western medicine and safeguarding of health. Zheng's political and economic literatures were far better known than his writings on physical condition and medication, but his thinking on medicine had a lasting impression on the Chinese.

First, Zheng condemned the charlatans of Chinese medicine and pointed out its weakness and shortcomings in terms of medical equipment, diagnostics, remedy, and others while identifying such advantages of Western medicine as scientific diagnostics, modern technology, and modern hospitals. After exploring the strength and weakness of Chinese medicine, Zheng revealed that Chinese medicine had to learn from Western medicine in five areas.[185] Zheng believed that promotion of Western medicine was to help not only improve Chinese medicine but also make the Chinese state rich and powerful and that social reforms were needed in a medical modernization of China.[186]

Second, Zheng was in favor of the establishment of modern medical schools in China. Zheng praised greatly Western medical schools where students were able to study chemistry, biology, anatomy, medical treatment, hygiene, and other subjects, which helped train good doctors. He encouraged Chinese merchants and nobles to raise funds to open Western medical schools in towns and cities in China, suggesting that only those students who passed the entry examinations and completed the study of all required courses taught by famous doctors were granted licenses by governments to practice medicine after their graduation. Zheng also urged the government to prohibit those medical doctors without medical licenses from practicing medicine and punish severely those doctors who mistreated their patients.[187] Zheng additionally stressed the importance of women doctors while condemning China's lack of women's education, especially women's medical education, in comparison with that in Western countries.[188]

Finally, Zheng was one of the first Chinese reformers to advocate amalgamation of Western and Chinese medicines. In a letter of 1880 to the progressive reformist Sheng Xuanhuai in connection with the establishment of the Shanghai Medical School, he wrote that both Western and Chinese medicines had their own advantages and disadvantages; each would learn from the other and get rid of its shortcomings and absorb the benefits of the other and that if such a combination happened, it would be very good for humanity.[189] Zheng also cited the case of Japan that the Japanese were learning Western medicine, although they had practiced Chinese medicine for many centuries, and that Chinese medicine would continue to develop and become more scientific only when it was strengthened by Western medicine.[190]

In brief, like other Cantonese reformers, Zheng's medical thinking under the impact of Western medicine was very valuable in helping not only the Chinese medical practitioners in overcoming the weakness of Chinese medicine, but also in helping the Chinese to realize the advantages of Western culture and science over theirs. For this reason and others, Zheng not only called for the establishment of state medicine but also social reforms in China.

State Medical Reform and Modern Hospitals in China

In the late 1890s, there was a transformation in the attitudes of the elite Cantonese toward state medicine in discussion of general modernization of Chinese society. They raised the issues of peoples' health, medical education, modern hospitals, and others and appealed for the establishment of modern and progressive state medical institutions. They advocated medical reform, which was becoming a part of the social reform they promoted in China.

Many of the Chinese elite shared the Cantonese reformers' feelings about the need for active state interest in medical improvements. Editorials appeared in reform-oriented journals, urging the government to adopt state medicine in the process of nation-building. Progressive reformers' newspapers published commentaries to condemn Chinese medicine and to advocate Western medicine, especially modern health concepts. They stated that the Western countries were powerful because they used modern medicine to cure diseases so the people had healthy bodies, which led to a strong nation and powerful state. Thus, if the Chinese wanted to have a strong state and establish a position in the world, they needed healthy bodies with the help of Western medicine, which would produce a healthy race. Reformer Liu Zhenling, for example, wrote in an article that people's healthy bodies resulted in a physically strong race, which would contribute to a mighty state, citing the case of England that a powerful Great Britain started with a strong Anglo-Saxon race because Western scientific medicine was excellent in curing diseases, healing sickness, and restoring to health, which helped create a strong race. Obviously, modern medicine was a means not only to cure the diseases of individual bodies but also was a method to save the Chinese nation, as Liu stated.[191]

Reform of Chinese medicine became a part of the Reform Movement of 1898. Kang Youwei's career climaxed in 1898 in a national catastrophe when the foreign powers were fighting for concessions within the Chinese empire. During the spring, Kang urged the Qing court for reform, including medical reform. Faced with these domestic calls for reform, the young Emperor Guangxu, fascinated by Kang's persuasiveness, announced a series of reform decrees on June 11 and interviewed him several days afterward. In August, Emperor Guangxu issued an imperial edict that a new imperial university, which had a medical school of both Chinese and Western medicines, be created so as to promote medical progress. Under Kang's direction, the imperial decrees continued for one hundred days until Empress Dowager Cixi suppressed the reform movement on September 21.

The reform movement of 1898 failed, but subsequently the Chinese government gradually adopted new policies to protect and support missionary hospitals and to set up Western hospitals in China. With the support of the Qing government, the Beijing Union Medical College was founded in 1906 by the American Board of Commissioners for Foreign Missions, the Board of Foreign Missions of the Presbyterian Church in the U.S.A., and the London Missionary Society.[192] For the first time in Chinese history, the central government established a Western medical college in cooperation with medical missionaries, which helped contribute to medical modernization in China in the twentieth century.

The performance of autopsies and dissections was formally legalized under the new Chinese laws. The Qing government approved in 1871 that lectures on anatomy could be offered at Tongwen guan (Foreign language school) in Beijing, but the Chinese still could not carry on anatomy in the late nineteenth century under the Qing laws. After the new Republic of China was born in 1912, in November 1913 the president of the Republic of China issued a decree, *Jiepo shiti guize* (Regulations of Dissection), which provided that postmortem examination was allowed at hospitals and medical schools and that parts of a dead body would be allowed to be displayed for teaching, the first central government document to legalize autopsy in China. This decree also established regulations for the dissection of human bodies, requiring that physicians had to first obtain the consent of the relatives.

As a result, one of the earliest dissections was made openly on the body of an executed criminal on November 13, 1913. A medical school in Jiangsu province carried out an autopsy, inviting to the scene government officials, Chinese and foreign doctors, and judges. Sixty-five persons were in attendance, pictures were taken of the corpse and the assembled company, and a published pamphlet claimed that this was the first dissection open to the public in China in the past 3,000 years, a first step to develop anatomy in

China in the future. In the following April, the rules were expanded authorizing all medical schools and hospitals to perform dissections.[193] Even then, in divided China, the status of such procedures remained unstable in remote and conservative regions, consequently holding up all medical research and teaching, with which dissection and autopsy would generally be concerned. As a consequence of the harsh cultural resistance to any abuse of the human body, the scarcity of corpses continued to be a major impediment for the medical schools in China in the first half of the twentieth century.[194]

Modern hospitals gained strength in China after the end of the Opium War in 1842. Mission hospitals started in Canton and began to spread to other parts of China, and Dr. Parker's ophthalmic institution was the decisive step in the spread of medical missions. After the War, the missionaries established more hospitals in China. In 1844, Dr. William Lockhart (1811-1896), the President of the London Medical Association, arrived in Shanghai and thereafter opened the Renji Hospital, the first Western Hospital in Shanghai, providing free medical care to people. In 1843, American doctor Daniel J. MacGowan founded a hospital in Ningpo, Zhejiang Province and opened up medical services. The Western hospitals had become popular in the cities on the coast in China by the 1870s, as an article on the Tongren Dispensary in Shanghai wrote:

> After the treaty-ports were established in 1842, more and more Western hospitals were opened in these cities. At the beginning, only the poor, helpless patients came to the hospitals. Due to the success of the treatments, rich and noble patients visited the hospitals when the Chinese medicine treatment failed. Consequently, more and more patients, poor or rich, appealed to Western doctors for therapeutic treatment due to the miracle and simplicity of Western medicine.[195]

There was one medical missionary in China in 1835, twenty-eight missionary doctors in 1859, and 214 medical missionaries in 1890, of whom one hundred were from America. The American Presbyterian Mission dispatched the largest number—thirty-four—while the American Methodist Mission was next with thirty-one. Of all medical missionaries, twenty-nine were in Guangdong Province.[196] Medical work in other parts of China had been greatly strengthened, following the Boxer rebellion of 1900 when various missionary bodies were unified. In 1905, there were 166 missionary hospitals, 241 dispensaries, 301 missionary doctors all over twenty-one provinces. After the Chinese government officially recognized Western medicine in 1911, 450 medical missionaries were working in China in 1913.[197] By the 1930s, the influence of American medical missionaries had spread through many cities and rural areas, partially helping contribute to the distribution of Western medicine in China.

In the first three decades of the twentieth century, China was still profoundly reliant upon foreigners, mainly missionaries, in constructing the system of modern medicine. In 1935, the Republic of China claimed to have 350 modernized hospitals, with a total number of 70,000 doctors (over 15,000 were modern medical practitioners). About one hundred hospitals belonged to private and government groups and 250 were mission hospitals with a total capacity of about 20,000 beds and $44,000,000 investment.[198]

Conclusion

The medical missionary movement that emerged in the nineteenth and twentieth centuries played a role in the progress of modern Sino-Western relations. American medical missionaries created the Canton Hospital and initiated the dispensary movement to provide medical services to the sick, which helped promote modern medical work in south China. American medical missionaries also founded the Medical Missionary Society, the first of its kind in the world, which played a part in the founding of a national medical association in China. With regard to medical journals, American doctors took a step ahead, and their journals enabled the Chinese physicians of modern medicine to have an organ for the first time, which also played a role in promoting Western medicine in China. The Canton Hospital took the lead in the development of modern surgery and modern medical technology, which had an effect on the development of medical science in China.

Mission hospitals started in Canton and began to spread to other parts of China; Dr. Parker's ophthalmic institution was the decisive step in the spread of medical missions. Prior to Dr. Parker, medical westernization was unsystematic and irregular in China. When the Canton Hospital opened its doors and operated productively, it gave impetus to the spread of the influence of foreign medicine on more modern hospitals in China. Many factors were responsible for medical modernization in China from 1835 to 1935, and the eminent achievements of American missionary doctors in Canton as well as in south China was one of them. American hospitals still have an impact on China now because after the Chinese government took over them in 1949, those hospitals have become the leading hospitals in Canton and in south China today.

Western medicine and surgery were becoming more popular with the common Cantonese. Their skepticism of and antagonism to Western medicine gradually faded away and their desire for physical relief had led them to appreciate the superiority of the knowledge and skills of American doctors. Those hospitals and dispensaries in the countryside in south China also became admired among the poor peasants, gentries, and merchants because of the medical mission's successful treatments. Efficient treatments helped many people in the city of Canton and in rural south China turn to Western medicine. Attention that was given at the missionary hospitals convinced many patients who came for medical aid that American doctors relieved their physical sufferings. Thus many Chinese began to take a positive attitude towards Western medical institution and Western medicine. The Canton Hospital and other missionary hospitals and dispensaries in south China facilitated good relations between American medical missionaries and the Chinese in general and the patients in particular. American doctors had an impact on the Cantonese because of their medical work rather than their missionary work, which had won them very few converts.

Western medicine also had an impact on the officials in Canton when their illnesses were successfully cured by American doctors at the Canton Hospital. Western medicine was one of the forces, if not the sole one, that encouraged the Qing officials in Canton to take a positive attitude towards the Canton Hospital. They first recognized and then protected it. They finally adopted more liberal policies towards other Western institutions in China, such as toleration of Christianity. Western medicine, to some extent, stimulated high-ranking officials in Canton to take a different attitude towards Westerners in general and Americans in particular and, in part, helped make them more tolerant and open-minded.

Western medicine had a more significant effect on the Cantonese progressive reformers than on the commoners and officials. Three progressive Cantonese reformers were not in good health and adopted Western medicine to regain their health in the late nineteenth century. The common people and government officials identified the efficiency of Western medicine, but the Cantonese progressive reformers realized not just the advantages Western medicine offered over native medicine in individual therapy, but also the importance of Western medicine to Chinese society and the nation at large. The enlightened Cantonese intellectuals began to voice the view that *guojia yixue* (state medicine) was essential for national strength and the survival of the Chinese race. In face of this "dying man" of the Chinese nation, the Cantonese reformers advocated the slogan, "To Rescue China with Western Medicine." They urged the reform and improvement of medicine in China so as to strengthen the race and, through it, the nation. Therefore, the reform of Chinese medicine constituted a part of their reform programs.

Western medicine, in some measure, helped make the Cantonese reformers realize not only the shortcomings of Chinese medicine and the advantages of Western medicine, but also the superiority of Western learning, as well as scientific ways and rational thinking of Western culture. As a result, Western medicine became one of the many agencies, if not the sole one, for removing prejudice and of enlightening the minds of the Cantonese reformers and helped them, in some way, change their attitude toward Western culture. Western medicine became one of the many factors in the formation of their reform ideology. They advocated social and political reforms because those reforms were more crucial than medical reform to the survival of China when they initiated the reform campaign in 1898. The reform movement of 1898 which included reform of Chinese medicine failed, but the Cantonese reformers' efforts were not in vain. Thereafter, the Qing government began to adopt new policies to protect and support missionary hospitals and to set up Western hospitals in China, and subsequently the new Republic of China formally legalized the performance of autopsies and dissections under the new Chinese laws. Thus Western medicine was one of the sources of inspiration to the Cantonese elite in the early modern transformation of China.

Contrasting American businessmen who came first before them, American medical missionaries to China were strong-minded enough to break through the cultural and political stumbling blocks, and the various restrictions imposed by the Chinese government, which had segregated the Chinese from Westerners for a long time. American medical missionaries used one of the most efficient tactics—the founding of hospitals and dispensaries—to promote Christianity in China. With such an approach, American medical missionaries, endowed with a means of social interaction with the Chinese, did break social barriers between the Chinese and American doctors. From the commencement of the work at the hospitals and dispensaries in Canton as well as in south China, American medical missionaries put emphasis on not only the healing of the body but also on the teaching of Christianity, and they worked as diligently for the latter as they did for their physical health.

The Chinese, however, were more interested in missions' medical work than their religious work. Many Chinese had a high regard for Western hospitals, but only a few of them were converted to Christianity. For this reason as well others, medical missionaries realized that it was crucial to first heal the wounds of the bodies of the Chinese before treating "infections" of their spirit—medical work first and religious work second. The formation of the Medical Missionary Society in 1838 indicated that American medical missionaries had to adjust themselves to Chinese society when implanting a Western institution in China—they had to put the medical work before the religious work because most Cantonese were more interested in Americans' medical arts than their sermons at the hospital. Since then, the Canton Hospital, as well as other missionary hospitals in China in the following decades, became mainly a medical center rather than a religious center, although it was performing those two functions. Thus, American medical missions were more successful in breaking technological barriers than converting many Chinese, bringing the benefits of Western medical science to the Chinese. They played a role, together with the Chinese elite, in promoting medical modernization in China. Medical modernization or Western medical modernity was a global cultural movement in the nineteenth and twentieth centuries, and American doctors were becoming transmitters in China of the globalization of medical technology.

Notes

1. For an overview of the beginning of the ABCFM movement in China, see Rufus Anderson, *History of the Missions of the American Board of Commissioners for Foreign Missions to the Oriental Churches*, 2 vols. (Boston, 1872). Rufus Anderson was the corresponding secretary of the American Board. See also Latourett, *A History of Christian Missions in China*, 218, 222; Samuel Couling, *Encyclopedia Sinica* (Shanghai, 1917), 424; and Harold Balme, *China and Modern Medicine: A Study in Medical Missionary Development* (London: London Missionary Society, 1921), 39-45.

2. Bridgman was instructed to remember that his main goal was to spread Christianity among the Chinese, a work for which "the providence of God may soon open a wide and effectual door." In 1832, Bridgman initiated to publish the *Chinese Repository*, an English-language magazine, and it soon became a main site for academic study of Chinese culture and an imperative tool for the encouragement of missionary work. See E.C. Bridgman and Eliza J. Gillett, ed., *The Pioneer of American Missions in China: The Life and Labors of Elijah Coleman Bridgman* (New York: Anson DF Randolph, 1864), 20-27.

3. Bridgman started to appeal vigorously in 1833 for the American Board to dispatch a physician in an attempt to open an ophthalmic hospital in Canton because they witnessed "old, blind, decrepit men, 'with staff in hand', led thither by their little grandchildren." See E. C. Bridgman, "Canton Dispensary," *Chinese Repository* 2 (October 1833), 276. See also E.C. Bridgman to R. Anderson, Canton, December 26, 1833, Papers of the American Board of Commissioners for Foreign Missions (ABCFM), Missions to China (ABC 16.3), Houghton Library, Harvard University, microfilm, reel 256, ABCFM.

4. Harold Balme, *China and Modern Medicine* (London: United Council for Missionary Education, 1921), 39.

5. Peter Parker was born at Framingham, Massachusetts on June 18, 1804, the son of Nathan and Catherine Parker. His father was a farmer, and Peter was the only boy in a family of three girls. He grew up in a Christian home of very ordinary economic conditions and accepted the common form of schooling given to kids of that time. Learning at the Amherst College in the beginning and moving to the Yale University afterward, he obtained his degree of doctor of medicine and his ordination as Presbyterian minister in 1834. As the first Protestant medical missionary appointed to China, Parker was dispatched by the ABCFM. The Board instructed him not to let his practice of medicine retard his preaching of the Gospel. His initial task would be to study the Cantonese dialect and accustom himself to the Chinese ways and habits. It was said that Mr. Olyphant had given a total of fifty-one free passages in his ships to missionaries and their families traveling to the Chinese empire. See George B. Stevens, *The Life, Letters, and Journals of the Rev. & Hon. Peter Parker, M.D.* (Boston: Congregational Sunday-School & Publishing Soc., 1896), 82-83.

6. Without Howqua's financial assistance, the hospital might never have been materialized. The Western merchants also were there for Parker devotedly. Mr. Olyphant, well known for his generosity, which included furnishing a house rent-free for the missionaries in Canton, provided most beneficial

assistance. He let Dr. Parker use one of his warehouses as a hospital, "so that patients could come and go without annoying foreigners by passing through their hongs, or excite the observations of natives by being seen to resort to a foreigners' house, rendered it most suitable for the purpose," according to Parker's report. See Peter Parker, "First Quarterly Report of Ophthalmic Hospital at Canton," *Chinese Repository* 4 (February 1836): 461. See also Wong K. Chimin and Wu Lien-Teh, *History of Chinese Medicine* (Tientsin, The Tientsin Press, 1932), 315.

7. "Walks About Canton-Extracts from a Private Journal," *Chinese Repository* 4 (May 1835): 45.

8. Peter Parker, "First Quarterly Report of Ophthalmic Hospital at Canton."

9. When the Hospital commenced to accept patients, no one came on the first day. The next morning only one woman dared to seek advice from the doctor about her eyes. As reports of Dr. Parker's remarkable expertise and accomplishment were distributed among the Cantonese, the Canton Hospital was swamped with scores of patients. On the word of his statement to the American Board, in merely several weeks after the hospital's opening, Dr. Parker wrote, "I have now three hundred patients, who, with few exceptions, have been afflicted with ophthalmic diseases." P. Parker to American Board, Canton, November 28, 1835, Papers of the American Board of Commissioners for Foreign Missions (ABCFM), Missions to China (ABC 16.3), Houghton Library, Harvard University, microfilm, reel 256.

10. Peter Parker, "Second Quarterly Report of Ophthalmic Hospital at Canton," *Chinese Repository* 5 (May 1836): 33.

11. C. T. Downing, *The Stranger in China,* vol. 2, (Philadelphia: Lea & Blanchard, 1838), 23. C. T. Downing, an American in China, who from time to time assisted Parker at the hospital.

12. Canton Mission to Anderson, Canton, March 7, 1837 and September 12, 1837, Papers of the American Board of Commissioners for Foreign Missions (ABCFM), Missions to China (ABC 16.3), Houghton Library, Harvard University, microfilm, reel 257, ABCFM.

13. "Twenty-Eighth Annual Meeting of the Board," *Missionary Herald* XXXIII (November 1837): 468-73.

14. P. Parker to Anderson, Canton, March 7, 1837, Papers of the American Board of Commissioners for Foreign Missions (ABCFM), Missions to China (ABC 16.3), Houghton Library, Harvard University, microfilm, reel 257, ABCFM.

15. Peter Parker and E. C. Bridgman, "Suggestions for the Formation of A Medical Missionary Society," *Chinese Repository* 5 (December 1836): 369-71.

16. Peter Parker, "First Quarterly Report of Ophthalmic Hospital at Canton," *Chinese Repository* 4 (February 1836), 461; *Twenty-Eighth Annual Report of the American Board of Commissioners for Foreign Missions* (Boston: 1837), 87; and Peter Parker, *Statements Respecting Hospitals in China, Preceded by a Letter to John Abercrombie* (Glasgow: Maclehose, 1842), 22-23.

17. Dr. Parker stated in his report of 1840, "though diseases of the eye still preponderate, and the original name of the institution is retained, yet it is no longer peculiarly an ophthalmic, but has become a general hospital."

Consequently, the "total number of patients that has been admitted and their names recorded, during the year 1839, has been 800, the aggregate number since the commencement of the institution in November 1835,—about 700." See "General Letter," *Missionary Herald* XXXVI (March 1840): 82 and *The Hospital Reports of the Medical Missionary Society in China for the Year 1839* (China: the Office of the Chinese Repository, 1840), 2-6.

18.   Medical Missionary Society, *Report of the Medical Missionary Society in China: The Fourteenth Report of the Ophthalmic Hospital, Canton* (Canton: The Chinese Repository, 1848), 3.

19.   John Glasgow Kerr was born in Duncansville, Ohio on November 30, 1824. Leaving Ohio at the time of his father's death, he lived with his uncle in Virginia until 1840 when he entered college in Granville, Ohio. He began studying medicine at Maysville, Kentucky in 1842 and graduated from Jefferson Medical College in Philadelphia in March 1847. While practicing medicine in southern Ohio, he listened to a lecture given by a Chinese who underscored the imperative want of Western medicine in China that many Chinese victims from curable sicknesses were given up or put out of action because the Chinese were completely dependent upon medicine without any surgery and that the mortality rate in China was higher than that in the whole Europe. The stirring appeal had an emotional impact on Dr. Kerr so greatly that he decided to be a medical missionary. Before leaving the United States, he married Miss Abby Kingsbury. Unfortunately, his young wife died in Macao in August 1855. See Wong and Wu, *History of Chinese Medicine*, 228-29.

20.   The London Missionary Society's hospital at Jinlifan in western Canton survived a little better. All the furniture and apparatus were taken off, but the walls remained standing. For more information on the London Missionary Society's hospital under the care of Dr. Benjamin Hobson, see *A Report of the Mission Hospital in the Western Suburbs of Canton under the Care of Dr. Hobson, 1853-1854* (Canton, 1855).

21.   John Glasgow Kerr, "History of Medical Missionary Society's Hospital, Canton," *China Medical Missionary Journal* 10, no. 1(1896): 55-7, 95-8.

22.   John Kerr, "Report of the Medical Society's Hospital at Canton for the Year 1860," *Report of the Medical Missionary Society in China for the Year 1860* (Canton, Friend of China Press, 1861), 5-6.

23.   Joseph Thomson of Scottish ancestry was born in Cincinnati, Ohio on April 10, 1853. He graduated from the Hanover College, Indiana in 1875, spent two years at Danville Theological Seminary in Indiana, and graduated from Union Theological Seminary in New York City in 1878. Later, he studied medicine at New York University and the Bellevue Hospital Medical College where he graduated in 1881. Ordained by the Presbytery of Cincinnati on September 14, 1881, Dr. Thomson organized several Sunday Schools for the Chinese at several churches in New York. While engaged in this work, he met Miss Agnes Louise Dornin, and they married on September 21, 1881. Appointed as missionaries of the American Presbyterian Board, they arrived in Canton on November 25, 1881, after a few weeks of sailing for China. See W.W. Cadbury, *At the Point of a Lancet*, 169-70.

24. In 1889, the Hospital reported the following statistics:

	Males	Females	Total
Outpatients	13,758	3,415	17,173
Inpatients	945	379	1,324
Operations	1,543	616	2,159
Patients Treated			40,300

. See *Annual Report of the Presbyterian Board of Foreign Missions* (New York: The Board of Foreign Missions, Presbyterian Church in the U.S.A., 1889), 140-41.

25. Dr. Swan was born in Glasgow, Ohio on September 11, 1860. Early in his life, he desired to engage in the study of medicine, but there were major barriers in the way before him. With the aim of realizing his aspiration, he worked in a grocery store during the day while spending his evenings in study under the guidance of a general practitioner. When he was ready to go into a medical college, he went to New York, where he lived a life of great frugality. It was his wish to serve humankind, and so he became interested in the work of medical missions. He lost no time making a decision and in the end applied to the American Presbyterian Board of Foreign Missions for a position. Once receiving a positive response, he and his bride sailed for China in the fall 1885. See *A Guide to the City and Suburbs of Canton* (Kelly & Walshi, 1904), 36.

26. Dr. Swan set up the hospital's entire antiseptic unit and laid great weight upon a proper routine in the operating room. Mrs. Swan, for the meantime, took over the supervision of the kitchen, leading to great improvement on dietetics of the Hospital. A lot of upgrading in the old buildings was made, much extra land was purchased, and new buildings were constructed. Slowly but surely, the Boji Hospital was developing into a modern institution under the leadership of Dr. Swan and his colleagues. See *The Hundred Years History of the Canton Hospital* (The Organization Committee of the Sun Yat-sen Medical College, Lingnan University, Canton, 1935), 12-15.

27. These rules were: 1) The foreign physicians of the hospital and college be the medical staff and they elected their chairman yearly; 2) Each member of the staff, after one year's study of the language in the field, should have an equal voice in deciding all medicinal work of the Society; and 3) The medical and surgical work of the Society be arranged into departments and each one of the physicians be assigned his department by the staff. Cadbury, *At the Point of a Lancet*, 209-10.

28. *China Medical Journal* 35 (1921): 347.

29. *China Medical Journal* 34 (1920): 106-107.

30. The medical staff included Dr. W. W. Cadbury, chairman and head of the Department of Internal Medicine; Dr. J. Thomson, head of the surgical service; Dr. A. H. Woods, neurologist; and Dr. H. J. Howard, head of the Eye, Ear, Nose, and Throat Department. See *The Hundred Years History of the Canton Hospital,* 16-17.

31. The Union was originally formed by the Medical Missionary Society, the Women's Board of American Baptist Mission (North), the American and Reformed Presbyterian Missions; afterward the New Zealand Presbyterian

Mission and the Canton Christian College enrolled, too. On December 19, 1916, a special meeting was held at the hospital to celebrate the eightieth anniversary of its founding. American Consul-General P. S. Heintzleman presided at the meeting, and British Consul-General J. W. Jamieson spoke of the early history of the hospital, both of whom were members the Canton Medical Missionary Society. So did the civil governor of Guangdong, Zhu Qinglan. They praised the work that had been done and spoke of the prospect. Even the president of Republic of China sent a telegram of congratulations. See *The Hundred Years History of the Canton Hospital*, 19-20.

32. The Canton Christian College did not enter the Union until 1919. Dr. W.W. Cadbury, the head of the Department of Internal Medicine, was appointed to represent the China Medical Board of the Rockefeller Foundation. J. M. Henry, the son of B. C. Henry, was chosen in 1918-1920 as chairman of the Board of Directors of the Union and was also a Trustee of the Society. He always maintained a vigorous interest in this organization, which consequently proved to be very efficient and well organized. He later was the provost of Lingnan University in 1935. See Charles C. Selden, "The Life of John G. Kerr: Forty-three Years Superintendent of the Canton Hospital," *The Chinese Medical Journal* 2 (1935): 364-76.

33. "Canton Hospital: Its Work in 1919," *South China Morning Post*, July 31, 1920, 8.

34. "Canton Hospital," *The Canton Gazette*, October 8, 1924, 6.

35. In 1926, the Canton Hospital's foreign staff was: Drs. W.W. Cadbury, C.A. Hayes and Mrs. Hayes, J. L. Harvey, F. Oldt, W.G. Reynolds, J.C. Thompson, J. M. Wright and ten Chinese physicians and surgeons.

36. Three years later, at the 90th annual meeting held on April 19, 1929, thirty-six members of the Society presented and adopted the following recommendations: The Board of Directors of the Canton Medical Missionary Union be authorized to reopen the hospital, and the Directors of Lingnan University be asked to appoint six persons to conduct the work of the Canton Hospital during the following year. This Board of twelve, six representing the hospital and six Lingnan University, met three times between April 29 and June 25, 1929. See *Guangzhoushi ge yiyuan yange* (History of the hospitals in Canton) (Guangzhou, 1934), 54.

37. The doctors of the Canton Hospital were:

William W. Cadbury	Head of Department of Medicine & Superintendent
J. Oscar Thomson	United Church of Canada, Head, Department of Surgery
Frank Oldt	United Brethren Mission, Director, Health Service
A. Clair Siddall	United Brethren Mission, Head, Department Gynecology & Obstetrics
Xu Gangliang	Head of Department of Pediatrics

.   Visiting Physicians: Dr. Zhou Guangming, Dr. Zhou Huoming, Dr. Zhou Jingtine; Resident Physicians: Dr. Xia Qiaoyun, Dr. Liang Xiguang;

Interns: Dr. Liu Wu, Dr. Guo Youchen.

. See Charles C. Selden, "The Life of John G. Kerr: Forty-three Years Superintendent of the Canton Hospital."

38. "Canton Hospital: Celebration of the Eightieth Anniversary." *The Hong Kong Daily Press*, December 21, 1916.

39. John Kerr, "Report of the Medical Society's Hospital at Canton for the Year 1860," *Report of the Medical Missionary Society in China for the Year 1860* (Canton, Friend of China Press, 1861), 8. See also *The Twenty-Fourth Annual Report of the Board of Foreign Missions of the Presbyterian Church in the United States of America* (New York, 1861), 71.

40. Named the First Municipal Hospital of Fushan, this hospital has 1,800 beds and 1,300 employees, serving a population of five million in the city today. See http://tech.sina.com.cn/roll/2006-07-27/102950764.shtml.

41. R. H. Graves, "Some Personal Reminiscences of Thirty Years' Mission Work," *Chinese Recorder* XVII (November 1886): 421-35.

42. John Kerr, "Report of the Medical Society's Hospital at Canton for the Year 1860," *Report of the Medical Missionary Society in China for the Year 1860* (Canton, Friend of China Press, 1861), 4.

43. Medical Missionary Society, *Report of the Medical Missionary Society for 1861* (Tung-Hing Office, Canton, 1862).

44. *Chinese Recorder* 7: 174-201.

45. Mary Alexander, *Seedtime and Harvest in the South China Mission of the Southern Baptist Convention, 1845-1933* (Richmond, Virginia: Foreign Mission Board Southern Baptist Convention, 1934), 36.

46. B.C. Henry, "Strategic Importance of Lien Chow," *The Church at Home and Abroad* 6 (September 1889): 244 and "Missions in China," *The Church at Home and Abroad* 15 (February 1894): 113.

47. Eleanor Chestnut, "Medical Work in Lien-Chow, Kwangtung," *China Medical Missionary Journal* 14, 2 (April 1900): 123.

48. *History of the South China Mission of the American Presbyterian Church, 1845-1920* (Shanghai: The Presbyterian Mission Press, 1927), 110-11.

49. J. Stewart Kunkle, "Report of the Lienchow Station: Medical work," Folder 3, Box 4, Record Group 82, Presbyterian Church in the U.S.A. Board of Foreign Missions. Secretaries Files: China Missions, 1891-1955, Presbyterian Historical Society, Philadelphia, Pennsylvania.

50. This hospital, named the People's Hospital of Lianzhou Municipality in the 1950s, has more than 600 employees and 450 beds. See http://www.lzsph.com/about.asp?newsid=5.

51. *History of the South China Mission of the American Presbyterian Church, 1845-1920* (Shanghai: The Presbyterian Mission Press, 1927), 54-5.

52. *Annual Report of the Presbyterian Board of Foreign Missions* (New York: The Board of Foreign Missions, Presbyterian Church in the U.S.A., 1891), 33.

53. Dr. Thomson left for Canada to take up work among the Chinese. In 1894, he was asked to go to Montreal, Canada to work with the Chinese who had come in by the thousands, and he was appointed superintendent of Chinese Mission work under the Canadian Presbyterian Church in Canada until 1919 when he returned to China. His son, Dr. J. Oscar Thomson, had been the resident physician and surgeon since 1910 and later was the

chief surgeon at the Canton Hospital, supported by the United Church of Canada. See *Annual Report of the Presbyterian Board of Foreign Missions* (New York: The Board of Foreign Missions, Presbyterian Church in the U.S.A., 1895), 35-36.

54. The Forman Hospital is called Yangjiang People's Hospital today. See *Yangchen wanbao* (Guangzhou evening daily), June 25, 2008, B5.

55. W. H. Dobson, " A Statement of the Medical Work off Yeung Kong station," September 5, 1913," Folder 5-6, Box 5, Record Group 82, Presbyterian Church in the U.S.A. Board of Foreign Missions. Secretaries Files: China Missions, 1891-1955, Presbyterian Historical Society, Philadelphia, Pennsylvania.

56. Report of the Yeung Kong Station, March 31, 1915, Folder 6, Box 5, Record Group 82, Presbyterian Church in the U.S.A. Board of Foreign Missions. Secretaries Files: China Missions, 1891-1955, Presbyterian Historical Society, Philadelphia, Pennsylvania.

57. *Annual Report of the Presbyterian Board of Foreign Missions* (New York: The Board of Foreign Missions, Presbyterian Church in the U.S.A., 1904), 53; *Annual Report of the Presbyterian Board of Foreign Missions* (New York: The Board of Foreign Missions, Presbyterian Church in the U.S.A., 1905), 55.

58. Dr. Dobson did not return to the United States until 1940, after serving the Chinese for forty years. He died in New York in 1965. Today his hospital is named the People's Hospital of Yangjiang Municipality, which has 700 beds and employs 800 people. It is a leading hospital in the city of Yangjiang. See http://www.cqhuashan.com/hospital/36476.html.

59. Notes on A Historical, Sketch of the American Presbyterian Mission Hainan China, 1899, Folder 7, Box 1 Record Group 129, Presbyterian Church in the U.S.A. Board of Foreign Missions-China Mission Secretaries' Files, 1893-1957, Presbyterian Historical Society, Philadelphia, Pennsylvania.

60. *First Annual Report of the American Presbyterian Mission in the Island of Hainan, China for the Year 1893* (Nodoa: Hainan Mission Press, 1894), 2-7.

61. *History of the South China Mission of the American Presbyterian Church, 1845-1920* (Shanghai: The Presbyterian Mission Press, 1927), 52-53.

62. *Annual Report of the Presbyterian Board of Foreign Missions* (New York: The Board of Foreign Missions, Presbyterian Church in the U.S.A., 1894), 67-68.

63. *The Isle of Palms, Sketches of Hainan: the American Presbyterian Mission* (Shanghai: the Commercial Press, 1919. Reprint,the Garland Publishing, 1980), 95-96.

64. Hainan Island is one of the provinces in China today. Named the People's Hospital of Hainan Province, this hospital has 1,200 beds and 1,800 employees, the leading medical and health center in Hainan now. See http://daj.haikou.gov.cn/Article/ShowArticle.asp?ArticleID=805.

65. For an account of the hospitals in Guangdong Province today that were established by American medical missionaries, see *Guangdong shengzhi: weishen zhi* (Annals of Guangdong Province: annals of the health administration) (Guangzhou: Guangdong renmin chubanshe, 2003), 22-34.

66. Zheng Entao, *Liangguangjinxinhui yiyuan baogaoshu* (Report on the two guang Baptist hospital) (Guangzhou: Liangguangjunhui yiyuan, 1946), 4-9.

67. During Japan's occupation of Canton from 1938 to 1945, Dr. Hayes came to Canton in 1938 with approval of the American consulate in Hong Kong. He, assuming the president of the Hospital, maintained functions of the Hospital and protected the Hospital's property. He opened a new dispensary in Canton providing medicine and medical treatment to the poor and the wounded. Due to the Pearl Harbor Attack, the United States declared war on Japan. As a result, Dr. Hayes was forced to leave Canton for the States in 1942. He died in 1946 at the age of 75 years old. See *Liangguang Jinxinhui yiyuan sanshi zoulien tekan* (The special issue of the two guang Baptist hospital's thirtieth anniversary) (Canton: *Liangguang Jinxinhui yiyuan*, 1947), 6-9.

68. His death occurred on January 16, 1939, and his funeral was a memorable occasion. See Canton Hospital, *Annual Report for the 104th year of Canton Hospital, 1938-1939* (Canton: the Canton Hospital, 1939), 12.

69. George B. Stevens, *The Life, Letters, and Journals of the Rev. & Hon. Peter Parker, M.D.* (Boston: Congregational Sunday-School & Publishing Soc., 1896), 135; "Medical Missionary Society: Regulations and Resolutions, Adopted at a Public Meeting Held at Canton on the 21st of February, 1838," *Chinese Repository* VII (March, 1838), 33; Address of Parker, Colledge, and Bridgman (April, 1838), quoted in the *Chinese Repository* VII (May 1838): 37-40.

70. Thomas R. Colledge, *The Medical Missionary Society in China* (Philadelphia, 1838), 3.

71. "Report of the Medical Missionary Society," *Chinese Repository* 12 (April 1843): 190-191.

72. John Kerr, "Report of the Medical Society's Hospital at Canton for the Year 1860," *Report of the Medical Missionary Society in China for the Year 1860* (Canton, Friend of China Press, 1861), 5-6.

73. Henry William Boone had been in China almost as long as John Kerr, but his medical experiences were somewhat different. In 1861 he was in China, where he stayed for only a few months, returning to America in 1862 to serve as a doctor in the Confederate Army. Wounded at the second battle of Bull Run, he abandoned the Confederacy in 1863 for another tour in China, where for the next two years he directed a hospital for Europeans and Americans in Shanghai. By 1865 his health had so deteriorated that he was forced back to the United States again, and he spent the next fourteen years in private practice in San Francisco. But in 1879 he returned to Shanghai once more, opened a hospital, started teaching a few medical students, and settled in for a thirty-year stay. It was largely at his initiative that in 1886 the Medical Missionary Association of China was organized. For a biographical sketch of Boone, see K. Chimin Wong and Wu Lien-Teh, *History of Chinese Medicine*, 236.

74. Ibid., 311-12.

75. After having faithfully served China for twenty-three years, Dr. Parker finally retired, taking up his residence in Washington, D.C., where, though in failing health, he still held such positions as regent of the Smithsonian

Institute, president of the Evangelical Alliance, and president of the Yale College Alumni Association until his death in 1888 at the ripe age of 84. Cadbury, *At the Point of a Lancet*, 63.

76. Mrs. Dr. J. J. Boggs, M.D., Drs. Mary Fulton, John M. Swan, Chas. C. Selden, E.C. Machle, Paul J. Todd, A. W. Hooker, Josiah C. McCracken, Frank Oldt, and J. Allen Hofmann attended the meeting. See John Kirk, "Canton Branch," *The China Medical Journal* 23, 3 (March 1909): 202.

77. *The Hundred Years History of the Canton Hospital*, 4-6.

78. Wong and Wu, *History of Chinese Medicine*, 607.

79. "Annual Meeting of the Canton Medical Missionary Society," *Canton Gazette*, January 23, 1924.

80. Dr. J. Oscar Thomson, "A Century of Medial Work in China," *Missionary Review of the World*, February 1935.

81. H.T. Whitney, " A Quarterly Medical Journal in Chinese, " *China Medical Missionary Journal* 2, 2 (June 1888): 59.

82. John Kerr, *The Western Medical News*, 92-1-442, The Archives of Guangdong Province, Guangzhou, China.

83. *China Review*, February 7, 1881, 9.

84. Jia Yuehan (John Kerr), "Lun Neizi," *Wanguo gongbao* (Global News), 629 (March 5, 1881).

85. *China Medical Journal*, 1911, 54; Ibid. XXVII (March 1913): 69-70; Ibid. XXVII (July 1913): 276; Ibid. XXXIX, 2 (March 1915): 102.

86. *Chinese Medical Journal*, April 1935, 372.

87. Peter Parker, "First Quarterly Report of Ophthalmic Hospital at Canton," *The Chinese Repository* 4 (February 1836): 461-73.

88. Peter Parker, "Thirteenth Report of the Ophthalmic Hospital at Canton, Including the Period from the 1st January, 1844 to the 1st July, 1845," *Chinese Repository* XIV, 10 (October 1845): 452-57.

89. John Kerr, "Vesical Calculus in Canton Province, including the Report of a Personal Experience in 894 Operations, "*China Medical Missionary Journal* 8 (March 1894): 104.

90. W. Hamilton Jefferys and James L. Mazwell, *The Disease of China* (Philadelphia: P. Blakiston's Son, 1910), 523.

91. Park performed operations on those tumors, some of which were so exceedingly huge that Parker was compelled to require "establishing other departments" and "supplying them with men of requisite qualifications." See Peter Parker, "Third Quarterly Report of Ophthalmic Hospital at Canton," *Chinese Repository* 5 (August 1836), 188; Peter Parker, "Fourth Quarterly Report of Ophthalmic Hospital at Canton," *Chinese Repository* 5 (November 1836): 332; and Peter Parker, "Seventh Quarterly Report of Ophthalmic Hospital at Canton," *Chinese Repository* 6 (January 1838): 438-39.

92. Cadbury, *At the Point of a Lancet*, 210-11.

93. *The Hundred Years History of the Canton Hospital*, 12-13.

94. For a study of China's first autopsies performed by Peter Parker, see Larissa N. Heinrich, *The Afterlife of Images: Translating the Pathological Body between China and the West* (Durham: Duke University Press, 2008), 118-19.

95. Harold Balme, *China and Modern Medicine: A study in Medical Missionary Development* (London: London Missionary Society, 1921), 156.

96. Medical Missionary Society, *Report of the Medical Missionary Society in China: The Fourteenth Report of the Ophthalmic Hospital, Canton* (Canton: The Chinese Repository, 1848), 13.

97. *Guangzhoushi ge yiyuan yange* (History of the hospitals in Canton) (Guangzhou, 1934), 20-24.

98. For a study of the first medical photography taken by John Kerr in China, see Larissa N. Heinrich, *The Afterlife of Images: Translating the Pathological Body between China and the West*, 78-81.

99. *The Hundred Years History of the Canton Hospital*, 19-20.

100. Peter Parker, "First Quarterly Report, from the 4th of November 1835 to the 4th of February 1836," *The Chinese Repository* 4 (February 1836): 462-63.

101. *Dong xi yang kao mei yue tong ji zhuan* (Eastern western monthly magazine, 1833-1838) (Canton, 1833-1838. Reprint, Beijing: Zhonghua shuju, 1997), 404-405.

102. "Case of Tumors, and other Morbid Growths," *Chinese Repository* 19 (1850): 271-72.

103. Yie Fangpu, "Biography of Medical Doctor John Kerr," *Yixue weishe bao* (Medical and hygienic daily) 4 (1908): 25-30.

104. Charles C. Selden, "The Life of John G. Kerr: Forty-three Years Superintendent of the Canton Hospital," *The Chinese Medical Journal* 2 (1935): 364-76.

105. Yie Fangpu, "Biography of Medical Doctor John Kerr," *Yixue weishe bao* (Medical and hygienic daily) 4 (1908): 25-30.

106. "Swan," *The China Medical Missionary Journal* 34 (1920): 106-107.

107. "From the Scholars and Merchants of the Entire Province of Kwangtung," *Chinese Repository* XVI (April 1847): 196.

108. Yie Fangpu, "Biography of Medical Doctor John Kerr," *Yixue weishe bao* (Medical and hygienic daily) 4 (1908): 25-30.

109. Cadbury, *At the Point of a Lancet*, 52.

110. Peter Parker, "Ophthalmic Hospital at Canton: The Fourth Quarterly Report, for the Term Ending on the 4th November, 1836," *Chinese Repository* V (Nov. 1836): 328-29; Peter Parker, "Ophthalmic Hospital at Canton: The Fifth Quarterly Report, from the Term Ending on the 4th of February 1837," *Chinese Repository* V (February 1837): 458-59.

111. "Letter from Dr. Parker to the Editor of the *Canton Register*," quoted in the *Chinese Repository* VII (March, 1839): 552.

112. For a detailed account of these cases, see Peter Parker, "Eleventh Report of the Ophthalmic Hospital at Canton for the Term Commencing 1st January and Ending 17th June, 1840," *Chinese Repository* XIII (May 1844): 240-43.

113. Medical Missionary Society, *The Hospital Reports of the Medical Missionary Society in China for the Year 1839* (China: the Office of the Chinese Repository, 1840), 6.

114. Peter Parker, "Ophthalmic Hospital at Canton: The Fourth Quarterly Report, for the Term Ending on the 4th November, 1836," *Chinese Repository* V (November 1836): 328-29; Peter Parker, "Ophthalmic Hospital at Canton: The Fifth Quarterly Report, from the Term Ending on the 4th of February 1837," *Chinese Repository* V (Feb. 1837): 458-59.

115. J. M. Callery and Melchior Yvan, *History of the Insurrections in China with Notices of the Christianity, Creed, and Proclamations of the Insurgents.* (New York: Harper and Brothers, 1853), 132.

116. Jia Yuehan (John Kerr), *Qizheng lunshu* (On special illness) (Canton: Canton Hospital, 1886), 14.

117. For a study of Zhang Zhidong, see William Ayers, *Chang Chih-tung and Educational Reform in China* (Cambridge, MA: Harvard University Press, 1971) and Daniel H. Bays, *China Enters the Twentieth Century: Chang Chih-tung and the Issues of a New Age, 1895-1909* (Ann Arbor: University of Michigan Press, 1978).

118. W.W. Cadbury, *At the Point of a Lancet*, 169-70.

119. *History of the South China Mission of the American Presbyterian Church, 1845-1920* (Shanghai: The Presbyterian Mission Press, 1927), 67-8.

120. *The Hundred Years History of the Canton Hospital*, 15-16.

121. Jia Yuehan (John Kerr), *Qizheng lunshu* (On special illness) (Canton: Canton Hospital, 1886), 15.

122. There is not new in an account on the interactions between American doctors and high-level officials in the Qing Dynasty. Dr. Peter Parker's treatment of Lin Zexu, a key Chinese official during the Opium War, has been told in Jonathan Spence's book, *To Change China: Western Advisers in China 1620-1960* (Boston: Little, Brown and Company, 1969), chapter 2. Parker's association with Imperial Commissioner Qiying has been recounted in both Warren Cohen's *American Response to China: A History of Sino-American Relations* (New York: Columbia University Press, 1989), 10-15 and in Michael Hunt's *The Making of a Special Relationship: The United States and China to 1914* (New York: Columbia University Press, 1983), 27-35. These great scholar books, however, discuss in detail only the medical impact on the Chinese officials, rather than the Chinese officials' attitudes toward Western religion and Westerners after they were treated by American doctors with Western medicine.

123. Lin was in an extensive range of positions in Yunnan, Jiangsu, Shaannxi, and Shangdong provinces. As a governor of Jiangsu, he began an anti-opium campaign, submitting a petition in 1833 to the emperor that opium was killing many peoples and taking a lot of money from the people. As governor-general of Hubei province from 1837-38, he launched vigorous campaigns against opium smokers. During that time Lin made great efforts to close the opium houses, confiscate opium drugs, and destroy opium pipes so as to suppress entirely the opium addicts. In 1837, in a petition to the emperor Lin suggested that all smokers of opium should be strangled while pushers and producers should be beheaded. For a study of Lin's life, see Chang Hsin-pao, *Commissioner Lin and the Opium War* (Cambridge: Harvard University Press, 1964).

124. "Chou ji bian," in Qi Shihe, ed., *Choban yiwu shimo, daoguan chao*) (The history of the foreign affairs during the reign of Daoguan) (Beijing: Zhonghua shuju, 1964), 1.

125. "Chouyi yanjin yapian zhangchen jie," (Memorial on prohibition of opium) Qi Shihe, ed., *Choban yiwu shimo, daoguan chao*) (The history of the foreign affairs during the reign of Daoguan) (Beijing: Zhonghua shuju, 1964), 1.

126. By mid-May 1839, over 1,600 Chinese had been took into custody and about 35,000 pounds of opium and 43,000 opium pipes had been taken away. For a study of the background of the Opium War, see James Polachek, *The Inner Opium War* (Cambridge, MA: Harvard University Press, 1992) and Arthur Waley, *The Opium War Through Chinese Eyes* (London, England: George Allen & Unwin, 1958).

127. "Lin's Letter to Lianyu on May 1, 1839," in Lin Zexu, *Lin Zexu quanji* (Lin Zexu's works), vol. 7 (Fuzhou: Haixia wenyi, 2002), 3445-46.

128. *Chinese Repository* 8, 12 (April 1840): 634-35.

129. Peter Parker, *Statements Respecting Hospitals in China*, 15.

130. Medical Missionary Society, *The Hospital Reports of the Medical Missionary Society in China for the Year 1839*, 14.

131. "General Letter," *Missionary Herald* XXXVI (1840), 82; Peter Parker, *Statements Respecting Hospitals in China*, 110.

132. Peter Parker, *Statements Respecting Hospitals in China*, 15.

133. Qi Shihe, ed., *Choban yiwu shimo, daoguan chao*) (The history of the foreign affairs during the reign of Daoguan) (Beijing: Zhonghua shuju, 1964), 1: 171, 195 96, 282, 298-300, 531.

134. Indeed, although China imposed trade embargo again the British, trade in Canton by no means came to a standstill. The Americans especially were delighted to profit from the new opportunity to operate as middlemen for the British. See James Polachek, *The Inner Opium War* (Cambridge, MA: Harvard University Press, 1992).

135. It was true that when Lin asked all foreign merchants to promise not to be engaged in opium trade, Americans did promise but the English refused and threatened to stop trade with China. American Vice-Consul Warren Delano let his countrymen sign bonds in early July promising not to violate Chinese regulations. When Lin asked all foreign merchants and officers to go to the site to see the burning of opium confiscated by the Chinese government in Canton in June 1839, Americans went to the site and listened carefully to Lin's instructions without any opposition to Chinese government's actions, but the British refused to go and condemned the burning of opium. See James Polachek, *The Inner Opium War* (Cambridge, MA: Harvard University Press, 1992).

136. Letter of Peter Parker, Canton, November 29, 1839, American Board of Commissioners for Foreign Missions, South China, 1838-1844, Letters and Papers of the Board, vol. 130, item 123, Houghton Library, Harvard University.

137. For a study of Qiying's role in negations with Americans and the French after the Opium War, see Jonathan Spence, *The Search for Modern China* (New York: W.W. Norton, 1990), 160-64.

138. *Chinese Repository* 13 (January to December 1844): 302-3.

139. Ode of Qiying, quoted in the general letter from the Canton Mission, July 20, 1843, *Missionary Herald* XL (July 1844): 217-18

140. Letter of J. H. Temple, quoted in Theodore Parker, *Genealogical and Biographical Notes of John Parker of Lexington and His Descendant* (Worcester, Mass.: Press of C. Hamilton, 1893), 301. See also Edward V. Gulick, *Peter Parker and the Opening of China* (Cambridge, Mass.: Harvard University Press, 1973), 118, 121-4.

141. George B. Stevens and W. Fisher Markwick, *The Life, Letters, and Journals of the Rev. and Hon. Peter Parker, M.D., Missionary, Physician, and Diplomatist, the Father of Medical Missions and Founder of the Ophthalmic Hospital in Canton*, 328-9.

142. "Letter from Doctor Parker, August 1, 1844," *Missionary Herald* XLI (Feb., 1845), 53.

143. Kenneth S. Latourette, *The Chinese: Their History and Culture* (New York: The Macmillan, 1929), 279.

144. *Chinese Repository* 14, 10 (October 1845): 539-40.

145. Qi Shihe, *Choban yiwu shimo, daoguan chao*) (The history of the foreign affairs during the reign of Daoguan) (Beijing: Zhonghua shuju, 1964), 6: 2877-80, 2898-2900, 2948-54.

146. Ibid., 6: 2954.

147. Cadbury, *At the Point of a Lancet*, 80.

148. "A Form of Prayer to the God of Heaven with Preface, by Qiying, Governor of the Two Kwang Provinces," translated by Sixensis, *The North China Herald*, April 12, 1851, 146.

149. Ibid.

150. For a study of Kang Youwei, see Kung-chuan Hsiao, *A Modern China and a New World: K'ang Yu-wei, Reformer and Utopian, 1858-1927* (Seattle: University of Washington Press, 1975).

151. Kang Youwei, *Kang Nanhai zibiannianpu* (A self-compiled chronological biography of Kang Youwei) (Beijing: Zhonghua shuju, 1992), 13.

152. Lo Jung-pang, ed., *K'ang Yu-wei: A Biography and a Symposium* (Tucson: University of Arizona Press, 1967), 42.

153. Chang Po-chen, *Nanhai Kang xiansheng quan* (Biography of Mr. Kang Nanhai) (Beijing, 1932), 7.

154. Kang Youwei, *Datong shu* (Great Harmony) (Zhengzhou: Zhongzhou guji shubanshe, 1998), 256-58.

155. Laurence G. Thompson, ed., *Ta T'ung Shu: The One-World Philosophy of K'ang Yu-we* (London: George Allen & Unwin, 1958), 202.

156. Ibid., 41.

157. Ibid, 256-57. See also Kang Youwei, *Datong shu* (Shanghai, 1935), 428.

158. Kang Youwei, *Kang Youwei qunji* (Works of Kang Youwei), vol. 3, ed. Jiang Yihua, (Shanghai: Guji chubanshe, 1992): 619-21.

159. Ibid.

160. Ibid., 583-88.

161. Tang Zhijun, *Kang Youwei zhenlun–shangji* (Political Essays of Kang Youwei, volume 1) (Beijing: Zhonghua shuju, 1981), 151-52.

162. Kang Youwei, "Riben shumu zhi" (Japanese bibliography), in Kang Youwei, *Kang Youwei qunji* (Works of Kang Youwei), vol. 3, ed. Jiang Yihua (Shanghai: Guji chubanshe, 1992).

163. Frank Dikötter, *The Discourse of Race in Modern China* (Stanford, Calif.: Stanford University Press, 1992), 111.

164. Jiang Yihua, *Lixing quefa de qimeng* (The Irrational Enlightenment) (Shanghai: Sanlian chubanshe, 2000), 6.

165. Kang Yuwei, *Kang Nanhaizibian nianpu* (A self self-compiled chronological biography of Kang Youwei), in Jian Bozhang. ed., *Wuxu bianfa* (The reform movement of 1898) (Shanghai: Shengzhou guoguan she, 1953), vol. 4, 115-18.

166. For a study of Liang Qichao, see Hao Chang, *Liang Ch'i-ch'ao and Intellectual Transition in China, 1898-1907* (Cambridge, MA: Harvard University Press, 1971); Philip C. Huang, *Liang Ch'i-ch'ao and Modern Chinese Liberalism* (Seattle: University of Washington Press, 1972), and Joseph R. Levenson, *Liang Ch'i-ch'ao and the Mind of Modern China*, 2d ed. (Berkeley: University of California Press, 1970).

167. Li Xisu, *Liangqichao chun* (Biography of Liang Qichao)(Beijing: Renmin zhubianshe,), 17-24.

168. Ding Wenjiang, *Liang jiangong xiansheng nianpu chugao* (The first draft of a chronological biography of Liang Qichao) (Taipei, 1959), 1: 16-17.

169. Liang Qichao, "Kang Youwei Chuan" (Biography of Kang Youwei), in Chen Weiliang, ed. *Liang Qichao wenji* (Liang Qicha's works) (Beijing: Yanshan Chubanshe, 1997), 466; Xia Shaohong, *Laing Qichao wenxuan* (Liang Qichao's selected works), vol. 1 (Beijing: Zhongguo guangbodianshi chubanshe, 1992), 287.

170. Liang Qichao, "Xixue shumubiao"(A list of Western books), in Liang Qichao, *Yinbingshi heji* (Writings from the ice-drinker's studio) (Beijing: Beijing daxue chubanshe, 2005), 1121-1158.

171. Liang Qichao, "Du xixueshu fa," (On reading books of Western learning) in Liang Qichao, *Yinbingshi heji* (Writings from the ice-drinker's studio) (Beijing: Beijing daxue chubanshe, 2005), 1159-1170.

172. Wang Xincai, *Liang qichao dushu shengya* (Liang Qichao reading books) (Wuhan: Changjiang wenyi, 1998), 36.

173. Liang Qichao, "Yixue shanhui xu," *Shiwu bao* 38 (August 11, 1897).

174. Liang Qichao, "Biography of Six Martyrs," in Chen Yinci, *Liang Qichao's Academic Works* (Shanghai: East China Normal Press, 1998), 449.

175. Ding Wenjiang, *Liang Qichao nianpu changbian* (Chronicled biography of Liang Qichao) (Shanghai: Shanghai renmin chubanshe, 1983), 1079-88 and *Wu limin, Liang Qichao he ta de er numen* (Liang Qichao and his children) (Shanghai:Shanghai renmin chubanshe, 1999), 9-11.

176. Liang Qichao, "Yixue shanhui xu," *Yinbingshi heji* (Works of the ice cream house), vol. 2, (Beijing: Zhonghua shuju, 1989), 69-72.

177. Liang Qichao, "Yixue shanhui xu," *Shiwubao* 38 (August 11, 1897).

178. Liang Qichao, "Baoguohui yanshuoci," in *Yinbingshi heji* (Works of the ice cream house), vol. 3, (Beijing: Zhonghua shuju, 1989), 27-28.

179. Xia Dongyuan, *Zheng Guanying chuan* (Biography of Zheng Guanying) (Shanghai: Huadong shifan daxue chubanshe, 1985), 275-81.

180. Ibid.

181. Zheng Guanying, *Zheng Guanying ji* (Works of Zheng Guanying), vol. 2 (Shanghai: Shanghai chubanshe, 1988), 197.

182. Ibid., 197.

183. Volume 5 of *Zhongwai weisheng yao zhi* was not completed until 1895. See "Beiji yanfan" in *Zheng Guanying ji* (Shanghai renmin chubanshe, 1982) 2:1168.

184. For a study of Zheng Guanying, see Albert Feuerwerker, *China's Early Industrialization: Sheng Hsuan-huai (1844-1916) and Mandarin Enterprise* (Cambridge, Mass.: Harvard University Press, 1958).

185. They are: 1). Chinese medicine had to establish a medical examination system like the Western one in order to improve the quality of Chinese

medical practitioners; 2). Chinese medicine had to learn dissection; 3.) Since some Chinese medical theories were unfounded in terms of physiology and pathology, Chinese medicine needed to do more research; 4.) Chinese medicine needed to learn from the West in terms of medications; 5.) Chinese medicine needed to have more medical instruments. He advocated using modern technology to examine Chinese medical theory, diagnostics, and remedy in order to improve and modernize traditional Chinese medicine. See Zheng Guanying, *Zheng Guanying ji* (Works of Zheng Guanying), vol. 1 (Shanghai: Shanghai chubanshe, 1988), 520-4.

186. "Fushenggongbao lun chuanjian yi yuan shu," in *Zheng Guanying ji* (Shanghai Renmin chubanshe, 1982) 2: 197-8.

187. Zheng Guanying, *Zheng Guanying ji* (Works of Zheng Guanying), vol. 1 (Shanghai: Shanghai chubanshe, 1988), 520-4.

188. Zheng Guanying, "Nujiao,"(Women education) in *Zheng Guangyin ji* (Shanghai Renmin Chubanshe, 1982) 1: 287-8.

189. Zheng Guanying, *Zheng Guanying ji* (Works of Zheng Guanying), vol. 2 (Shanghai: Shanghai chubanshe, 1988), 197.

190. "Yidao," in *Zheng Guanying ji* (Shanghai Renmin chubanshe, 1982) 1: 520-24; 2: 197-8

191. Liu Zhenling, "Fuqiang shi yu weisheng lun,"(On strength and prosperity coming from hygiene) *Zhixinbao* (November 11,1897).

192. *Daqing dezong (Guangxu) huangdi shilu* (The record of Emperor Guangxu of great Qing), vol. 6 (Taipei, Huawen shuju, 1960), 879.

193. Wong and Wu, *History of Chinese Medicine*, 2nd ed., 556-572.

194. See He Xiaolian, *Xi yi dong jian yu wen hua tiao shi* (Introduction of Western medicine to China and cultural accommodation) (Shanghai: Shanghai gu ji chubanshe, 2006).

195. "On Tongren Dispensary in 1877," *Shen bao* (Shanghai daily), December 22, 1877.

196. R. H. Graves, *Forty Years in China or China in Transition* (Baltimore: Woodward, 1895. Reprint, Scholarly Resource at Wilmington, Delaware, 1972), 246-48.

197. *China Year Book, 1913* (London: H. T. Montague Bell & H. B. W. Woodhead, 1913, Kraus reprint, 1969), 457.

198. Wu Lien-teh, "A Hundred Years of the Modern Medicine in China," *The China Medical Journal* 50, 2 (February 1936).

2

Western Medical Education in Canton and Its Influence in China, 1835-1935

American medical missionaries started training the Chinese at the Canton Hospital and initiated Western medical education in China. This chapter examines how American doctors established Western medical education in Canton and what role the medical students trained by Americans played in medical modernization in Canton as well as in China. This chapter also explores how the Cantonese medical students started to develop Chinese nationalism and to carry out political and social reforms in China.

Medical Education at the Canton Hospital, 1837–1912

American medical missionaries from the beginning of their practice of medicine in China realized the significance of "the education of young Chinese in those branches of science that belong to medicine." They believed, "The [Chinese] young men thus instructed will gradually be dispersed over the empire, traveling for pleasure, honor, or reward, and will dispense the benefits of a systematic acquaintance with the subject where they go."[1]

Medical Assistantship, 1837–66

As early as May 1837, two Cantonese boys were studying English with Peter Parker so as to become doctors, and by the end of 1837, Dr. Parker had three native assistants. One of them held the office of dispenser, and all of them helped Parker take care of patients and the hospital. Parker started instruction in medicine with the intention of training native Chinese to be doctors who would lend him a hand. The instruction of the Chinese pupils took much of Dr. Parker's time because he was trying to educate them in both medicine and the basics of Christianity in English. Four native pupils were receiving medical training from Dr. Parker between 1848 and 1849, the beginning of modern medical education in China. His native pupils helped him exceedingly in his medical work.[2]

With the introduction of medical education to train Chinese assistants, several doctors who came after Parker carried on this type of education. During the early period, medical training was performed along with the normal routine of the hospital, but as that expanded in size and scope, a structured and formal medical training became necessary. In 1862, American doctors regarded medical education as a principal part of the objectives of the hospital to teach young men in the science and art of surgery. The following year, they started formal training of three regular pupils and four other pupils who were connected with a German Missionary Society, the Rhenish Mission. These pupils had to supply themselves with surgical instruments, several of which made by Chinese craftsmen copying the model of those instruments used in the hospital. In 1864, the pupils had the unusual experience of a post-mortem when one of them removed a stone, to which a bean stalk adhered, from the bladder. Dr. J. H. Lockhart spoke of these pupils with high praise, "several of them, on leaving the hospital, have established themselves as surgeons in private practice in distant parts of the Canton province."[3]

South China Medical School, 1866–1902

Dr. Kerr played a significant role in the introduction of Western medical education into Canton. Emphasizing medical training of the Chinese, Dr. Kerr hoped that the Chinese students would help him in medical work. The regular class of medical instruction with eight students began in 1865 under Kerr. In this year, the pupils had a chance to do a post-mortem on a new-born child with a congenital deformity of the head, who was left in the street to die. After Dr. Kerr was told of this, the child, still alive, was brought to the hospital but soon died. As a result, a careful examination of the dead body was made at the hospital.

After moving into the new hospital building in 1866, Kerr lost no time starting to teach a medical course, and the South China Medical School was formally opened in which systematic instruction was given to the Chinese pupils. Kerr hoped that this would be the germ of a medical school that would send its people into all parts of the Chinese empire in the future, as he wrote,

> It is of the utmost importance that a thoroughly equipped school of medicine should be established for the vast multitudes of the empire, and it is believed that opportunities for instruction in the healing art will be as much appreciated as we know the healing art is.[4]

Four medical students were at the South China Medical School. Dr. Kerr was assisted by the faithful Guan Yadu, who was very helpful and immensely lightened Dr. Kerr's load. During Kerr's sickness for several weeks, Guang took charge of the patients. Dr. Kerr was also aided by Dr. Huang Kuan. In the 1867 report, Dr. Huang provided detailed information about the significant achievements of the medical pupils and patients' confidence in those Chinese doctors who had been educated in the art of modern medicine and surgery. During that time, Dr. Huang gave instruction in anatomy, physiology, and surgery; Dr. Kerr in materia medica (therapeutic properties of substances), chemistry, and physiology for the first time; and Dr. Guan gave instruction in practical and Chinese medicine. In 1868, twelve pupils were at the medical school, among whom were several old-style practitioners and sons of physicians of Chinese medicine. Two students, after studying at the hospital for two years, were about to start private practice.[5]

Training of students was conducted systematically in 1869. Apparatus for practical work in chemistry was obtained and taken into use; anatomy, physiology, chemistry, practical medicine and materia medica were taught. By 1871 more than twelve young men had spent at least three years or more as students in the hospital and started to practice medicine independently. In 1874, courses were offered in anatomy using the dissection of dogs. It was unfeasible to study anatomy from dissections of human beings, but what the students obtained from dissecting the animals was very remarkable. Dr. Kerr also was able to make a post-mortem examination of a man who died in October from aneurysm of the aorta. In 1876, the school had eleven students, and a collection of preserved surgical specimens was started. In 1885, the days for teaching and practice were increased, but the years required for graduation were the same—three years. Gradually, the class was assuming the character of a regular medical school when suitable instructors came forward for all the different subjects. When the number of pupils was increased, the school assumed the title of "The Canton Medical College." Beginning in 1886, the students at the Canton Hospital received no aid and needed to pay $20, although in some cases only half of it was collected. The students were also required to purchase their own books. The payment of tuition reduced the numbers in attendance, but it had the effect of making an unquestionable improvement in the class.[6]

Kerr praised the achievements of the South China Medical School in comparison with those of the Hong Kong Medical College founded in 1887. He claimed the South China Medical School had three advantages over the counterpart in Hong Kong: cheaper tuition, teaching in Chinese, and female students. He believed that the model of his medical school would contribute significantly to modern medical science in China.[7] Kerr repeated the significances of medical education in China, as he wrote in 1889:

> I maintain that the teaching of medicine is one of the duties devolving on us as Medical Missionaries, and one which will become more

important as the appreciation of Western medicine becomes general and the prejudice in favor of native practice passes away."[8]

In 1890, the School had twenty students. Daily class on five days of the week were held, and each student read in two or three branches of study every day; Saturday was given to demonstrations, experiments, the use of the microscope, and other practical subjects. During that time, Kerr was ready to admit the qualification problem of his students and wrote in an article of 1890 that insignificant outcome had been measured in terms of medical students' competence due to "no public opinion requiring any standard of qualification in those who profess to cure disease." He, however, concluded that this difficulty had to be taken into account only when the question concerned what could be expected of Chinese medical students once they had left the mission hospitals and schools where they were trained.[9]

The school was expanded when a new building (more wards) was erected in 1891. The new building enabled the students to set apart a room where classes were held, and the apparatus, models and plates for illustrations were maintained and were at all times within reach. The increased equipment and the recruitment of gifted teachers were signs of unambiguous improvement in the training of the medical students, becoming year by year a more important part of the work of the hospital. The school was to be prepared to give a high quality of instruction to a larger class of students. In his article of 1896, Dr. Kerr highly praised a number of pupils, who had made commendable progress.[10]

In 1897, the School had twenty-five male and six female students, and the period of study was lengthened from three to four years. The Medical Missionary Society was determined to free Dr. Kerr from the routine of the hospital and appointed Dr. Swan in charge of the hospital so as to enable Kerr to focus on scholarly work and instructions, although he remained available to perform critical operations. In 1898, the class had thirty-seven pupils, and by that time, the senior students were able to observe operations, and the Chinese literary language was used exclusively. An important change took place in 1899: Dr. Kerr left the Canton Hospital to take charge of the newly opened asylum for the insane. He took his male students with him to finish their medical courses there, but not the female students.[11]

South China Medical College, 1902–12

The founding of the medical college in Canton was largely due to the great efforts of Dr. Swan, the superintendent of the Canton Hospital, who had a large interest in medical education. In 1901, forty students, as well as two foreign and eight Chinese teachers, were at the Canton Hospital. It was not until 1902 that, three years after Dr. Swan had been in charge of the hospital, a design for a medical college was really created, when circumstances were encouraging enough and suitable for the formation of a medical college. A special report, submitted to the Medical Missionary Society, wrote, "It is therefore proposed to establish a properly organized medical college for men in connection with the hospital and to use every possible means to make it of a high standard." On January 15, 1902, under Dr. Swan's leadership, the Canton Medical Missionary Society took part in a ballot to set up the South China Medical College; a special committee on organization and equipment was created with American Consul Robert M. McWade as chairman. The new medical college, like the hospital, was administered by the Society; Dr. Swan thereafter was appointed the first president of the college.[12]

A piece of land next to the hospital on the river front was contributed by the viceroy of Guangdong, and a total of fifty thousand dollars was required for such a project. All members of the Medical Missionary Society and those people keen on medical work conducted by the Society in the past were asked to give all possible donations, but the main part of the cost, over $16,000, was presented by particular donations, by and large from the Cantonese.[13]

The building included classrooms, laboratories, and a lecture theatre to seat one hundred students. The ceremonial opening of the building did not happen until November 1, 1904 when the medical classes first moved out of the hospital and into the new building. In February 1909, a new dormitory was completed, a substantial four-story building sufficient to house seventy students. The college building and dormitory buildings, bordering the hospital compound, proved of great value. The college, well-equipped, was administered on a self-financing basis and was completely independent of hospital funds; the Medical Missionary Society was the owner of the buildings and took charge of the educational work.[14] After many years of devoted, educational work, carried out by late Dr. John G. Kerr, this branch of the Society's work was put on a more permanent foundation by the creation of an impressive and spacious college.

The first course commenced on September 1, 1904, and fifty students were enrolled, twelve of whom were in regular attendance. The Cantonese dialect was used as the means of teaching; a set of courses of four years was adopted. Ten professors were employed for a school where only fourteen students were in one graduating class.[15] In 1909, there was a graduating class of fourteen pupils, with thirty-six students enrolled, and eleven physicians on the staff. All fees, tuition, rent, and other expenses were paid at the opening of the semester for the entire academic year. Attendance was required for all students; eight hundred hours of informative teaching, with the exception of clinical work, were contained in the courses. The course of Chinese Materia Medica was offered at the School. In 1910, there was a graduating class of fourteen pupils with thirty-six students admitted and eleven physicians teaching.[16]

It was a promising year, but before long the professors became so worn-out that many of them left the college. To make things worse, internal conflict occurred within the college. As a result, after training a lot of medical students, the Canton Hospital was obliged to shut down its medical college in 1912 on account of having insufficient teachers. In 1913, the college building was sold to the South China Christian Book Company for a Central Missionary Business Agency, and the dormitory was used as a ward for the Canton Hospital.[17]

Medical Contribution of American Doctors' Students

Dr. Parker's most notable student was Guan Yadu, who treated many patients in Parker's absence from 1839 to 1842 and returned to study further under Parker's direction. Guan performed several minor surgeries after learning to do many operations. In 1843, he, a great help to Parker, performed many surgeries at the hospital, acquiring a reputation as surgeon and oculist almost as extensive as Parker's. By the year 1847, he had performed several difficult operations and was performing the majority of the surgeries on the eye, an area of expertise that carried him to other places in China. Guan was then competent to maintain the hospital's operations when Parker was not present in the short term. As indicated by Parker in 1847, "Guan Yadu [Kwan Taou]…is now able to render important assistance in the duties and labors of the Hospital."[18] In 1851, Guan performed effectively many operations—extirpating tumors, extracting teeth, removing diseased bones, and treating dislocations and fractures. He obtained a large amount of both medical theory and practical experience and became an accomplished practitioner, as both an oculist and a surgeon. In addition to his medical work, Guan was in charge of tutoring medical students. Thanks to Guan's important assistance in the duties and labors of the hospital, the Medical Missionary Society decided at its annual meeting on February 21, 1857 to pay money to Guan, a stipend of $10 per month during the year 1857, and voted thanks to Guan for his services.[19] In 1860, enlisted as surgeon to the imperial forces, Guan was sent from Guangdong Province to fight the rebels in Fujian Province. On one occasion, he barely escaped with his life when the rebels enclosed a city where he had opened a military hospital. His services were rewarded by receiving the crystal medal granted by the emperor, with the title of a mandarin of the fifth rank.[20] Guan Yadu remained in the Canton Hospital assisting Dr. Kerr until 1864, and thereafter began practicing with the government of Fujian Province. He was one of Parker's best students.[21]

Dr. Kerr, during his forty-four years at the Canton Hospital, trained one hundred and fifty students who took the full three years' courses of his instruction and fifty students who had less than three years studying under him. Su Daoming (1847–1919) was one of Kerr's best students. As a small boy, he came to the attention of Dr. Kerr because he might have lost his way or have been kidnapped. Whatever happened, Dr. Kerr identified, accepted, and raised him, later teaching him in medicine, when he became one of the eight students under Dr. Kerr's direction in 1865. After graduating from the Canton Hospital's medical school in 1865, Dr. Su became a valuable assistant to Dr. Kerr. In 1880, Su was teaching the courses of anatomy and practical medicine with Dr. Benjamin Hobson's textbooks. Su, the chief anesthetist, won high admiration for the period of his activities in the hospital. As a resident doctor from 1866 to 1886, he took care of outpatients and was in charge of administering chloroform to more than 10,000 patients without a single death. He continued to work as a regular assistant, serving on the staff of the hospital for twenty-three years. Unfortunately, he died in 1919, a devoted supporter of the Hospital.[22]

Ni Xipeng was another example. He was the son of Gideon Ni and his Chinese wife, whose father was an American merchant and the vice president of the Canton Medical Missionary Society from 1845 to 1888. Ni entered the medical college under Dr. Kerr in 1888 and gradated four years later, immediately joining the hospital staff until 1911, with brief intervals in which he was engaged in private practice. The Canton Hospital almost certainly was indebted more to Dr. Ni than to any of its graduates because he had wide-ranging clinical experience and worked in the position of native house physician.[23]

The students of the Canton Hospital not only practiced medicine in Canton but also in rural areas in south China as well as in other places. According to Dr. Kerr's 1871 report, most of his students worked in country towns, but some of them were in the cities, and they often sent patients to the Canton Hospital when surgery was necessary, which they could not perform. The most difficult thing at the commencement of practice was to win the confidence of the patients, it was said.[24] As indicated by Kerr in 1894, as many as 100 Chinese physicians who trained at the Medical Missionary Society's hospital successfully practiced medicine all over Canton and in larger inland towns not so reachable to the missionaries.[25] As stated by Dr. Kerr's 1896 report, one of the Chinese instructors at the South China Medical School was called to a professorship in the Tianjin government's medical college close to Beijing. Two graduates of the School successfully passed an examination organized by the Medical Board at Honolulu and started in private practice there. Most of Dr. Kerr's students practiced medicine in south China. For example, while working as a pastor of a local church, Zhang Yunwen practiced medicine at the city of Zaoqing in Gaoyao County in West River valley in Guangdong Province; Pan Yunhe practiced medicine at the city of Shaoguan in North River valley in Guangdong Province, too.[26]

The Canton Hospital was the mother of modern medical education in China. The Canton Hospital's medical institution, representing the medical education work of the Canton Medical Missionary Society, was a local, independent, self-supporting missionary organization, but it first introduced Western medical science into China and trained China's first doctors of modern medicine, promoting modern medical education for the Chinese and contributing to the spread of Western medicine in China. More significantly, American doctors adjusted themselves to Cantonese society and modified their medical training of the Cantonese students when they used the Cantonese dialect as the means of teaching, an important approach to remove the technological barriers so as to promote the medical technology in China in modern medical globalization.

The Gongyi Medical Institution, 1909–1935

The South China Medial College connected with the Canton Hospital was shut down by reason of a students' strike in 1908. Due to the crisis, a noteworthy enterprise built on enthusiastic collaboration between the Cantonese and Americans began to operate in 1909 in Canton, under the name of the Gongyi Medical College. Sent out by the American Presbyterian Board, Dr. Paul J. Todd came to the Canton Hospital as physician and surgeon in 1902 and left the Canton Hospital in 1907 to open a private Bethesda Hospital, which had an eighteen-bed ward in a rented building in Canton. His efforts to buy land to construct a hospital of his own were abortive, but he received prompt response when appealing to his Chinese friends for support of this new college.[27]

About fifty Cantonese merchants, professional people, businessmen, and officials made an endeavor to start with a new learning institution to help the forty medical students, who had been in the Canton Hospital's medical classes, continue their studies. They attended a meeting held in the winter 1908, each of whom pledged $100 towards the foundation of a medical college. They thereafter launched a campaign to collect donations for the formation of the college, a strategy brought to fruition. After getting sufficient endowments, the Gongyi Society began to operate. Guangdong Gongyi Medical School was established in 1909, a medical institution supported entirely by the Cantonese but run with the assistance of American experts.[28]

The Gongyi Medical School, 1909–23

Pan Peiru was appointed the first president of the Gongyi Medical School. Since the students applied to Dr. Paul Todd for further instruction, he was appointed as the president of the Gongyi Hospital, affiliated to the School, and Dr. Su Daoming was employed as proctor. The medical school was financed by the Chinese and administered by a Chinese board of directors. The Chinese directors at first did not ban their missionary professors from their religion, but they did not require religious education. Medical missionaries working at the local hospitals were employed to teach at Gongyi. Instruction started early in the year 1909 with forty-two students and thirteen teachers.

A residential house was rented in western Canton. In 1910, a building near the Canton Hospital site was rented for classrooms, and the school provisionally moved to it, the real beginning of the Gongyi Medical School. In 1911, Gongyi's new modern hospital with sixty beds was opened to the public, and the deanship was taken over by Dr. Louis Hugh, a Chinese graduate of the University of Oregon.[29]

Since the medical teaching and work had gone beyond Gongyi's own accommodation, the Canton government got in touch with Gongyi and willingly awarded a well located place outside the East Gate of Canton in December 1912. By the year 1913, the Gongyi Medical School had 184 students and twenty-six faculty members, including four Americans—Drs. Todd, W. W. Cadbury, J. A. Hofmann, and E. C. Machle. In 1914, the Board of Trustees of the School was founded, of which Pan Peiru was the first president. More improvements were made during 1914–1915 when land next to the School beyond the city was purchased, making the School up to ninety Chinese acres or nearly fifteen English acres. The School soon obtained authorized recognition from the Board of Education of Canton and thereafter raised the criterion for admission.[30]

In 1916, Dr. J. A. Hofmann was fully appointed the dean of the School and Dr. John Kirk began to teach on a part-time basis. There were five American physicians associated with this hospital and medical school and a staff of seventeen Chinese, most of whom were physicians. The Gongyi Hospital provided for a large proportion of patients: in-patients, 1,443 men and 88 women; outpatients, 8,425 men and 2,030 women.[31] Thus, it was a good time to upgrade the standard of the men's college. In the fall of 1917, a pre-medical year was added to the curriculum, increasing the set of courses to five years. Two Chinese graduates from America, one from Tufts Medial College, Boston and the other from University of Tennessee Medical School, joined the faculty of the School. Dr. C. A. Hayes gladly assumed responsibility for the instruction of diseases of the eye, ear, nose, and throat. Drs. J. M. Wright, H. W. Boyd, and J. O. Thompson offered unpaid part-time teaching. Preparations were made for clinical training at the Canton Hospital and John Kerr's Refuge for the Insane.[32]

In 1918, after twenty-six months of construction, students moved into the new buildings erected at a cost of approximately $180,000 on the location near the East Gate. The college had a college building, an anatomy building, a hospital building housing seven general wards and forty-six private patients, and an out-patient building. All together, the authorization for dissection, long hoped for, was accorded, and scholarships adding up to $2,000 were granted by the provincial government of Guangdong.[33]

In the spring of 1921, the Board approved Dr. Li Shufen, then a foremost doctor in Hong Kong, to travel to America to seek funds from the Chinese Americans. After a most successful campaign and a term of study in Europe,

Dr. Li retuned in the summer of 1922 with a sum well in excess of $100,000. It was thus possible not only to free the Gongyi Society from all financial burdens but to make new plans. In 1921, fifty-one students of the government medical school were transferred to Gongyi to finish their learning, and their fees were paid by the provincial bank accounts.[34] The School thus changed its policy significantly with such modifications:

- it was resolved to invite the best teachers available, irrespective of nationality;
- the faculty executive was re-instated;
- the curriculum was extended to six years, comprising a pre-medical course, four years of medical study, and one year of internship at recognized hospitals.[35]

The enlargement of the school demanded extra accommodation for students. A new dormitory with accommodation for 100 students was constructed, which opened at the end of 1921. A small dormitory for nurses was opened. Dr. R. M. Ross assumed responsibility for training in psychiatry on behalf of Dr. Selden, on home leave at that time. The hospital, under Dr. Todd, continued to be in the black, submitting part of its gains to the school.[36]

Sun Yat-sen was in support of the Gongyi Medical College. During the military campaigns against the warlords, Gongyi was called up to care for a daily average of over 300 wounded and sick soldiers of Sun Yat-sen's revolutionary armies, significantly helping Sun's revolutionary course. After defeating the warlords and establishing his new revolutionary government in Canton in early 1923, Sun instructed Sun Ke, the mayor of the Canton, to appropriate a piece land of forty *mu* in eastern Canton to the Gongyi Medical School on July 12.[37]

The Gongyi Medical University, 1923–35

For some years, the Gongyi Society had made great efforts to have the college work recognized by the Ministry of Education of the Republic of China as meeting the criteria for a medical college. To realize this goal, a committee led by Dr. Li Shufen was selected. The Committee successfully improved the medical education of the School to meet the national standard. Thus the Goying School was temporarily registered by the Beijing government as having university status and was granted the name of Gongyi Medical University. The Gongyi Society then passed a resolution to change its name formally in September 1923, and the faculty executive would be replaced with the faculty senate.[38]

When the school opened on September 15, 1923, the majority of old students were admitted into the new curriculum, but they were required to fill in any gaps between the new and the old. Dr. Li Shufen, unselfishly giving up his lucrative practice in Hong Kong, assumed the deanship of the University.

Dr. Lu Jinghui, whose full-time services had been secured, was appointed proctor to replace Dr. Li Duo, who had resigned as the dean and proctor.[39]

A full-time professor of anatomy was appointed in 1924 to make possible the anatomical work expected by the new curriculum, which was significantly practical. The anatomy building was appropriately renovated, and an agreement was reached, with the support of Procurator-General Lu Xingyun, to get hold of all available dead bodies from the prison.

The new medical university had thirty-six faculty members, nineteen of whom were full-time professors. With the assistance of the Reformed Presbyterian Mission, Dr. James M. Wright was employed as professor of pathology and bacteriology in the 1925–26 academic year. The school had 189 students in attendance, including twenty-nine women, and the total number of graduates reached 252.[40]

Condition in Canton, however, was progressively becoming more troubled when anti-Christian propaganda was greater than ever, which had an impact on Gongyi. After the Nationalist-Communist alliance in Canton was established in 1924, the year 1925 witnessed the rise of nationalism in Canton. The Nationalist-Communist coalition was mobilizing the masses behind for abolition of the "unequal treaties." Recognizing the missionary school as symbols of Western imperialism, the Nationalists encouraged the Cantonese to call for "educational right recovery," and attempted to impose "secularism" on all religious institutions in Canton. Both the Communist and Nationalist leaders in Canton employed anti-imperialism and anti-religion as their slogans; and the missionary hospitals were seen as physical representations of the slogans because they were exciting and compatible to the strategies of mass mobilization. Early in 1925, Chinese debates about education sovereignty were opened. Most of Gongyi students took part in this anti-imperialism campaign to bring about increase government participation in the school's affairs. They strongly condemned President Li Shufen of attempting to let American financiers and bankers control this medical college by securing Rockefeller Foundation's donations during the financial crisis in Gongyi. They denounced cultural imperialism at Gongyi because American medical missionaries were teaching at and administering the college. Nationalism brought about consensus among the great majority of Gongyi students that the government should control and operate the school. They appealed to the government to take over Gongyi.As a result, the Guangdong government, supported by the great majority of the Gongyi students, controlled the Gongyi institution and made it a part of the National University of Guangdong in 1926.[41] The president of the National University of Guangdong explained the causes of the affiliation of Gongyi with his university:

> The remote causes: (a) the handicap and the insolvency incurred
> by contracting debts of more than $100,000, thus bringing it to a

standstill; (b) the indifferent attitude of the remaining members of the Kung Yee Society after death had carried away its majority, rendering no more zealous service to the work.

The immediate cause: (1) the appealing for a fund to the Rockefeller Foundation allowing the latter to nominate foreigners to shape theeducation policy of the work; (b) the petition of the whole body of the students to the Central Executive Committee of the Kuomintong, the Head Quarter of the Generalissimo, and the National University of Kwongtung.[42]

It was clear that in 1926, under the influence of the Nationalists and Communists, the major interest of the students at Gongyi to dominate the Chinese medical college was nationalism against the American financial institution—the Rockefeller Foundation. The Gongyi students played an imperative part in the affiliation of Gongyi with the government.[43]

Gongyi was reopened in 1927 as the Medical Department of the National Guangdong University, called the Sun Yat-sen University Medical School after 1927. The school had a five-year curriculum, two years of which were dedicated to pre-clinical instruction. Provision was made for post-graduate work as interns or assistants.[44] By 1935, the Gongyi medical institution, including Gongyi Medical School (1909–1923), Gongyi Medical University (1923–1925), Department of Medicine of National Guangdong University (1925–1926), and the Medical College of Sun Yat-sen University (1927–1935), had graduated a total of 523 students. After their graduation, most Gongyi students practiced medicine in Guangdong as well as in other provinces in China. They contributed to medical modernization in China.[45]

Ironically, Western medicine was one of the forces that aroused the Cantonese elite to learn from the Westerners to carry out social reform in China in the late nineteenth and early twentieth centuries, but Western medicine was becoming one of the forces that prompted the Cantonese medical elite to challenge American medical missionaries at the medical college in Canton and took Gongyi out of missionary hands entirely. Many reasons explained the rising of strong nationalism at Gongyi, such as the Communist propaganda, the Nationalist mass-mobilization strategy, and others, but Western medicine was one of them because the Cantonese medical elite had realized the significant role Western medicine played in China's modernization and did not want foreigners to monopolize medical education in China. Dr. J. Allen Hofmann of the Canton Hospital commented on the 1925 anti-imperialism campaign in Canton: "The rising of the people is a good omen, even though we may not approve of their methods. After all they are doing what Western nations have taught them."[46]

The Guanghua Medical College, 1908–1935

The Guanghua Medical College was founded by the Cantonese nationalists. In 1907, a Chinese sailor was beaten to death for no reason by an Indian policeman on a ship sailing between Hong Kong and Canton. After an autopsy on the corpse, the Chinese physicians claimed the Chinese sailor's death had resulted from violence, but the foreign physicians argued that his heart disease contributed to his death and denounced the Chinese doctors' poor knowledge of Western medicine. Since foreigners enjoyed immunity in China, coupled with the corruption and incompetence of the Qing government, the Indian policeman was not brought to justice. This case promoted strong national sentiments in Canton and angered many Cantonese doctors, especially Liang Peiji, who was Dr. Kerr's student and graduated from the South China Medical College of the Canton Hospital.[47]

The Cantonese medical elite believed that the Chinese had to make their own great efforts to promote modern medicine and to make good progress in medical science in China. Thereafter, Liang and several Cantonese businessmen and medical professionals decided to organize the Guanghua (Revive China or Glorify the Chinese Nation) Medical Association to set up a medical school and a hospital in order to win medical sovereignty and the right to medical education in Canton. Liang then was elected the first president of the Association. The objectives of the Guanghua Medical Association were as follows:

> to study the most modern medical science in the world and to introduce into China new medicines invented by foreigners while contributing Chinese medical achievements to the world; to unite Chinese medical professionals so as to promote China's medical standing in the world while restoring Chinese medical rights in China and reforming China's medical science; and to promote medical and sanitary knowledge among the Chinese.[48]

This statement indicates that the Cantonese elite not only encouraged the Chinese to study Western medicine, but also tried to reform Chinese medicine with the help of Western medicine.

After the founding of the Guanghua Association, Guanghua Medical School and Guanghua Hospital were founded in March 1908, the first Western medical school in China where the Chinese doctors taught medicine in Chinese language and the first Western medical hospital in China administered by the Chinese. The objective of this new medical school was to promote modern medicine, train medical doctors, take care of the sick, provide medical care to the poor, and to end foreign domination of medical institutions in China.[49]

Dr. Zheng Hao was appointed the first president of the College. Born in Zhongshan County in Guangdong Province, Zheng graduated from a medical school in California in 1904, the first Chinese who had a Western medical license. After his graduation, he returned home, serving as general instructor of the Guangdong Army Medical School. Dr. Chen Yanfen, after resigning from the position of the superintendent of a hospital in Hong Kong, was appointed in 1908 as the first superintendent of the Guanghua Hospital and the dean of the Guanghua Medical School. On March 1, the Guanghua Medical School began to offer courses to students. Each medical professional donated 500 yuan in order to collect sufficient funds to buy a big building in Canton as a medical school and a hospital. In 1909, the school opened with sixty new students in a four-year curriculum and had access to the Canton Hospital for clinical training.[50]

The Guanghua institutions made significant progress in the following years. The minister of education of the Nationalist Government in Nanjing officially recognized in 1929 the private Guanghua Medical College with a six-year term and its nursing school, which had thirty-three professors and 292 students. The standard of the Guanghua Medical School was superior to that of the private medical schools in Shanghai, but the hospital facilities were quite deficient and only one big room was used for all laboratory instruction. Dr. Zheng was the president of the Guanghua Medical College for twenty-two years without being paid until he died in 1931. After Dr. Zheng's death, Dr. Chen Yanfen was appointed the president of the medical college.[51] By 1935, the Guanghua Medical Association had recruited 1,990 members, whilst it had had only 400 members in 1929.

The Guanghua Medical College was nationalistic. During the Sino-Japanese conflict in Shanghai in January 1932, the Guanghua Hospital students, angered by the Japanese invasion of China, organized a medical team led by Professor Cen Entao to Shanghai to take care of the wounded Chinese soldiers for three months. Their courageous and heroic activities and dedicated service saved many lives and won the praise of the Chinese, and they received a great award—an ambulance granted by the International Medical Association.[52]

The Guanghua Medical College had 155 students and seven full-time and eleven part-time professors in 1935.[53] By that time, Guanghua had trained roughly 454 doctors and 80 nurses and treated nearly 500,000 patients.[54] Guanghua, a major private medical college in Canton, not only provided medical service to the Cantonese but also contributed significantly to medical modernization in Canton.

The Guanghua Medical School was a product of Chinese nationalism. The Cantonese medical elite of Western medicine, recognizing the importance of modern medical education in China's nation-building, considered that the Chinese had to own their medical education, rather than allow it to be dominated by foreigners. They thus established China's first Chinese-style medical school run by the Chinese, where the Chinese taught in Cantonese dialect. Many reasons motivated the Cantonese medical elite to do this, but Western medicine was one of the sources.

Western Medical Texts and Schools and Western Medicine Doctors in China

Western Medical Texts

Western medical texts were first translated into Chinese in Canton. After running a dispensary for a short time at Hong Kong, Dr. T. T. Devan, a medical missionary of the American Baptist Mission, settled in Canton with a dispensary in 1845. He was compelled by ill-health to retire to the United States in 1847. His activity was very noteworthy because he published a book in 1847, *Beginner's First Book in the Chinese Language*, in Canton vernacular in Hong Kong, which contained anatomical terms as well as a list of diseases and medical terms in both Chinese and English. This book, a first attempt to create a Chinese medical classification, was published in a modified and enlarged version in 1858 and appeared in a third edition supervised by William Lobscheid in 1861.[55]

After modern medical education started in Canton, the need for medical textbooks was urgent. As a result, besides teaching, Dr. Kerr translated more than thirty-four medical textbooks between 1871 and 1899, providing sufficient texts for medical students. In addition to translation, Dr. Kerr published many articles on medicine in journals and pamphlets. In 1873, for example, he published a small brochure: *The Method for Restoration of the Drowning* and *A Manual of Skin Diseases*.[56] These books, while differing greatly in the quality of the work, were exceedingly practical, and they were the only books available in many branches of medical science at that time in China.

As medical educational work at Canton was vigorously making good progress, more medical books were required to add to Kerr's series of medical textbooks in Chinese. Kerr's books were not the only medical works appearing visible in China during that time; some Chinese doctors of modern medicine were translating Western medical books into Chinese. Yin Duanmo was the first Chinese doctor to translate Western medical books. Born in Guangdong, Yin graduated from Beiyang Medical College in the city of Tianjin and later worked at Dr. Kerr's Canton Hospital. When Sun Yat-sen was a student at the Canton Hospital, Yin was Dr. Kerr's assistant. Under the influence of Dr. Kerr, Yin published in 1884 *Yi xue bao* (Medical Journal), the first Western medical journal edited by a Chinese doctor in China.[57] Dr. Yin himself, in addition to helping Dr. Kerr translate medical texts into Chinese, translated medical books into Chinese independently, such as *Bingli cuoyao* (Summary of Pathology) in 1892, *Erke Cuoyao* (Summary of Pediatric) in 1892, *Yili lueshu* (Outline of Medical Theory), and *Taichan juyao* (Summary of Pediatrics) in

1893. Dr. Yin continued working for many years under the auspices of the Canton Medical Missionary Society, taking part in the preparation of Kerr's medical vocabulary with Dr. H. T. Whitney and compiling one of his own in 1898.[58]

As a result, more Western medical books were translated into Chinese. Dr. Elliott I. Osgood's *Anatomy*, for example, was translated into Chinese in 1881, a book on internal medicine, and *Exhortations to Abandon Opium Smoking* (containing a chapter on the medical aspects of the opium cure and several prescriptions) was translated by both Rev. D. Hill and Dr. C. C. Daly in the city of Hangzhou in 1884.[59] In 1892, Dr. Wen Tianmou translated Mitchell Bruce's *General Therapeutics*.[60] Thus, a considerable amount of medical literature in Chinese was available to medical students in Canton as well as in other cities. Dr. Kerr played a significant role in translating modern medical books into Chinese, which helped remove one of the obstacles to modern medical education in China by breaking the language barrier.

Western Medical Schools

Western medical education in Canton led to the beginning of modern medical education in China. Before 1866, medical education in China was on the apprentice—practitioner level, which was effective for practical clinical skills but lacking in theory and laboratory work in such subjects as chemistry and anatomy. After the South China Medical School, the first modern medical school in China, was founded in Canton in 1866, more and more missionary medical schools were created in the following decades. By 1935 eighteen had been founded. On the whole, the medical missionaries were disappointed with the criteria of their schools when comparing them to the medical schools in Europe and America. With their own inadequate resources, they made every effort to elevate the level of ability of their students.

The development of the missionary medical schools helped produce men and women competent to become lecturers at private and public medical colleges. Accordingly, more modern medical schools were opened in China. A medical school was established in the north China seaport of Tianjin in 1881 by a Scottish physician, John Kenneth MacKenzie, the Hong Kong College of Medicine for Chinese in October 1881, the Union Medical College in Beijing in 1906, a medical school of twenty medical students in Changsha in 1908, the South Manchuria Medical College in 1911, the Mukden Medical College in March 1912, and the Nantong Medical School by progressive entrepreneur Zhang Yin in the city of Nantong in late 1912. In 1934, the total enrolment of twenty-eight medical schools in China was 3,616, of whom 2,978 were men and 638 were women. The number of graduates from the year 1934 was 532, of whom 453 were men and 79 were women. The geographical dissemination of the medical colleges and schools was not even: they were located in thirteen of the eighteen provinces, seven of them in Shanghai.[61]

New official regulations on medical colleges were published shortly after the Canton government broke new ground, publishing regulations on medical education. The Beijing government created new rules that were of immense importance for the medical life of the Chinese. The first of these regulations was the establishment of a standard for the set of courses of medical schools in China in 1912, and the regulations for medical and pharmaceutical tests were issued in 1916. Notwithstanding official endeavors to put standards into effect, the training of doctors differed very much from school to school. A number of colleges had to depend on charts and models for the instruction of anatomy; specifications were not published for corpse dissection. Only the Union Medical College in Beijing and National Sun Yat-sen University in Canton had enough autopsies. By the mid-1930s, such national medical schools as the National Shanghai Medical College and the National Sun Yat-sen Medical College had gone beyond some mission medical schools in terms of human resources, apparatus, and facilities, but the medical missionary schools continued to uphold quite rigorous entrance policies and still educated their share of doctors for Chinese patients.[62]

Western Medicine Doctors in China

At the end of the nineteenth century, most Chinese still consulted Chinese medicine, but many of them had accepted Western medicine, as Dr. E. P. Thwing of the Canton Hospital commented in 1890, "The conservatism of the Chinese was a great barrier to advancement in the knowledge and practice of medicine, but it was being overcome slowly but surely."[63] In a survey of a sample of 5,390 physicians in 1935, 4,638 (87 percent) were Chinese. Of this Chinese group, 3,843 (83 percent) were graduates of medical schools in China.[64] Even if the number of physicians who graduated from the Chinese medical schools was still insignificant with reference to the population of 400 million, it was an imperative start. In terms of the number of physicians trained in modern medicine, only 918 were registered with the government in 1929, but 9,098 were registered in 1937, a tenfold increase.[65]

The statistics were not so cheering because geographical distribution of these physicians was uneven. The results of the 1935 report verified those of a parallel survey conducted in 1932 and 1933, both of which demonstrated the uppermost intensity of modern doctors: Jiangsu province had the record in the number of physicians, then Guangdong, Hebei, Zhejiang, Shangdong, and others.[66] The two coastal provinces of Jiangsu and Guangdong comprised about half of the modern trained physicians. Physicians gathered together in such large cities as Shanghai, Canton, Nanjing, and Beijing. Shanghai had 1,182, or 22 percent of the 5,390 physicians in China in 1935; Canton had 5.6 percent; and Nanjing 5.1 percent, extraordinarily insufficient medical service for the tremendously large number of the populations, especially the peasants in the countryside.[67] One of the reasons for this unequal allocation of modern-trained physicians was that those provinces had the intensity of the large metropolitan, political, industrial, and commercial centers where medical schools and hospitals were situated. The noticeable intensity of doctors in Jiangsu province was for the most part by reason of the two large cities, Shanghai and Nanjing.[68]

Canton had only seventy male modern-trained physicians and twenty-eight female in 1919.[69] In 1922, there were about 1,300 registered Chinese medicine doctors and 228 registered Western medicine doctors, which included nine Americans and one British.[70] In 1934, there were 208 Western medicine doctors and 598 Chinese medicine doctors in Canton, according to the Canton government's statistics.[71] Dr. Oldt also stated that the number of doctors in Canton reached 984 and that there was one physician to every 905 people in the metropolitan city of Canton.[72] It seems that although Western medicine gained its strength in Canton, most Chinese patients still consulted Chinese medicine doctors for treatments, and Western medicine had not dominate Cantonese society in the 1930s.

In brief, the establishment of the South China Medical School resulted in the creation of several medical schools in Canton, making Canton one of the modern medical education centers in China. The graduates of the medical schools in Canton resulted in the spread of Western medicine in China when they practiced medicine in Canton and in other places. Western medicine was gradually but incontestably moving forward in China generally, and in Canton particularly, between 1835 and 1935. American medical missions in Canton played a part in China's medical transformation.

The Campaign for the Sino-Western Medical Convergence

The Cantonese physicians were the first to call for Sino-Western medical intercourse. Due to the spread of modern Western medicine in Canton, the contact between Western and Chinese medicines increased. Some Cantonese physicians of Chinese medicine tried to compare and contrast the methods of Western and Chinese medicines in order to deal correctly with both medical systems in the mid-nineteenth century. The challenge posed by the arrival of Western medicine in China urged some Chinese physicians to reject the shortcoming of traditional Chinese medicine and to assimilate the beneficial aspects of Western medicine without abandoning their national heritage. This tide of thought was known as *Zhongxi huitong pai*, or school of Sino-Western convergence. American doctors in Canton and the Cantonese medical elite of Chinese medicine took the lead in this new trend.

Dr. Kerr encouraged medical missionaries to study Chinese medicine. He published an article in 1887, titled "Chinese Materia Medica," believing that Chinese patients were familiar with Chinese medicine and often took Chinese medicine first and then consulted Western medicine only after Chinese medicine failed and that with the help of Chinese medicine, Western doctors would cure some cases of illnesses more efficiently. To Dr. Kerr, if Western medicine practitioners knew about the function of Chinese medicine and its chemical elements and physiological reaction, they would provide better treatments to their patients.[73] Thus, at the Canton Hospital's medical school, courses of Chinese medicine were offered, where Chinese medicine physicians were welcomed to teach Chinese remedy. Chinese physicians were admitted to study Western medical arts at the Canton Hospital.[74]

Since Canton was the first city in China to be acquainted with Western medicine, the Cantonese traditional physicians became the pioneers doing research on the integration of Chinese and Western medicines in the first half of the nineteenth century. Chen Dingtai was one of the pioneers of this comparative study. Born in the town of Xinhui, one hundred miles from west of Canton, Chen studied Chinese medicine when he was young. In 1829, when he was visiting Canton, his friend, a Western physician, took Chen to a missionary clinic. As a result, Chen became interested in Western medicine, especially modern anatomy. Later, he visited missionary hospitals in Canton several times, including Dr. Parker's Canton Hospital. According to his account, he watched the whole surgical process at the hospital, such surgeries as craniotomy, cataract, enema, and other eye procedures. After many years communicating with Western physicians and studying anatomy, Chen wrote a book, *Yitan chuanzhen* (Truth of Medicine) in 1844 to challenge Wang Qingren's medical theory.[75]

The nineteenth-century anatomist Wang Qingren (1768–1831) was a famous physician of Chinese medicine. His influential treatise on anatomy emphasized the importance of the eyewitness observation of internal organs in order to describe their location accurately. After observing and studying several corpses, Wang published his book in 1830, *Yilin gaicuo* (Correction of Medical Theory), correcting a lot of wrong interpretations of Chinese medical theories and pointing out a new interpretation of anatomy.[76] Without a shred of doubt, Wang's book greatly influenced Chinese traditional doctors, without being challenged for many years until Chen. Chen cited sixteen Western anatomical drawings in his book, although he did not know how to read books in English. While studying the essence of the viscera in Wang's book, Chen compared the visceral map in Wang's book with the Western anatomical drawings. Chen's book disagreed with traditional visceral theory, questioned the collateral theory in terms of anatomy, and documented a case of glaucoma decompression. Chen was the first Chinese to study very carefully Western anatomical atlases and to cite them in a Chinese medical book, although he did not study and have a good understanding of Western medicine. Despite his limited knowledge of modern anatomy, he realized the errors in the Chinese theory on viscera and criticized Chinese medicine while using Chinese medicine in treatments of patients. Chen was one of the pioneers of the school of the Sino-Western medical intercourse.

Chen's son Chen Xiangjing continued his father's work and published a book, although he did not contribute significantly to his father's scholarship. By the end of the nineteenth century, Dr. Kerr's hospital as well as other missionary hospitals became well known in Canton. Under the influence of Western medicine, Chen's grandson Chen Zhen'ge developed his father's theory more thoroughly. After comparing Wang Qingren's anatomical drawings with Western's, Chen Zhen'ge identified a lot of differences between two ones. He thought that the differences probably came from different physical characteristics between the Chinese and Europeans. Thus, in 1882, he went to Singapore to study Western medicine at the British Royal Medical College and participated in the surgical operations, believing that internal organs of both Chinese and European people, such as hearts, livers, spleens, lungs, kidneys, stomachs, galls, intestines, and bladders were the same. After spending three years studying and practicing, he mastered the theory of modern Western medicine, publishing *Yigang zongshu* (On General Medicine) in 1890. This book, condemning Chinese medicine for lacking a study of physical anatomy, supported Chen Dingtai's theory. It discussed both Chinese and Western internal medicine, and combined together Western and Chinese medical treatments by using Chinese medicine. This book used Western medical terminology and pathology to discuss internal diseases, the first Chinese medicine book adopting Western medical terminology. Chen Zhen'ge's book testified to his concern that tradition Chinese medicine had to be reformed, significantly contributing to the school of Sino-Western convergence and intercourse in the nineteenth century. Under the influence of the missionary doctors in Canton, in just fifty years three generations of the Chen family had developed their medical theory which reached a higher level and took the lead in the new trend in the integration of Chinese and Western medicine during that time.[77]

Western medicine also had an impact on the Imperial Examination System in Canton. The Imperial Examination in China lasted for 1,300 years from its founding in the seventh century to its abolition near the end of the Qing Dynasty in 1905, a system to determine who among the population would be permitted to enter the state's bureaucracy. Examination takers were tested on their proficiency in arts (such as music, arithmetic, writing, and knowledge of the rituals and ceremonies in both public and private life) and five studies (military strategy, civil law, revenue and taxation, agriculture and geography, and the Confucian classics).[78] Since more Cantonese scholars and traditional physicians became interested in Western medicine, in 1887 the subject of medicine was introduced into the official metropolitan examinations in Canton. The metropolitan examinations were administered in the provincial capitals every three years. For the first time in Chinese history examination takers were tested on their proficiency in medicine. Two traditional physicians, Kong Peiran and Zhu Peiwen, passed the medical test and earned the

Jìnshì degree (presented scholar). Both of them became very interested in studying Western medicine. Kong later became a student at the South China Medical School of the Canton Hospital. After graduation, he continued his studies at the Liangguang Medical School. In 1912, he assumed the position of the physician-in-chief of the Guangdong Military Academy in Canton. Kong used Chinese medicine to treat his patients, but he adopted some Western medical medications and technologies to take care of his patients. He became one of the pioneers of the early Sino-Western medical integration.[79]

Zhu Peiwen was also a pioneer of the school of the Sino-Western convergence and intercourse. Born to a traditional doctor's family between 1851 and 1861 in a town of Foshan, ten miles west of Canton, Zhu was fond of reading both Chinese and Western medical books when he was young. Canton gave Zhu an opportunity to learn modern medicine. After he earned his *Jinshi* degree, he became more interested in Western medicine and even went to the missionary hospitals to observe anatomy and surgery. He could read the medical books in English and was regarded as the one Chinese physician to understand Western medicine better than other physicians of Chinese medicine at that time. He became distinguished in the circle of Chinese traditional medicine. After comparing Western medicine with Chinese medicine, he published a book, *Huayan zangxiang yuezuan* (The Drawings of Viscera of the Chinese and Europeans), in three volumes in 1893. In his book, Zhu believed that Chinese medicine attached importance to discovery of symptoms while Western medicine distinguished between illnesses. As indicated by Zhu, the aim of discovering symptoms was to localize the source of the illness and treat the illness with the appropriate drugs. He stressed studying Western medical anatomy in order to compensate for the lack of a study of human anatomy by the Chinese physicians, promoting modernization of Chinese medicine so as to raise the level of traditional medicine.[80]

Zhu, valuing tradition without ever being in its thrall, totally opposed abandonment of Chinese medical theory, and advocated the study of Western medicine to identify the different methods and theories of both Chinese and Western medicines. He called for convergence and intercourse because both approaches had its shortcomings to abandon and had its advantages to conserve. Zhu, a passionate supporter of Sino-Western medical exchange, justified such a system by referring to the necessity of calculating the advantages of the ancient and new, and of weighing up the pros and cons of what was the Chinese and foreign. He believed that the ideal solution was to combine the strong points of each, bringing together two different medicines to form one system, the reconciliation of Chinese and Western medicine.[81]

Thanks to the Canton Hospital to some degree, the Cantonese physicians of Chinese medicine played a significant role in developing the early Sino-Western medical convergence school. More importantly, American doctors in Canton realized that Western medicine had absolute advantages in medical fields like surgery, diagnosis of organic diseases, and others, but Chinese medicine took the lead in the treatment of some illnesses. Thus they tried to adopt some Chinese medical methods in the treatments of patients so as to make Western medicine more efficient.

The Combination of Chinese and Western Medications in Pharmaceutical Industry

Most Cantonese patients were still in favor of taking traditional Chinese medication at the beginning of the twentieth century, although Western medicine began to gain its strength in Canton. Many Cantonese still took Chinese therapies and used Chinese medicine in traditional preparations, such as pastes, pellets, creams, and others, and had little confidence in Western medications. The Cantonese, however, took the lead in taking the advantages of both Chinese and Western medications by combining both medications together to produce a new form of tablets.

Liang Peiji (1875-1947) was the founding father of the combination of traditional Chinese and Western medications in China. Liang, alumnus of the South Chain Medical School, practiced medicine after his graduation, but his patients were small in number at the beginning, only a few visiting his dispensary. He then successfully cured the illness of a rich family's son, and his reputation increased in Canton. At that point, Liang was trying to produce a new and efficient medication to overcome the malaria epidemic that had prevailed in south China for many years. Caused by a parasite that was transmitted by the bite of infected mosquitoes, this infectious disease was characterized by recurring chills and fever. Liang thus used Western okinawa quinine as the main material, together with Chinese licorice powder, to manufacture pellets. Named "Liang Peiji Chill Pill," these pellets, a combination of the Chinese and Western medications, were successful in curing malaria diseases and in relieving patients' suffering. By reason of their very effective medical results, these pills became popular and well-known in south China and gradually more and more Chinese were willing to take such kinds of medications. Since then, many Chinese have been taking this kind of medications until today.[82]

Liang Peiji was the first Chinese to open a national pharmaceutical plant in China. English John Strickland erected a pharmaceutical plant in Shanghai in 1900, but the Chinese did not open anyone until 1902 when Liang opened a small pharmaceutical factory in Canton, manufacturing chill pills, cough pills, toothache waters, anti-smoking waters, and others. His business expanded very fast, and his drugstores soon appeared in Hong Kong, Malaysia, South Pacific islands, and even the China towns in the United States in the 1920s. After the opening of Liang Peiji factory, other cities in China gradually began to open more pharmaceutical companies. In 1912, the China Pharmaceutical

Company was opened in Shanghai; by 1936 Shanghai already had fifty-eight pharmaceutical factories, 1,500 employees, and nearly three million yuan of capital, although most of the Chinese pharmaceutical companies were generally small, poorly equipped and funded at that time. Canton had about thirty pharmaceutical companies and produced more than one hundred different types of drugs, combining Western medications with Chinese ones, becoming the birthplace of China's national pharmaceutical industry.[83]

Tang Shiyi (1874-1939) was another pioneer of the modern pharmaceutical industry in China. Born in July 1874 at a town in Sanshui County, thirty miles west of Canton, Tang was raised by his grandmother because his parents died when he was a child. A clever student, Tang had excellent academic achievements when studying Western medicine at the Canton Hospital. After graduating from the school, he opened a medical dispensary in Canton in 1912, and his excellent treatments of patients with coughs helped make him renowned in Canton. As a result, like Liang, Tang began manufacturing cough tablets and asthma pills at home. To keep secret the prescription of his drugs, he refused to hire any helpers. To promote the sale of his new drugs which combined both Chinese and Western medications, Tang spend a lot of money on advertising his pills in the newspapers and named them as Tang Shiyi pills. When going out to see patients, he sat in his sedan, which was painted with big Chinese characters, "Great Doctor Tang Shiyi." Since his pills and tablets were excellent in the treatment of patients, they became famous in Canton, and the demand increased greatly. Consequently, Tang expanded both his dispensary and drug factory and hired helpers to work at his pharmaceutical plant. Tang assumed the position of general manager of his business and hired his elder son as assistant manager, both taking charge of the plant named as Tang Shiyi Father-Son Factory.[84]

To promote the sale of his medications in China, Tang opened another medical dispensary in Shanghai in 1919. As he did in Canton, he spent a lot of money on advertising his pills and tablets in the newspapers. As a result, more and more patients came to see him and took more and more his drugs. Accordingly, he established another bigger pharmaceutical company in Shanghai in 1924. In the following years, sales of his drugs extended to such cities as Tianjin, Hankou, Hong Kong, and others. Shanghai became the headquarters of his enterprise.[85]

Since a key to the expansion of the pharmaceutical industry was to renovate the equipment of the pharmaceutical plant, in 1931 Dr. Tang took the lead installing machines in his plants in both Shanghai and Canton. In addition, he was successful in developing new drugs, "chill pill" and "malnutrition remedy." To reduce the cost of his products, Tang began experiments at his factory to extract hydrochloride from traditional Chinese medical materials. During that time some of the main raw materials, such as ephedrine hydrochloride, were used to make his drugs, which were very expensive because they were imported from other countries. When the malaria epidemic prevailed in south China, Tang's drugs were efficient in treatments of this disease. Consequently, Tang's chill pills, cough pills, asthma pills, and others were becoming progressively popular all over China as well as in Southeast Asia because his drugs were cheaper and easier to carry than other drugs. More importantly, his drugs were contained in boxes that had instructions in Chinese. Tang became a famous doctor and a rich man in China in the 1930s. In 1931, he built another new factory to increase medicine production due to the increasing demand for his products. Later, he opened new factories in Hong Kong, Tianjin, and Shanghai, and his business extended all over China. His most popular products, Xiaochuan wan (asthma pill) and Keshu wan (cough pill), remained popular after he died in Shanghai in 1939, and is still very well-liked in China today. He was one of the pioneers of the Chinese national pharmaceutical industry.[86]

Canton established not only China's first national pharmaceutical industry but also China's first pharmacy store run by the Chinese, owing to the increasing demand of the Canton Hospital as well as other Western hospitals in Canton. In 1870, British merchants opened the first Western pharmacy store in Canton. As the demand for Western pharmacy increased, six medical doctors of the Canton Hospital contributed 600 yuan and appointed a Cantonese American merchant Luo Kaitai to open in 1881 the Tai'an Drugstore close to the Canton Hospital. This was first Western pharmacy store run by the Chinese, ending foreigners' monopoly on Western pharmacy markets in China. Several branches of the Tai'an Drugstore were opened in the city afterward.[87] Several years later, a Chinese, Gu Songquan, opened Zhongxi dayaofang (Sino-West Drugstore) in Shanghai in 1888, the first Western pharmacy store run by the Chinese in Shanghai. In 1894, there were eight or more modern pharmacy stores in Canton, such as Guang'an xiyaofang founded in 1890, selling Western pharmacies.[88] By 1936, Canton had eighty-four modern pharmacy stores owned by the Chinese, such as Bidesheng yaofang opened in 1906. Shanghai had ninety-seven in 1936 and Beijing had 130 in 1936. As a result, the control of Western pharmacy markets in China shifted from foreign merchants to the Chinese. National pharmaceutical industry and stores started in Canton and spread to other major cities in China during the Republic era, and Dr. Kerr's students played a significant role in this movement.

In brief, the combination of Chinese and Western medications facilitated localization of Western medication and effectively fulfilled the cultural and social needs of the Chinese people. In this process, Western medicine was becoming culturally reinterpreted as it moved from one cultural venue to another in a global medical modernization.

The Canton Hospital's Students and Reform in China

American Doctors' Comments on Reform

While in China, American medical missionaries were practicing medicine in an attempt to promote the spread of Christianity. They also hoped that through a gradual evolutionary process of education, industrial development, construction of communications, and regeneration, China would ultimately become a modern nation with the help of foreigners. Dr. Parker believed that medical missionaries would be agents in a reformation movement in China, a process of the transformation under the influence of Christianity. After arriving in China, Parker wrote in his journals:

> This time is coming when her people will be delivered from their burdens of perpetual disease, and when they will no longer be debarred the privileges of education and the pleasures of intellectual life, and when, under the rule of Jesus, China will be wonderfully different from China of today.[89]

In 1841, Parker's conversations with various organizations in the United States portrayed the backwardness of Chinese society and emphasized the need to open the country to the effects of Christian civilization. Speaking at the First Presbyterian Church in Philadelphia, Parker examined the condemnation of the established social and political structure in China, asserting that the "Tartar race" currently in control of the country "despise and insult the aboriginal Chinese," and "their attachment to old customs is strong and inveterate, which leads them to defend ancient practices, however absurd."[90] Parker wanted to convince American listeners that the great majority of the Chinese people were living in a situation of political subjugation by the Manchu conquerors who at the time occupied the government.

Dr. John Kerr also believed that medical physicians should play a role in social and political reforms in China. He claimed in 1878 that the physician's science explained why, in all "civilized and enlightened nations," his profession had "attained to a position of honor" and unrivaled "power" wherever sound knowledge had been diffused. Medicine, John Kerr told his listeners, gave its physicians and its patients "a perception of the natural causes which are in operation around and within them, and which are controlled by the Supreme Being." With that insight, Americans and Chinese both could be expected to abandon all "injurious and foolish customs."[91]

When Dr. Kerr regarded physicians as prominent persons in their societies as a result of the integrity of their conception of natural laws, he was appealing to a vision that assumed a social order previously formed in line with the tenets of the natural order. This assumption could not be easily conveyed to the Chinese world where, as he sternly pronounced, the missionary physician found himself "living among a people of a strange language, uncongenial customs, and with whom it is impossible to form intimate and elevating association."[92] At this juncture Dr. Kerr entailed that American general practitioners needed to help the Chinese abandon their hostile customs and adopt Western culture so as to build a new Chinese society in accordance with the tenets of the natural laws.

In May 1890, Dr. Kerr, together with Drs. Thomson and Fulton, attended the China Medical Missionary Association in Shanghai, which afforded an opportunity for many medical missionaries in China to meet together for the first time. At the conference, Dr. Kerr "spoke strongly of the hopelessness of expecting anything from the Chinese Government or the mandarins" and claimed that "the only resource is the introduction of Christianity."[93]

Dr. Kerr repeated the role medical missionaries played in the renovation of the world at the conference on May 19, 1890. Kerr said:

> Shall our profession do its part in this great work of renovating the world? Our Association and this meeting here today answer this question. We represent a movement which had its origin fifty years ago, and which in recent years has been progressing with ever-increasing volume and force.[94]

Like Parker and Kerr, Dr. R. H. Graves who had been practicing medicine in south China for more than forty years by the end of the nineteenth century regarded medical missions as forces for change in rejuvenation of traditional China under Western culture and Christianity. He wrote in 1895:

> The foreign medical missionary...will be an influential factor in the work of China's regeneration. He often has intercourse with the high officials, he has men of influence among his patients, and is generally looked up to by the masses of the people. Thus, by his personal influence he may accomplish much.
>
> [W]e may consider medical missions among the most far-reaching and hopeful of the forces brought to bear upon the ancient empire of China, tending to bring her under the influence of Western progress and of Christian civilization.[95]

Dr. H. W. Boone, the president of the China Medical Missionary Association, wrote that missionary physicians should promise to be an agency whose influence would extend "into other departments of life," thereby helping China "along philanthropic, moral, yes, political lines."[96]

Medical missionaries took to China not only Western medicine but Western values and culture, which had an impact on their patients and students. Western influence could be seen by those students' earliest determinations to study Western medicine. Western inspiration could be seen when the Cantonese medical students were interested in many features of Western learning and many aspects of the Western society, such as missionary perceptions on religion, family, society, and politics. Some Chinese students absorbed, to some extent, Western thoughts while studying modern medicine and began to develop their reform ideas. The Canton Hospital's medical school was one of examples, which helped cultivate several famous reformers and revolutionaries in modern China.

Sun Yat-sen

Sun Yat-sen (1866–1925) was one of Dr. Kerr's students. Cuiheng, the village where Sun was born in November 1866 was situated in the Pearl River Delta, and the port of Macao was only forty miles to the south. Sun's father had possession of too little land to sustain his family and was forced to add to his inadequate resources by various incomes. He worked as a tailor in Macao, a journey man, and a porter while his wife was working hard on the small piece of land. After spending his first thirteen years in Cuiheng, Sun ended his peasant childhood when Sun Mei, his elder brother, delightedly returned with his great fortune from Honolulu to the village to visit his parents. Sun decided to see his brother in Hawaii the following year. Impressed with Western influences, Sun found a new world in the process of transformation and later was admitted into a missionary boarding school sponsored by the Anglican Bishop Alfred Willis. In the fall of 1882, in company with other missionary schools' students, Sun began to study at the Oahu College supported by American Congregationalists, keeping on his inquiry into Western learning, especially the subjects of medicine and law. Nevertheless, Sun Mei decided to stop his support of Sun Yat-sen and sent him back to Cuiheng in 1883 because he was irritated by his younger brother's objective to religious conversion, giving up devotion to their ancestors and throwing out their Chinese uniqueness, as indicated by Sun Mei. In the spring of 1884, Sun was studying at the government central school, a secondary school for middle class children, where both the English and Chinese curriculums were adopted.[97]

As stated by his biographers, Sun Yat-sen was fascinated by two fields of study—science and religion—during that time. Sun was christened by American Congregationalist Dr. Charles Hager, a new settler in Hong Kong. On one occasion, he visited a Chinese missionary and suddenly saw some medical books on the book shelf. He asked the missionary why he put those medical books in his study, although he was not a doctor. To answer Sun's question, the missionary cited the renowned motto of the eminent scholar of the Song Dynasty, Fan Zhongyen, "If one cannot be a fine premier, then be a fine physician." It seems that the Chinese missionary's reply had an effort on Sun, and he thereafter decided to study Western medicine so as to serve the Chinese people. As Sun later made clear, "he decided to go to the Canton Hospital to study medicine because he believed that he would practice medicine for the benefits of the Chinese."[98] To let the Chinese enjoy the benefits of medical science was one of the reasons that Sun later chose to study medicine. To Sun, to become a doctor would help many Chinese.

After the Sino-France War of 1883–1884, the Qing court was forced to sign a treaty with France in 1885, which brought humiliation to the Chinese and prompted Sun and other reformers to distrust the corrupt Manchu bureaucracy and to carry out social and political reforms in China. Sun assumed that the medical school was a good place to discuss and promote reform ideas and that the study of medical art was a means to exchange ideas with other students at the school. He also believed that a general practitioner would have more opportunities to promote reform ideas because he would see many patients every day and nobody would regard a physician as a revolutionary. His aim was to prepare for reform under the cloak of a doctor's activities.[99] Sun's dream of reform in China was another reason that he took up the study of medicine. With the help of a recommendation letter from Dr. Hager, Sun was admitted into the South China Medical School of the Canton Hospital in 1886.

The South China Medical School provided a place where open-minded students could exchange their ideas. Since the Qing government did not control the mission school, students had freedom to discuss their reform ideas. Sun was joined there by his old village friend Lu Haodong while becoming friendly with another fellow student and a baptized Christian, Zheng Shiliang. The three students seemed to have discussed China's fate repeatedly, even if not reaching any unambiguous conclusions.[100] Dr. Li Jiliang studied at the Canton Hospital for three years and worked for eight years at the out-patient department without pay, aside from what the patients might turn out to make payments. He recollected that Sun was an extremely bright student and that he had already started his plans for the reform of China while he was at the Canton Hospital. Li also claimed that Sun Yat-sen later left Canton for Hong Kong because he was regarded as a dangerous person by reason of his relentless discussion about his ideas of to cause the downfall of the Qing government at the Canton Hospital.[101] Dr. J. O. Thomason of the Canton Hospital also wrote afterward in his article of 1935 that much of Dr. Sun's disappointment with China's current conditions and his new thoughts were nurtured at the Canton Hospital from where those reform inspirations spread all the way through the Chinese empire.[102] In his own book, *Kidnapped in London,* Sun mentioned his year at the Canton Hospital where he first began to put together his ideas for a new Republic of China. It was apparent that this year of training in Canton wielded an imperative effect on the noble mission of his life, and his experience at the Canton Hospital laid down the foundation of his reform thoughts.[103]

Sun Yat-sen did advocate reform of the School's regulations when he became apprenticed to Dr. John Kerr at the Canton Hospital. At that time in the classroom sixteen male students and four female students were seated separately with a heavy curtain, and male students were not permitted to participate in the clinical practice of gynecology. Dr. Kerr implemented such rules and regulations because he understood that Confucianism discouraged any contact between male and female in public places. Sun, however, felt uncomfortable with such regulations, arguing that male students would have to see female patients in the future after their graduation and that Confucian teaching had a strong bias against women. Urged by Sun, Dr. Kerr abandoned those regulations, removing the curtains separating male students from the female students in the classroom and allowing male students to participate in the clinical practice of gynecology.[104]

After one year in Canton, Sun enrolled in the College of Medicine for the Chinese in Hong Kong in October 1887, which had just opened under the direction of Dr. James Cantlie that year. This newly established college relating to the Alice Memorial Hospital was opened as a project of the London Missionary Society and was under the benefaction of one of the most eminent representatives of the anglicized elite of Hong Kong. Sun, one of twelve students in the first batch, wrote in late life that he decided on the transfer because the Hong Kong Medical College could give him a better education and in Hong Kong he could have better chances and greater liberty to be engaged in his revolutionary work, particularly propaganda activities.[105]

In his five years at the college, Sun mastered the foundation of medical science and practice and developed his comprehension of both Western and Chinese cultures. He also got in touch with more reformers, talking about the indispensable renovation of China. In a letter of 1890 to a professional man from his home town, Zheng Zhaoru, Sun advocated learning from the West, to carry out political reforms, promote agriculture, prohibit opium, and establish a public education system.[106] More importantly, during his study at the Hong Kong Medical College, Sun began to realize that a good doctor would help cure the disease of patients but have limited resources to save a lot of people's lives and that the evil Manchu bureaucracy had a lot of power and resources and abused its authority, contributing significantly to the sufferings of the Chinese people. Sun also recognized that hundreds of thousands of Chinese lives would not be saved if the oppressive regime was not overthrown.[107] In view of the fact that physicians could only save a few people's lives rather than all the Chinese, Sun decided to abandon his medical careers and to participate in the revolutionary cause to save the Chinese nation. As indicated later by Sun, his revolutionary thoughts were cultivated in Hong Kong.[108]

Sun was the first graduate from the college in 1892, receiving a diploma signed by Dr. Cantlie, but neither the British Hong Kong authorities nor the Portuguese Macao government accepted Sun's documentation. During the short time, Sun, in fact, practiced medicine, first in Macao, then in Canton, using both Western and Chinese medicines. Sun did not expect to turn out to be one of the Chinese pioneers of Western science and technology because the specific, restricted, and slow effect of a doctor was not the kind of effect that Sun wanted to see on the masses of the Chinese. Therefore, Sun was determined to commit himself to a revolution movement. After the failure of the 1895 Canton rebellion plotted by Sun, he sneaked into Canton Hospital's medical school when the Qing armies were trying to arrest all the revolutionaries. With help of the medical students of the school, Sun successfully fled from Canton to Japan.[109]

Sun became the first president of the Republic of China in 1912, but never forgot the revolutionary cradle. He returned to visit the Canton Hospital several times, giving financial support and demonstrating his interest in the Canton Hospital. It was at his wish that his son, Sun Ke, the mayor of Canton, donated 120 mu (1/6 acre) of land to the hospital for a new location. The mayor wrote on April 24, 1924, "In recognition of the distinguished services it has rendered to the community of the city of Canton, this government approves in principle the plans for the construction of a new plant upon the site granted by the government."[110] In the same year, a year before his death, Dr. Sun's name took precedence on a donation list with his charitable endowment of $1,000 for a dispensary on the Lingnan University campus, later the division of the Canton Hospital, Sun's last connection with his medical school in Canton, in which he never lost interest.[111]

Zheng Shiliang

Zheng Shiliang (1863–1901), a son of a rich Shanghai merchant, had been educated at a German missionary school in Canton and had connections with the secret organization of eastern Guangdong Province. He participated in the Tri-society, a secret anti-Qing society in eastern Guangdong, in order to bring down the Manchu government and restore the Ming dynasty of the Chinese.[112] At the medical school, Sun Yat-sen and Zheng became good friends. During their conversation, Sun learnt that Zheng was a high-ranking Triad celebrity and realized the significance of Zheng's secret society as a reform force in the future. Sun also believed that this kind of secret organization would be very useful in mobilizing all kinds of the people, an inspiration that prompted Sun to establish a political party for revolutionary cause ten years later.[113] Interested in Sun's attention to the revolutionary potential of the secret societies, Zheng turned out to be a kindred spirit. Both started to discuss at the Canton Hospital the need for reform in China and the future of the Chinese in the face of increasing Western influence. Both gradually came to the conclusion that Western cultures had advantages over the Chinese traditional cultures to some extent and that the Chinese had to learn from the Western countries to carry out political and social reforms so as to salvage China.[114] Under Sun's reform influence, Zheng agreed with Sun's ideology of disrespecting the Qing government and often discussed with other students about how to rescue, enrich, and strengthen China and how to establish a republic. Zheng informed Sun that he was a leader of the anti-Qing Tri-Society but did not have any reform ideology which Sun had and that he would follow Sun's noble course in the future.[115] Zheng was becoming a reformer at the Canton Hospital's medical school under Sun's influence.

After Sun left the South China Medical School in 1887 for Hong Kong, Zheng dropped the School in 1888 and returned to his home town. He opened several medicine stores and was engaged in recruiting members more aggressively to expand his tri-Society. Sun and Zheng were not classmates after 1886, but they maintained close relations, often discussing how to reform China with Western political systems. In November 1894, Sun created a revolutionary association, Revive China Society, in Honolulu to lead the Chinese to put an end to the Manchu rule. In January 1895, Sun, Zheng, and others set up the headquarters of the Revive China Society in Hong Kong, and Zheng became one of Sun's chief lieutenants during that time.[116] In 1895, Zheng Shiliang, Sun Yat-sen, Lu Haodong and others established Nongxue hui (Agricultural Study Society) in Canton to study how to explore new lands and to fertilize soil so as to increase agricultural production. This was the first society in Canton to advocate scientific research and to promote modern science, one of the early scientific societies in China. Given that the members of the society were radicals, the organization was banned by the Canton government before long.[117]

Zheng helped Sun recruit fighters to engage in the Canton uprising of 1895. After the collapse of the uprising, Zheng took refuge in Japan, together with Sun, but soon returned to Hong Kong, where he continued working with the secret societies. During the Huizhou uprising of 1900, Zheng again acted as liaison between Sun and the Triads and directed military operations in the field in eastern Guangdong where he started off the secret society. When the uprising failed, Zheng fled to Hong Kong again and died soon after. Zheng played a role in the reform and revolutionary movement before the 1911 Revolution.[118]

Kang Guangren

Kang Guangren (1867–1898), the famous Cantonese Reformer Kang Youwei's younger brother, studied medicine under Dr. John Kerr for three years at the Canton Hospital's medical school. After graduation, he went to Shanghai with a plan to open a medical school of Western medicine, but his plan failed. Kang soon became a progressive reformer when he and his brother, Kang Youwei, established an Anti-Footbinding Association in Guangdong in 1895. The activities of the association reached the city of Shanghai where, with the support of the renowned Shanghai people, the Cantonese reformers inaugurated a larger association, with Kang Guangren and Liang Qichao in charge. In 1896, Kang Guangren served in Zhejiang Province, becoming a an assistant, where he worked for less than a year to his great aversion.[119]

Since the progressive reformers understood that journals and newspapers were important to promote reformers' ideologies and programs, Kang Youwei decided to publish a newspaper in south China to inspire more people to participate in the reform movement. He traveled to Macao with his brother Kang Guangren. Supported by both Kang Youwei and Liang Qichao, Kang Guangren was ready to publish a periodical, *Zhixin bao* (New Knowledge Journal), in Macao. The purpose of the this progressive journal was, as said by Guangren's letter of November 30, 1896 to his friend Wang Kangnian, to introduce Western learning to the Chinese and to help educate the Chinese because if the Chinese did not learn Western science and technology, they would not know how to open factories, build railroads, and manufacture machines.[120]

On February 22, 1897, the first issue of *Zhixin bao* was published in Macao with the financial support of a Macao merchant. *Zhixin bao*, at first a five-day periodical, later appeared once every ten days. Under the management of Kang Guangren, one of the two managers of the newspaper, *Zhixin bao* soon became a major propaganda tool of the Chinese progressive reformers and a key source of Western learning, becoming a very popular reform newspaper not only in China but also in Japan, the United States, and Singapore. As Macao was a Portuguese colony, it was hard for the Qing government to ban any progressive and radical articles published in the newspaper. With this advantage, the reform journal published many articles to condemn the Qing government and advocate political and social reforms in China, especially promoting the progressive and radical reform ideologies and programs of both Kang Youwei and Liang Qichao.[121]

This radical journal also published many foreign articles translated into Chinese on Western political systems and ideologies, sciences, and technologies, which helped awaken the Chinese to see the great material progress of Western countries and realize the backwardness of Manchu China. Since the progressive reformers were debating the possibility of the Sino-Britain alliance against both Japan and Russia, Kang Guangren himself wrote an article, entitled "An Alliance with Britain against Japan," in the journal, advocating establishment of the Sino-British alliance against both Russians and Japanese because Britain was the most powerful country in the world.[122] In addition, this reform newspaper published translations of approximately thirty Western articles on modern medicine and hygiene between 1897 and 1898 so as to promote a modern medical and hygiene revolution in China.[123]

Since books on Western laws, political systems, economic models, and sciences and technology were vital in the reform movement and Kang Guangren's *Zhixin bao* was becoming popular, Kang was asked by the reformers to open a translation company. In November, 1897, Datong Translation

House was opened in Shanghai. Kang Guangren became a manager of the new company and had a plan to translate into Chinese foreign books on Western reform programs, laws, constitutions, sciences, and technologies. The first thirty books were published in early 1898, including Kang Youwei's *On Confucius' Reforms.*[124]

In that year, the foreign powers were staking out "spheres of influence" in China, and the partitioning of the country by the imperialists seemed imminent. Kang Youwei was inspired by this renewed threat to new re-form endeavors, submitting in January 1898 "Overall Coordinating under the Emperor's Order." Won over to the need for reform by then, Emperor Guangxu ordered Kang to elaborate his reform proposals. As Kang Youwei was very busy receiving reformers in Beijing during the daytime and writing books and composing reform memorials at night, Kang Guangren, in support of his brother, helped to receive reformers and progressive scholars in the morning, contacted other officials of the imperial court, and helped modify and draft reform memorials at night. When working on the reform memorials, Kang Guangren often gave suggestions to Kang Youwei that the most important task in reform was to abolish the eight-part essay (literary composition prescribed for the imperial civil service examination, known for its rigidity of form and poverty of ideas) and the civil service examination system so as to attract talents and promising scholars to the government and to promote political, economic, and social reforms thereafter. Without abolishment of this examination system, it would be impossible to carry out any reforms in China, as Kang Guangren maintained.[125]

On June 12, Emperor Guangxu issued the "State Affair Edict," a historic document proclaiming a new national policy of "Reform and Self-strength-ening." The imperial rulings were issued, but traditionalists in the central bureaucracy refused to go along with any reforms, especially the empress dowager. During that time, Kang Guangren realized the difficulties the re-formers were facing, and asked Kang Youwei and Liang Qichao to return to Canton to train new reformers because at that moment it was not the best time to carry out comprehensive reforms in Beijing. He said to Kang Youwei, "You have to leave Beijing as soon as possible because now all the power is concentrated in the hands of the empress dowager who hates reform."[126] Kang Youwei, however, refused to accept his brother's suggestion. During the crisis before the imperial coup on September 21, Kang Guangren and other reformers were trying to rescue Emperor Guangxu who was arrested by the empress dowager. They also attempted to organize the secret societies in Hunan Province to revolt against the empress dowager, encourage warlords' armies to march on Beijing, and persuade the British and U.S. governments to intervene, but all these plans failed.[127] Guangren refused to flee when the empress dowager sent three hundred mounted officers to arrest him and other reformers. Six of reformer leaders, including Kang Guangren, were executed on September 28 after their arrest. Reform was terminated in 1898, but Kang Guangren, one of the major reform leaders, played a significant role in the reform movement.

Liang Peiji

Liang Peiji (1875–1947) was a student of the South China Medical School of the Canton Hospital from 1894 to 1897. After graduating from the School, he taught medical courses while practicing medicine. Liang had become a nationalist by the beginning of the twentieth century when he helped open a medical college in Canton. Liang asserted the establishment the Guanghua Medical School not only put a stop to foreign domination of medical institutions in Canton to regain Chinese medical rights, but also revitalized the Chinese nation and reawakened Chinese national consciousness because he had realized the significance of Chinese control of modern medical science in modern transformation in China.[128]

Liang strongly criticized foreign domination of modern medical education in China. At the first meeting of the Guanghua Medical Association on December 15, 1908, Liang alleged that modern medicine came to Guangdong earlier than it was introduced into Japan, but it made much greater progress in Japan than in China by reason of foreign domination of modern medical institutions in China, a tragedy when the Chinese lived under the control of the foreigners. Liang also claimed that if the Chinese wanted to make great progress in medical science, they needed to establish and run their own modern medical institutions by themselves rather than relying on foreigners. He further pointed out three major goals of foreigners' medical institutions in China: the first one was to promote political influence in China of their states, the second was to carry out medical experiments on the Chinese in order to seek new medical findings, and the last one was to promote charitable enterprise.[129]

Liang supported Sun Yat-sen's revolutionary course. During the Canton Revolt in March 1911, Liang helped the revolutionaries put arms and ammunitions at his house. After the rebellion failed, many revolutionaries were killed, and dead bodies lay on the streets. Liang was nearly arrested by the Manchu armies when they were searching his home, but he escaped. Liang later helped bury many dead revolutionaries. After Sun established a provisional revolutionary government in Canton in 1921, he tried to appoint Liang as the director of the Department of Health in his government, but Liang refused to take the position.[130]

Liang was very vigorous during the anti-imperialism campaign in Canton in 1926, promoted by both the Nationalists and Communists. He was engaged in propaganda work for the revolutionary government in Canton. In the 1930s, Liang became a renowned nationalist business leader in China, opening new national companies owned by the Chinese, such as tobacco and soda, to compete with the British and American companies. There is no doubt that medical education at the Canton Hospital helped nurture Liang's reform ideas and helped make him an anti-imperialism nationalist.[131]

Conclusion

American doctors in Canton played a role in promoting modern medical education in China. They took the lead in the establishment of China's first modern medical college, trained China's first doctors of Western medicine, and first translated Western medical textbooks into Chinese. The establishment of the South China Medical School resulted in the creation of several medical schools in Canton, making Canton one of the modern medical education centers in China. The graduates of the medical schools in Canton affected the spread of Western medicine in China when they practiced medicine in Canton and in other places. Western medicine and surgery were gradually but incontestably moving forward in China generally, and in Canton particularly, between 1835 and 1935. American medical missions in Canton played a part in China's medical transformation.

American doctors criticized the backwardness of Chinese society, condemned the evil customs and manners of the Chinese, and advocated transformation of China into a modern state under Christian influence. They came to China with not only medical arts but alsoWestern values and culture. It is not clear how the Cantonese students received progressive ideas or adopted the new Western concepts from their American teachers, along with their training in Western medicine, but it was clear that the Canton Hospital was a foreign missionary hospital where it was hard for the Qing government to ban any progressive and radical ideas. Thus the missionary hospital provided a new public sphere to the Cantonese. With this advantage, the medical students had the opportunity and freedom to discuss their ideas of reform and revolution. Their disappointment with China's current conditions and their new thoughts were nurtured at the Canton Hospital where their experiences laid down the foundation of their reform thinking, which later turned them into reformers and revolutionaries. After their graduation from the Canton Hospital, while practicing medicine, they gradually realized that Western medicine alone could not cure the ills of Chinese society and that only social and political reform would rescue the Chinese nation. They thus became engaged in the reform and revolutionary movements with an agenda to modernize China's traditional society. It is not surprising that the Canton Hospital became one of the cradles of the reform and revolution movements in modern China. The Canton Hospital's medical school not only trained China's first physicians but also generated China's earliest reformers and revolutionaries, such as Sun Yat-sen, Zheng Shiliang, Kang Guangren, and others.

Ironically, Western medicine, in some measure, was one of the sources of the rising of Chinese nationalism in Canton. Since China was still under the oppression of imperialism in the first half of the twentieth century, it was natural that Chinese intellectuals first developed their nationalism and then tried to awaken national consciousness among the Chinese people. The Canton Hospital's medical school helped nurture Chinese nationalism to some degree. The Canton Hospital's students and alumni began to realize that Western medicine was unusually important not only to individual health but also to the Chinese nation and that if China's modern medical institution was monopolized by Western nations, Chinese lives would be in the hands of Westerners.

The Guanghua Medical School was a product of Chinese nationalism. Liang Peiji, Kerr's student, and other Cantonese medical elite of Western medicine recognized the importance of modern medical education in China's nation-building. They considered that Chinese had to own their medical education, rather than let it be dominated by foreigners. They therefore established China's first Chinese-style medical school in 1908 run by the Chinese, where the Chinese taught medicine in Cantonese dialect. Many reasons motivated the Cantonese medical elite to do this, but Western medicine was one of the reasons.

The shift of administration of the private Gongyi Medical College to the Cantonese government was a good example in point of Chinese nationalism. Promoted by both the Nationalists and the Communists, the medical students in Canton launched an anti-imperialism and anti-religion campaign in the 1920s in order to develop Chinese-controlled modern medical education and services. They claimed that a Chinese-controlled modern medical college would be a victory in a fight for control of modern medical education in China, regaining sovereign rights lost in the treaties of the nineteenth century. The private Gongyi Medical College where American medical missionaries were teaching experienced this kind of agitation, especially when the students organized strikes and protests against Rockefeller Foundation's financial contribution to the Gongyi Medical College in 1925. Under the pressure of the Gongyi students, the Cantonese government took over Gongyi entirely. Many reasons explained the rising of strong nationalism at Gongyi, such as the Communist propaganda, the Nationalists' mass mobilization strategy, and others, but Western medicine was one of them because the Gongyi medical elite had realized the significant role Western medicine played in China's modernization and did not want foreigners to monopolize medical education in China.

American medical missionaries played a role in modern medical globalization in China, a process of interaction and integration between American doctors and Chinese doctors. American doctors were interested in the Sino-Western medical convergence and the study of Chinese medicine at the Canton Hospital. American doctors tried to adopt some Chinese medical methods in the treatment of Chinese patients so as to make Western medicine more efficient. American doctors also adjusted themselves to Cantonese society and modified their medical training of the Cantonese students when they used the Cantonese dialect as the means of teaching, an important approach to remove the technological barriers and promote medical technology in China. At the Canton Hospital, some Chinese traditional doctors were not only teaching students Chinese medicine but also studying Western medicine, which helped them learn Western medicine to treat their patients. The Cantonese doctors trained at the Canton Hospital successfully combined Chinese and Western medications to facilitate the introduction of Western medicine and to fulfill effectively the cultural and social needs of the Chinese people. As a result, in both processes, Western medicine was becoming culturally reinterpreted as it moved from its original cultural location to China.

Table 2.1 The Distribution of Physicians by Provinces in China in 1935

Province	Number	Percentage
Jiangsu	2,010	37.3
Guangdong	606	11.2
Hebei	387	7.2
Zhejiang	350	6.5
Liaoning	352	6.5
Shangdong	244	4.5
Hubei	192	3.6
Fujian	153	2.8
Jiangxi	85	1.6
Sichuan	71	1.3
Anhui	63	1.2
Hunan	56	1.0
The rest of China	284	5.6
Unknown	537	10.0

Sources: His-Ju Chu and Daniel G. Lai, "Distribution of Modern-Trained Physicians in China," *Chinese Medical Journal* 49 (1935): 533–46.

Notes

1. Medical Missionary Society, *The Medical Missionary Society in China: Address, With Minutes of Proceedings* (Canton, The Chinese Repository, 1838), 25.
2. Medical Missionary Society, *Report of the Medical Missionary Society in China: The Fourteenth Report of the Ophthalmic Hospital, Canton* (Canton: The Chinese Repository, 1848), 15.

3. Wong K. Chimin, and Wu Lien-teh. *History of Chinese Medicine* (Shanghai: National Quarantine Service, 1936), 200, 260, 332.

4. Medical Missionary Society, *Report of the Medical Missionary Society in China for the Year 1866* (Canton, China: The Medical Missionary Society, 1867), 9.

5. Dr. Huang Kuan was a noteworthy Chinese doctor, the first Chinese to receive a degree in medicine abroad. A native of a county in Guangdong, a few miles inland from Macao. Huang, a pupil at the school of the Morrison Education Society under Samuel R. Brown, and other two Chinese students, went together with their teacher to America. After receiving a degree in literature, Huang proceeded to Edinburgh where he studied medicine from 1848 to 1853, supported by the generosity of some foreign businessmen at Hong Kong. After completing his studies, Dr. Huang returned to Hong Kong and opened a dispensary. Huang remained there until 1860, during which time he consistently helped Dr. Kerr with all critical surgeries and became more and more directly associated with the Canton Hospital. When Dr. Kerr was forced to leave China in April 1867 owing to health, the hospital for the lasting months of the year was put under the care of Dr. Huang so that the Boji Hospital was run exclusively by Chinese personnel during those months, and the number of surgical operations carries out in that period was possibly greater than in any equivalent period of time. See *The Twentieth Annual Report of the Board of Foreign Missions of the Presbyterian Church in the United States of America* (New York, 1857), 72-76 and J. C. Thomson, "Medical Missionaries to China," *China Medical Missionary Journal* 1 (January 1887): 45-49.

6. *The Hundred Years History of the Canton Hospital* (Organization Committee of the Sun Yat-sen Medical College, Lingnan University, Canton, 1935), 9-10.

7. John Kerr, "Opening of the Hong Kong College of Medicine for Chinese," *China Medical Missionary Journal* 1, 4 (December 1887), 169.

8. J. G. Kerr, "Training Medical Students," *China Medical Missionary Journal* 3, 2 (1889): 135-40.

9. John Glasgow Kerr, "Training Medical Students," *China Medical Missionary Journal* IV (1890), 137.

10. John Kerr, *China Medial Missionary Journal* 10, 1 (1896), 55.

11. *The Hundred Years History of the Canton Hospital*, 21-28.

12. Ibid.

13. Ibid.

14. Ibid.

15. Dr. Swan taught surgery, Dr. Paul Todd, who had come as an assistant to the hospital in 1902, gave clinical lectures, Dr. Mary Niles lectured in gynecology and obstetrics, Dr. F. Oldt gave lectures in public health and hygiene, Dr. H. W. Boyd in the diseases of the eye, ear, nose, and throat, and Dr. Ni Xipeng taught minor surgery. Dr. Antou Andersson, dedicating his entire time to the college, taught several courses, assisted by several foreign-trained native physicians; Dr. E. C. Machle and Dr. John Kuehne of the Rhenish Mission assisted in teaching on the teaching staff, too. See *The Hundred Years History of the Canton Hospital*, 13-14.

16. It was extraordinarily disappointing for the medical students at that time to have no appropriate dissections for their study of anatomy, although they did have a skeleton, and used papier-mâché models. See John M. Swan, "South China Medical College," *The China Medical Journal* 23, 5 (September 1909): 303-306.

. The faculty of the Canton Hospital's medical school was:

Dr. John Swan	Surgery, Medical and surgical Clinics
Dr. J. Webb Anderson	Gynecology
Dr. Chas. C. Selden	Nervous Diseases
Dr. F. Oldt	Materia Medica, Hygiene and Sanitation
Dr. Yie Chendeng	Physiology, Obstetrics
Dr. Ni Xipeng	Theory and Practice, Medical and surgical clinics
Dr. Qi Dadeng	Materia Medica and Therapeutics
Dr. Su Daoming	Eye Diseases
Dr. Huang Kuan	Anatomy
Dr. Liu Deye	Chemistry

. See Canton Hospital, *Annual Report of the Canton Hospital Report for 1916* (Canton: Too Leung Printing Press, 1917), 73.

17. W. W. Cadbury, *At the Point of a Lancet: One Hundred Years of the Canton Hospital, 1835-1935*, 183.

18. Medical Missionary Society, *Report of the Medical Missionary Society in China: The Fourteenth Report of the Ophthalmic Hospital, Canton* (Canton: The Chinese Repository, 1848), 13-15.

19. Medical Missionary Society, *Minutes of the Annual Meeting of the Medical Missionary Society in China* (Macao: N. P. 1857), 8.

20. Medical Missionary Society, *Report of the Medical Missionary Society in China for the Year 1860* (Canton, Friend of China Press, 1861), 14-15.

21. Wong and Wu, *History of Chinese Medicine*, 233, 380-81.

22. Wong and Wu, *History of Chinese Medicine*, 382, 384.

23. Canton Hospital, *Annual Report of the Canton Hospital for the Year 1916* (Canton: Too Leung Printing Press, 1917) and Canton Hospital, *Annual Report of the Canton Hospital for the Year 1917* (Canton: Too Leung Printing Press, 1918).

24. *The Hundred Years History of the Canton Hospital*, 9-10.

25. John Kerr, "The Bubonic Plague," *China Medical Missionary Journal* 3 (1894): 178-80.

26. *Liangguang Jinxinhui yiyuan sanshi zoulien tekan* (The special issue of the thirtieth anniversary of two guang Baptist hospital (Canton: Liangguang Jinxinhui yiyuan sanshi, 1947), 2.

27. *A Brief Sketch of the History of Kung Yee* (Hong Kong: Victoria Printing Press, 1925).

28. *Guangdong gongyi xiaoyuan di ba, jiu zhou nian bu gao* (Report on the eighth and ninth anniversaries of Gongyi medical school) (Guangzhou: Guangdong gongyi, 1918), 12-13.

29. O. J. Todd, "Co-Operation with the Chinese in Medical Education Work," *China Medical Journal* XXVII (May 1913): 143-47.

30. T. Z. Koo, "Educational Conditions and Student Life in China Today," in T. T. Lew, *China Today through Chinese Eyes* (London: Student Christian Movement, 1926), 104.

31. "Abstract from Chinese Report of the Kwangtung Kung Yee Medical College and Hospital, 1914-1915," *China Medical Missionary Journal* 30, 6 (1916).

32. William Warder Cadbury, "The 1918 Pandemic of Influenza in Canton," *China Medical Journal* 34, 1 (January 1920): 1-17.

33. In 1920, the executive power of the faculty was cancelled, bringing about the termination of the dean, Dr. J. A. Hofmann. Dr. Wang Kentang became the new dean but resigned soon, and Dr. Li Duo was appointed interim dean. See Li Duo, "History of Guangdong Gongyi Medical College and its Hospital," *Guangzhou wenshi ziliao* (History and literature of Guangzhou) 21 (1980): 169-174.

34. *Guangdong gongyi xiaoyuan di shi yi, er zhou nian bu gao* (Report on the eleventh and twelfth anniversaries of Gongyi medical school) (Guangzhou: Guangdong gongyi, 1924), 5-9.

35. *A Brief Sketch of the History of Kung Yee* (Hong Kong: Victoria Printing Press, 1925), 11-14.

36. *Guangdong gongyi xiaoyuan di shi yi, er zhou nian bu gao* (Report on the eleventh and twelfth anniversaries of Gongyi medical school) (Guangzhou: Guangdong gongyi, 1924), 5-9.

37. Sun Zhongshan, *Sun Zhongshan quanji* (Beijing: Zhonghua shuju, 1985), 8: 23-24.

38. *Guangda yike zhou nian ji nian hao* (The special issue of the first anniversary of the Medical Department of Guangdong University) (Guangzhou: Guangdong yike da xue yi xue yuan, 1926), 5-10.

39. J. Oscar Thomson, "The Medical Educational Situation in Canton," *China Medical Journal* 40 (1926): 790-97.

40. *Guangda yike zhou nian ji nian hao* (The special issue of the first anniversary of the Medical School of Guangdong University) (Guangzhou, Guangdong yike da xue yi xue yuan, 1925), 2-3.

41. "Kung Yi Hospital and Medical school," *China Medical Journal* 39, 9 (September 1925), 853.

42. J. Oscar Thomson, "The Medical Educational Situation in Canton."

43. *Guangda yike zhounian ho* (Report on the first eleventh and twelfth anniversaries of Gongyi medical school) (Guangzhou: Guangdong gongyi, 1924), 5-9.

44. *The China Year Book, 1929-30* (Kraus reprint, 1969).

45. *Guangdong Gongyi yixue zhuanmen xuexiao, Guoli Guangdong daxue yike, Zhongshan daxue yixueyuan biyeshen mingce* (1909-1955) (the Graduate Register of Guangdong Medical School, Medical Department of National Guangdong University, and Medical College of Zhongshan University, 1909-1955) (Guangzhou, 1962).

46. Dr. J. Allen Hofmann to Our friends at First Church, September 20, 1925, Folder 16, Box 27, Record Group 82, Presbyterian Church in the U.S.A. Board of Foreign Missions. Secretaries Files: China Missions, 1891-1955, Presbyterian Historical Society, Philadelphia, Pennsylvania.

47. *Guanghua yishi hui tekan* (The special issue of the Guanghua Medical School) 7 (1929): 1-2.
48. Ibid., 87-88.
49. *Yixue weisheng bao* (Journal of Medicine and Hygiene) 7 (1909): 58-60.
50. Ibid.
51. *Sili Guangdong Guanghua yixue yuang gaikuang* (The outline of the history of the private Guangdong Guanghua Medical College) (Guangzhou, Guanghua yixueyuan, 1936), 1-10.
52. "A Short History of the Private Guanghua Medical College," *Guangzhou wenshi ziliao* 26 (1982): 139-154.
53. "Prospectus of Medical Colleges and Schools," *Chinese Medical Journal* 49 (1935): 998-1034.
54. *Guanghua biye tongxuehui tekan* (The special issue of the Alumni of Guanghua) (Canton, 1935).
55. J. C. Thomson, "Medical Missionaries to China," *China Medial Missionary Journal* 1 (January 1887):45-49.
56. The most popular of Kerr's books were: *Material Medica and the Therapeutics* (4 vols., 1871), *Essentials of Bandaging* (1872), *Treatise on Syphilis* (1872), *Symptomatology* (1873), *Treatise on Diseases of the Eye*, *Treatise on Eye Disease* (1880), *Manual of Operative Surgery* (7 vols., 1881) *Tract on Hernia and Intermittent Fever, Treatise on Fevers* (1881), *Treatise on Inflammation* (1881), *Principles of Chemistry* (4 vols., 1881-85), *Treatise on Diseases of Different Organs* (1882), *Theory and Practice of Medicine* (6 vols., 1883), *Manual of Physiology* (4 vols., 1884), *Surgery* (1891), *Manual of Cutaneous Diseases, Anatomical Plates, Hospital Materia Medica, Practical Chemistry for Medical students*, and *Vocabulary of Medicines*, and *Tract on Vaccination*. See Cadbury, *At the Point of a Lancet*, 281-286 and *The Hundred Years History of the Canton Hospital*, 19-25.
57. This journal published only two issues and then was closed because few readers could read this journal. See Wong, *History of Chinese Medicine*, 296.
58. John Kerr, "History of the Medical Missionary Society's Hospital," *China Medical Missionary Journal* X, 1 (March 1896), 55.
59. J. C. Thomson, "Medical Publication in Chinese," *China Medical Missionary Journal* 1, 3 (September 1887), 115.
60. John Kerr, "History of the Medical Missionary Society's Hospital," *China Medical Missionary Journal* X, 1 (March 1896).
61. Lee T'ao, "Some Statistics on Medical Schools in China for the Year 1933-1934," *Chinese Medical Journal* 49 (1935): 894-902.
62. Ibid.
63. Dr. E. P. Thwing wrote a paper titled "Medical Science in China" and sent it to Dr. Henry S. Drayton, who read it before the Academy of Anthropology on April 1, 1890. See "Absurd Chinese Notions: Remarkable Ignorance of Medicine and Surgery in China," *The New York Times*, April 2, 1890.
64. Hsi-ju Chu and Daniel G. Lai, "Distribution of Modern-Trained Physicians in China," *Chinese Medical Journal* 49 (1935): 544-46.
65. Jin Baoshan, *Zhangshi defang weisheng xingzheng gaiyao* (The local health administration during the war) (Chongqing: Zhongyang xunlian tuan dang zheng xunlian ban, 1940), 21; *Weisheng tongji* (Health statistics) (Chongqing: Neizheng bu, 1938), 34.

66. William G. Lennox, "The Distribution of Medical School Graduates in China," *Chinese Medical Journal* 46 (1932): 406; Zhongguo Guomindang zhongyang tongjichu (Central Statistical Bureau of the Guomindang), *Minguo ershier nian zhi jianshe* (The reconstruction in 1933) (Nanjing: Central Statistical Bureau of the Guomindang, 1934), 68-69.

67. Hsi-ju Chu and Daniel G. Lai, "Distribution of Modern—Trained Physicians in China," *Chinese Medical Journal* 49 (1935): 547-50.

68. See His-Ju Chu and Daniel G. Lai, "Distribution of Modern-Trained Physicians in China," *Chinese Medical Journal* 49 (1935): 533-46.

69. *Guangzhou zhinan* (Guide to Canton) (Shanghai: Shanghai xinhua shuju, 1919).

70. Huang Yanpei, *Yisui zhi Guangzhou* (One-year old of the city of Guangzhou) (Guangzhou: Shanwu, 1922), 60-61.

71. *Guangzhou Zhinan* (Guide to Canton) (Guangzhou: Guangzhoushi zhen fu, 1934).

72. F. Oldt, "Scientific Medicine in Kwangtung," *The Chinese Medical Journal* 48 (1934): 663-71.

73. John Kerr, "Chinese Materia Medica," *China Medical Missionary Journal* 1, 2 (June 1887): 79-80.

74. Ibid.

75. See http://www.chinamtcm.com/html/51730.htm.

76. Qingren Wang, *Yilin gaicuo* (Correction of medical theory) (Canton, 1830. Reprint, Beijing: Zhongguo zhongyi yao chubanshe, 1995).

77. See http://www.chinamtcm.com/html/51730.htm.

78. For a study of the examination system in China, see Benjamin Elman, *A Cultural History of Civil Examinations in Late Imperial China* (London: University of California Press, 2002) and Iona Man-Cheong, *The Class of 1761: Examinations, the State and Elites in Eighteenth-Century China* (Stanford: Stanford University Press, 2004).

79. Zheng Hong, "Wanqing zhongxi yi de weitong yu lunzheng" (Discussion on the Sino-Western medical integration during the late Qing dynasty), *Nanfang dushi bao* (South China city daily), October 21, 2009, B14. See also Zheng Hong, *Guoyi zhishang: Bainian zhongyi chenfu lu* (Tragedy of Chinese medicine in the past one hundred years of ups and downs) (Guangzhou: Guangdong keji chubanshe, 2010), 11-12.

80. *Huayan zangxiang yuezuan* (The drawings of viscera of the Chinese and Europeans) (Foshan, 1893).

81. See http://chinadoctor.org/doctor/oldtcm/story/616.htm.

82. See http://liyizhuang.blshe.com/post/4282/130653.

83. http://www.gzzxws.gov.cn/gzws//cg/cgml/cg6/200808/t20080826_4260_1.htm.

84. Huang Zhongye, "Tang Shiyi yaochang jianshi," *Guangdong wenshi ziliao* (History and literature of Guangdong) 20 (1980): 65-104.

85. Ibid.

86. Ibid.

87. Ye Nezhen, "Record on Guangzhou's New Drug Industry and Anya Drug Factory," *Guangzhou wenshi ziliao* (History and literature of Guangdong) 30 (Guangzhou): 152-160.

88. John Kerr, "The Bubonic Plague," *The China Medical Missionary Journal* 3 (1894): 178-80.

89. George B. Stevens and W. Fisher Markwick, *The Life, Letters, and Journals of the Rev. and Hon. Peter Parker, M.D., Missionary, Physician, and Diplomatist, the Father of Medical Missions and founder of the Ophthalmic Hospital in Canton* (Boston: Congregational Sunday School and Publishing Society, 1896), 127-8.

90. Quotations are from an account of Parker's talk presented in *The Christian Observer* (Philadelphia, 1841).

91. J. G. Kerr, *Medical Missions at Home and Abroad* (San Francisco: A. L. Bancroft, 1878), 89.

92. John Glasgow Kerr, "Medical Missionaries in Relation to the Medical Profession," *China Medical Missionary Journal* 4 (1890), 89.

93. *North China Herald*, May 16, 1890, 603.

94. J. G. Kerr, "Introductory—Medical, Missionaries in relation to the Medical Profession," *The China Medical Missionary Journal* 6, 3 (1890): 87-99.

95. R. H. Graves, *Forty Years in China or China in Transition* (Baltimore: Woodward, 1895. Reprint, Scholarly Resource at Wilmington, Delaware, 1972), 252-53.

96. Henry William Boone, "Medical Mission Work at Shanghai," *China Medical Missionary Journal* XV (1901), 24-5.

97. For a study of Sun Yat-sen's bibliography, see Marie-Claire Bergere, *Sun Yat-sen* (Stanford, California: Stanford University Press, 1994).

98. Sun Zhongshan, *Sun Zhongshan quanji* (Works of Sun Yat-sen), vol. 1 (Beijing: Zhonghua shuju, 1981): 547-9.

99. Sun Zhongshan, *Sun Zhongshan quanji*, vol. 6 (Beijing: Zhonghua shuju, 1985): 228-9.

100. See Lo Hsianglin, *Sun Yat Sen's University Days* (Taipei: The Commercial Press, 1954).

101. W.W. Cadbury, *At the Point of a Lancet*, 195.

102. Dr. Thomson quoted in the speech of the mayor of Canton in May 1912. On May 9, 1912, the Canton Hospital was honored by a visit from a former student, Dr. Sun Yat-sen, the first president of the Chinese Republic, for whom a reception was arranged in the hospital compound, permitting the many friends of this institution to meet Dr. Sun. When laying the corner stone of new building for the Canton Hospital, the mayor of Canton gave a speech praising Sun's revolution achievement. See J. O. Thomson, "A Century of Medial Work in China," *Missionary Review of the World* 2 (February 1935): 55-59.

103. Sun Yat-sen, *Knapped in London* (London: China Society. Rereprint, 1969), 7-9.

104. *Guangdong wenshi ziliao* (History and literature of Guangdong) 25 (1979): 276-79.

105. L. T. Ride, *Sun Yat-sen* (Hong Kong: Hong Kong Press, 1970).

106. Sun Zhongshan, *Sun Zhongshan quanji*, vol. 1 (Beijing: Zhonghua shuju, 1981): 1-3.

107. Sun Zhongshan, *Sun Zhongshan quanji*, vol. 2 (Beijing: Zhonghua shuju, 1982): 359-60. See also James Cantlie and C. Sheridan J Jones, *Sun Yat-sen and the Awakening of China* (London: Jarrold and Sons, 1912), 41-43.

108. Sun Zhongshan, *Sun Zhongshan quanji*, vol. 1 (Beijing: Zhonghua shuju, 1985): 584-5.
109. James Cantlie, *Sun Yat Sen and the Awakening of China* (New York: Fleming H. Revell Company, 1912), 27-35.
110. Cadbury, *At the Point of a Lancet*, 232.
111. *The Hundred Years History of the Canton Hospital*, 11-15.
112. Zou Jincheng, "Zheng Shiliang chun lue" (A short biography of Zheng Shiliang), *Guangdong wenshi ziliao* (History and literature of Guangdong) 63 (1986): 127-133.
113. "Zheng Shiliang Shi lue" (A short biography of Zheng Shiliang), in Feng Ziyou, *Geming yishi* (Informal history of the revolution) (Beijing: Zhonghua Shuju, 1981), vol. 1: 26-28.
114. Sun Zhongshan, *Sun Zhongshan quanji*, vol. 7 (Beijing: Zhonghua shuju, 1985): 115-16.
115. Wang Yilian, *Xiagu zhongyun: Zheng Shiliang chun* (Biography of Zheng Shiliang) (Taipei: Modern China, 1983), 25.
116. Chen Xiqi, ed. *Sun Zhongshan nianpu changbian* (A chronicle record of Sun Yat-sen's life) (Beijing: Zhonghua shuzhu, 1991), 84-100.
117. Marie-Claire Bergere, *Sun Yat-sen* (Stanford, California: Stanford University Press, 1994), 32-38.
118. Sun Zhongshan, *Sun Zhongshan quanji*, vol. 6 (Beijing: Zhonghua shuju, 1983): 297-300.
119. Liang Qichao, "Kang Youwei zhuan" (Biography of Kang Youwei), in Chen Weiliang, ed. *Liang Qichao wenji* (Liang Qichao's works) (Beijing: Yanshan chubanshe,1997), 466; Xia Shaohong, ed. *Liang Qichao wenxuan* (Liang Qichao's selected works), vol. 1 (Beijing: Zhongguo Guangbodianshi chubanshe, 1992), 287.
120. *Wang Kangnian shiyou shuzha* (A collection of Wang Kannian's letters), vol. 2 (Shanghai: Guji chubanshe, 1986): 1669-70
121. Liang Qichao, "Kang Guangren zhuan," (Biography of Kang Guangren) in *Yinbingshi heji* (Liang Qichao's works) (Beijing: Zhonghua shu ju, 1989), 96-97.
122. Kang Guangren, "Sino-British Alliance against Japan," *Zhixin bao* (China Reformer) 41 (March 3, 1898).
123. With regard to the articles on modern medicine and sanitation, See *Zhixin bao*,1897-1898.
124. Liang Qichao, "Kang Guangren zhuan," (Biography of Kang Guangren) in *Yinbingshi heji* (Liang Qichao's works) (Beijing: Zhonghua shu ju, 1989), 96-97.
125. Ibid.
126. Ibid.
127. Ibid.
128. Pan Zhuo'an, "Sili Guangdong Guanghua yixue yuan shilue" (The outline of the history the private Guangdong Guanghua Medical College), *Guangzhou wenshi ziliao* (History and literature of Guangzhou) 26 (1982): 139-155.
129. Liang Peiji, "On the Purpose of Foreigners Practicing Medicine in China," *Guanghua yishi weisheng zazhi* (Guanghua medial and health journal), 1 (August 1910), 5-14.
130. See http://liyizhuang.blshe.com/post/4282/130653.
131. Ibid.

3

The Hackett Medical College and the Modern Women's Rights Movement, 1899–1935

Some work has done on the Hackett Medical College for Women, focusing on the origins and development of the College, but little has been written on the social and political role of this institution and its alumnae.[1] This chapter examines the history of China's first medical college for women founded by American medical missionaries and its contribution to medical modernization in China. This chapter also studies the social and political role of the women doctors educated by Americans and their impact on the modern women's rights movement in China.

Women's Medical Attendance and Education in China

Chinese women received less medical care than men in traditional China. The Chinese social construct created a medical dilemma for Chinese physicians. Given that a woman was not supposed to meet men not in her family, and she could not be thoroughly examined—even touched—by a general practitioner, the Chinese sought a way to solve the problem: they had a male relative there, either a husband with his wife, a son with his mother, or a brother with his sister.[2] Another answer was to train women comprehensively in medicine so they could treat female patients. Consequently, some upper-class women, born into medical families, learned Chinese medicine, and after being tested by other physicians, they started practicing medicine, although most of these women were midwives.[3] Due to such obstacles, most Chinese women were unwilling to apply for medical advice, as Dr. R. H. Graves commented, "Female complaints go almost entirely unrelieved, as prejudice and their ideas of propriety forbid them calling in even their own ignorant male doctors, and they have no female physicians except a few women who deal in what we call 'old women's remedies.'"[4]

The women of the better classes even endured a vast amount of suffering, rather than submitting to what modern medical science required for the diagnosis and treatment of disease. The women of the respectable class consulted physicians in grave emergencies, but they demonstrated substantial unwillingness before they would state their cases. If a male physician was called to treat a lady of the upper-class family, he could see only her wrist without her body. The woman had to lie behind a bed curtain, with only her hand and arm exposed to the doctor, stretching out between the curtains of the bed.[5] Anything further than this was unacceptable. Some women took this to excess, prohibiting their doctors from grasping their wrists to take pulses, and the doctor could only tie a thread firmly round a woman's wrist, pull it tight, and feel her pulse through the thread. Frequently, women showed to their physicians where their ache was by identifying it on a doll.[6]

Women also received less education, not mentioning medical training, than men because until the nineteenth century China was still a very neo-Confucian society. Women were discouraged from leaving the family home and courtyard, and only the poorest went anywhere unchaperoned. Women stayed at home to care for their husband's families and kept to a minimum any contact with men not in their immediate family (husband, brothers, and fathers). The women of the upper class might receive some education, but most women had little learning, if any at all. The best hope for a girl who desired to learn was to ask her father and brothers to teach her. Since a girl became a member of her husband's family upon marriage, it seemed an unwise investment to spend money teaching a daughter. Moreover, the objective of learning was to succeed in the exam to be appointed as government officials, but such jobs were closed to women, so it was therefore a waste of money to teach a girl to learn.[7]

Women Patients at the Canton Hospital

The Chinese social construct created more difficulties for the medical missionaries than for the Chinese physicians. The first medical missionaries, all male, knew about the limitations on Chinese women but had never seen them in practice. They both miscalculated and exaggerated how preventive the regulations were. They were astonished at how women were attended because the whole family had to agree before a Chinese woman could take such a big step as to visit a foreign hospital. They were exceedingly uneasy about treating the women who turned up in their clinics.

While in China, medical missionaries began to challenge Chinese attitudes toward women in the medical sphere and tried to remove obstacles to attending women and teaching female medical students. Dr. Parker believed that women should be elevated and treated not as the slaves but as the helpmates and companions of man.[8] When the Canton Hospital was first opened to receive patients, no one came on the first day. The next morning only one poor woman dared to seek advice from Parker about her eyes, a young blind woman becoming Dr. Parker's first patient. His second and third patients were women accompanied by their parents or relatives, too, all having eye diseases. Dr. Parker did the surgery on the third woman patient the next day. During the first three months of the Ophthalmic Hospital, 925 patients consulted the American doctor, including 270 female patients.[9] Dr. Parker was the first foreigner in China to challenge Chinese tradition against women in the field of medicine.

Shortly before Dr. Parker's departure to Japan in 1839, a woman was brought into the hospital with breast cancer from which she had suffered for six years. The breast was removed, the first time such an operation had been performed in China upon a Chinese woman. It was certain that the patient endured it with great strength during the operation. She was discharged and returned in good health to see the doctor later. Another woman in the same situation was operated upon and was discharged four weeks later.[10]

Female entry into foreign organizations was illegal and difficulty was anticipated in attending female patients at the Canton Hospital, but it seemed that the solution of having a male relative with the female patient worked well. The number of female patients visiting the Hospital after the first female patient increased significantly. The number of patients who visited the Canton Hospital in 1856 was 16,417, of whom 4, 096 were females.[11]

Female patients were received at the Canton Hospital, although often the more highly regarded class of Chinese women sought advice from its medical doctors only in severe situations. In spite of this, much to their disappointment, American doctors were not called until there was little chance for the patients' survival. One or two times, the patients died while the doctors were still on the road. In 1866, for example, Dr. Kerr was called on April 12 to see a woman in labor with her first child. The labor had already continued for eight days, and she was in a condition of great exhaustion. The only hope for her survival was active interference. The delivery was accomplished in a few minutes as the head was already at the os externum (a small, depressed, somewhat circular aperture on the rounded extremity of the vaginal portion of the cervix), and an immerse flow of urine instantaneously came out. The child's skull bones had been cracked by the efforts of the native midwives helping deliver the infant. In this instance, the woman was physically powerful and in good physical shape, and the presentation seemed normal. The cause of the labor, which was lengthened, was not clear, but a well-timed intervention would have saved the lives of both mother and baby. The father of the patient was a wealthy salt merchant, who lived adjacent to the hospital and was conversant in its function, and it was not the issue of a lack of knowledge. The excessive shyness of the Chinese women of the more reputable class was a great impediment to their search for medical attention, which Western science and skill afforded in such difficulties. In this case, the arrogance of wealth also put a stop to a request for a foreign physician until it was too late.[12]

The male doctors at the Canton Hospital accomplished prominent achievements in women's health work. In 1860, Dr. Huang Kuan assisted delivery on a Chinese woman. This was the second case of childbirth on record at the hospital.[13] The first stone operation was performed in a female patient in July 1874; the first lithotomy ever performed on a Chinese woman was carried out successfully, removing a stone of one inch by five-eighths. In 1875, John Kerr carried out an operation on a woman's huge ovary tumor, the first surgery on a woman's abdomen in China. In 1892, China's first caesarean birth was successfully carried out at the Canton Hospital.[14]

The male doctors' treatments of the Chinese women patients at the Canton Hospital, a challenge to Confucian teachings that *Nannu shoushou buqin* (to observe propriety between the sexes) and separate spheres (man: outer / woman: inner), which prevented female from entering the public and male-oriented sphere. American doctor established the Canton Hospital to create public healing sphere to challenge Chinese healing culture, but it was the Cantonese female patients who actively sought American male doctor's treatments. To restore to health, they were determined to overcome social and cultural challenges in China, which prevented Chinese female patients from entering the public and men-dominated spheres of healing, especially the foreign institutions. The Canton Hospital not only helped improve women's physical condition but also provided a place to the Cantonese women to challenge traditions in Cantonese society.

The True Light School and the First Women Medical Students, 1852–1879

Chinese women's desperate need for education was first recognized by Western missionaries in consequence of their outreach to the Chinese women. To Western missionaries, since oppressed women were more receptive to religious sermonizing, which helped to alleviate their miserable lives, they would become the major population for missionary work. Missionaries were excited to readjust Chinese women's established faiths through educational process as well as to present Christianity to them. After the opening of trade relations between China and Western countries in 1821, missionaries supported some education programs for Chinese girls, and American doctors in Canton were engaged in this educational process.

Happer's Dispensaries

Andrew P. Happer (1818–94) arrived in Canton in 1847 and then decided to start a dispensary, after realizing that the Cantonese liked the missionary medical institutions.[15] In 1847, Happer moved to the suburb of Canton, which subsequently became the place of his medical practice. Under the helpful Presbyterian medical missionaries, medical work was started in 1851 when Reverend Happer opened the Huiji (Charitable Relief) Dispensary. In the first four months of 1851, he saw 4,690 patients and cured about 5,000 patients in the whole year. He thus became one of the fourteen pioneer medical missionaries to China. By 1853, Happer was treating over 7,000 cases annually, including some females, who were attended by Happer's wife, the former Elizabeth Ball of the American Board of Commissioners for Foreign Missions. Medicine succeeded at dispensary over the next few years, but its scope and expansion was still greatly restricted by various other calls for Happer. As time went by, and more and more patients visited his dispensary, he employed a Chinese assistant, Chen Apeng. Chen, very good at cataract extraction, had worked for Dr. Benjamin Hobson for more than six years and carried out surgeries independently. In 1854, Happer opened a second dispensary in a chapel rented in the city's southern suburb and opened a waiting room for women at his dispensary because he understood that, according to Chinese culture, women were not allowed to stay with any men in public places. The number of the patients rose to 10,000. Happer was delighted with the progress: "The sufferings of many persons are relieved, and the Christian instructions addressed to them by their benefactors have been in many cases received with grateful attention."[16] In 1854, Happer's hospital treated 967 inpatients, 17,591 outpatients, and performed 1,218 surgical operations.[17] Since the practice of medicine was not his first interest but always a means to getting into Chinese hearts, Happer brought to an end his medical practice when John Kerr arrived in Canton on May 15, 1854 to help him, and thereafter let Dr. Kerr take charge of his dispensary.[18]

Dr. Happer was engaged in preaching, teaching, and social work while practicing medicine. Maintaining his pastoral and educational activities, he was the principal of a school for training priests and other workers for the Cantonese Christian community.[19] While working long hours as an ordained minister of the Gospel, his primary duties, Happer founded a day school in 1850 as an attempt to reach young Chinese from the higher classes. While running a school for Chinese boys, he started to pay attention to education for the Chinese girls. He suggested to the Presbyterian Board of Foreign Missions that a Christian girls' school be established in Canton. With the approval of the Board, Mrs. Lillie B. Happer, together with missionaries John Booth French and William Speer, who arrived in Canton in 1846, opened a boarding school for girls in 1852.[20] Due to the limited freedom and social restriction of the Cantonese women, only one student did go to the school, but Mrs. Lillie Happer made a great effort to recruit and in 1853 six students successfully passed the entrance exam. The school was offering reading, writing, and home economics courses.[21] With the purpose of improving the quality of the school's education, Happer hired a teacher to teach students not only how to read and to write but also how to sew clothing, make shoes, and embroider cloth. As a result, the girls learnt the skills to make money to support themselves. This school became the first boarding school for women in Canton.[22]

In 1856, in the absence of Dr. Happer, the girls' boarding school was under the superintendence of Mrs. French, the wife of John B. French. A part of every day was devoted to the study of Christian books, and the girls were studying earnestly. The Chinese girls were motivated to learn. As Mrs. French commented, "In diligence, aptitude to learn, and propriety of behavior, they will compare favorably with the majority of their own age in England or America."[23]

This girls' boarding school was not expanded until 1872 when Miss Harriet Noyes, sent out by the Presbyterian Board of Foreign Mission in the United States, arrived in Canton on January 14, 1868. Interested in the girls' boarding school, she wrote a letter in April 1871 to the Women's Board in Philadelphia, asking for financial support of a girls' school in Canton. The request was granted, thus making the seminary one of the first of the special projects taken up by the Women's Board established in 1870.[24] In June 1872, by means of the dedicated efforts of Miss Harriet Noyes and Mrs. Lillie Happer, the first building was completed, located across a narrow lane from the Canton Hospital. With the endorsement and reinforcement of the Presbyterian Board of Foreign Mission, this girls' boarding school, named Zhengguang (True Light) School, was formally established on June 16, 1872, a model of missionary schools in China and the first formal girls' school in south China at that time. The School offered free tuition, board, clothing, and other benefits to the students.[25]

The first days of True Light were challenging. Their feet were bound, but the girls tried to prove that their brains were by no means bound. The girls showed great appreciation of Miss Noyes and her dedicated assistants for having faith in their competence in learning. At the beginning, only Miss Noyes and Mrs. Happer were teaching six pupils. In 1873, Martha Noyes, Harriet Noyes's sister, was sent by the Presbyterian Board of Missions in the United States to the True Light Seminary to help Miss Noyes.[26] She later married Dr. John Kerr and opened a Canton Hospital School while teaching at the True Light, both schools close to each other.[27] The significance of both the day and boarding schools for the Chinese girls were summarized in Dr. Happer's a paper entitled, "Women's Work for Woman," presented at the first missionary conference in China, held in Shanghai on May 10–24, 1877.[28]

First Female Medical Students

It was not hard for the Chinese to understand what liberation from physical pain suggested and why they willingly visited the hospital, but it was not easy for them to understand why women should be well-informed, especially to become physicians. The medical missionaries, however, already realized the need for training female medical students and understood the significance of the Chinese women physicians. As Dr. R. H. Graves wrote, "The profound ignorance of the native faculty, and the seclusion and modesty of the female members of most families open an unlimited field in China for the lady physician, who combines the necessary physical endurance and moral courage with devotion to the self-denying exercise of her profession."[29] He also believed that "with Chinese women well qualified as physicians under the instructions of their sisters from the West, and imbued with a true spirit of Christian sympathy, there is a hope for a great improvement in the well-being of the sick in China in the future."[30] Their wish was fulfilled when the girls of True Light were admitted to the Canton Hospital's medical school.

In view of the fact that the True Light students were living near the Canton Hospital, they were able to realize what it would mean to Chinese women if there would be doctors of their own sex. The female students then approached Dr. Kerr who, an untiring man, founded the Canton Hospital's medical school, in addition to his ordinary duties as a doctor. After much conversation, he accepted their request.[31]

In 1879, the Canton Hospital broke new ground, this time by admitting two Chinese women at their own serious application to its medical classes, the first medical institution in China to do this. Chinese women's medical education began in the style of apprenticeship when the Canton Hospital admitted Chinese women students—an unprecedented new development in Chinese history. Although medical attention had been offered for women at the very commencement of the Canton Hospital, this was the first time that an opportunity for medical education was available to Chinese women.[32]

Kerr took the two female students into his medical class and gave them the same training and advantages as the male students received. The introduction of women medical students allowed John Kerr to treat non-emergency female patients among the Cantonese women at the hospital. In 1880, two of the female students proved to be very useful not only in the hospital, but also in taking care of the women of the gentry class in private families under Dr. Kerr's guidance in cases of illness unusual to women. Dr. Kerr then sent one of the female pupils to relieve a woman suffering from retention of urine, as it would be more appropriate to Chinese cultures of politeness to have a female attendant in such a case. This female pupil had become conversant in the surgical procedure in attending to one of the ovariotomy cases. This was probably the first case in point in which a surgery, so easy and so necessary in many cases, was ever performed by a Chinese woman. By that time, at least one of the medical students was considered to be capable enough to set off alone on house calls and execute minor operations on female patients. In 1882, there were three women in the class of twelve. To learn the medical arts, the students had to watch the physicians to treat the patients, and on the whole, they were excellent learners.[33]

The Canton Hospital hoped that the attendance of Chinese women medical students would be enough to bring in more respectable women patients, but it was soon clear that at any rate one Western woman physician was required on the staff because Chinese women and their men folk remained hostile to the opinion of male physicians treating female patients. To Dr. Kerr, a woman physician meant much to Chinese women because they were still unwilling to allow a man to attend them. He asserted "The work of our lady physicians in the families was an important factor in gaining favor for Western medicine."[34] Realizing the significance of women physicians, Dr. John Kerr and Martha Noyes suggested to the Presbyterian Board of Foreign Missions to send female missionary doctors to Canton. Indeed, as early as ten years before, Dr. Happer had this request. Between 1872 and 1874, Dr. Happer had already written about twenty letters to the Presbyterian Board, requesting female missionary doctors to be sent to Canton in an attempt, rather than working at the Canton Hospital, to establish a new hospital for women.[35]

American Women Doctors at the Canton Hospital, 1882–1899

Women physicians began to appear in the United States in the mid-nineteenth century. In 1848, Samuel Gregory initiated a school for the attention of women in childbirth in Boston. Gregory's Boston school, launched as a medical college for women, was actually restricted for the most part to the instructions of hygiene, physiology, obstetrics, and the diseases of women. The first medical degrees given to women in Boston were awarded in 1854, and a small number of women continued to graduate as physicians for the next two decades. Before 1880, thirteen regular schools of medicine were opened to women in the United States. The small medical school of the State University of Iowa was coeducational from its commencement in 1870 when it admitted eight women. Michigan became the first prominent university outside Europe to receive women on an ongoing basis in medicine; its decision in 1870 to enlist women was applauded as the true inauguration of medical coeducation in the United States. Consequently, female physicians began to come into sight in the United States in the 1870s, which paved the way for women medical missionaries to China in the following years. The isolation of most of the Chinese women and their lack of knowledge opened an unrestricted sphere in China for American female physicians, who would combine the essential physical strength and honorable bravery with dedication to the unselfish tasks of their medical practice.[36]

Mary West Niles

In 1882, the Canton Hospital welcomed its first woman physician, Mary Niles (1854–1933), who began teaching and practicing women's and children's medicine in China. After arriving at Canton on October 19, 1882 as a medical missionary of the American Presbyterian Board of Foreign Missions, North, she lived with Miss Harriet Noyes at the True Light Seminary where she started leaning the Cantonese dialect and gave some assistance to Dr. Kerr in her spare time.[37]

Dr. Niles started working at the Canton Hospital in 1883 and superintended the women's wards when Dr. Kerr was forced to retreat to Hong Kong for a short time while Drs. J. C. Thomson and Wales were in charge of the Hospital. The female patients were pleased about the advantage of having a lady physician, to whom they could state their problems. Four cases of instrumental delivery were recorded in 1883. Dr. Nile attended three of them, and in the last case, the newborn was saved after the patient had been in labor for twenty-four hours before receiving Dr. Kerr's attention. Dr. Niles performed a post-mortem in 1883 on a woman, who died from an ovarian tumor, and assisted an ovariotomy, which was successful and the woman was restored to health after staying at the hospital for two months.[38] At the time, the terrible sufferings undergone by women when producing their babies were widespread in China.

Due to Dr. Nile's excellent accomplishments, at a meeting of the Canton Medical Missionary Society on January 1, 1885, Dr. J. C. Thomson recommended that Dr. Niles be appointed lady physician to the hospital, a suggestion that would not only increase the efficiency of the hospital, but also relieve the physician in charge of many burdens imposed upon him. Convinced of the suitability of this recommendation, the Medical Missionary Society appointed Dr. Niles as a formal doctor in charge of women and child patients at the Hospital.[39] At the meeting, Dr. Thomson also claimed that if an increased number of female patients came, as the Canton Hospital expected, more accommodations would be considered necessary and that an amount of $300 was approved to be spent for new wards.[40]

To attend more women patients, Dr. Niles created a dispensary for women and children in a building belonging to the Presbyterian Missions in 1885. The number presented at this dispensary remained small during almost four years, and it was forced to put up the shutters in June 1888.[41]

Since native doctors of Chinese medicine knew little about obstetrics and, in fact, were never called in such cases, except for feeling the pulse, in order to provide skilled assistance, the Canton Hospital sent doctors to the families. By 1889, Dr. Niles had done a great deal of good in her visits to many homes, as an author wrote, "Dr. Niles had visited, by invitation, and treated patients in the families of nearly all the high officials residing in Canton. In such ways, medical skill avails to open doors which are otherwise barred to the introduction of Christianity."[42] Dr. Niles activities were described in the 1890 annual report:

She has performed 683 surgical operations and 164 patients have been visited in their homes, 275 calls having been made. She has thus reached many firesides of the poor, and also of the wealthy and influential [including the wife of the provincial governor] always carrying the Gospel message.[43]

The hospital reports showed six calls in 1884, thirteen in 1885, and 162 cases in 1894. By 1894, Dr. Niles's practice with families had become one of the most important parts of the work of the Society. In 1896, Dr. Niles and her assistants visited 508 patients, half of whom producing babies.[44]

After returning to Canton in 1899, Dr. Niles resigned from the staff of the Canton Hospital. By that time, Dr. Niles had taken charge of the women's department of the Canton Hospital for fifteen years, assisting Dr. Kerr and devoting herself chiefly to obstetric work. Dr. Niles' experiment proved a success: the number of women patients and students at the Canton Hospital increased significantly, and by the end of the 1890s, Dr. Niles had three women medical missionaries. She healed many Chinese women and children in a modern medical way; her work improved the health condition of many Cantonese women and contributed considerably to the medical care of the patients, as historian G. Thomson Brown commented:

> In China, a women physician conforms with the high ideals of Chinese propriety. When Niles arrived, she was immediately put in charge of the female ward. In seven years, Niles did 683 surgical operations and visited 164 patients in their homes. She treated everyone from the very poor to the wife of the provincial governor.[45]

Dr. Niles also gave considerable time to the work of translation and revision of medical books. The most important of these were David James Evans' *Obstetrics: A Manual for Students and Practitioners* and John Kerr's *Practice of Medicine.*[46]

Mary H. Fulton

Mary H. Fulton was the second woman physician sent to China by the Presbyterian Board. After receiving her M. D. degree in 1884 from the Women's Medical College of Pennsylvania, a school eminent for its missionary women, she arrived in Canton in the same year, where her brother, the Rev. Albert Fulton and his wife had been living as missionaries for four years. No sooner had she arrived than she was introduced to Dr. Niles. Dr. Fulton recalled, "As Dr. Mary Niles is the only other lady physician in this province, I was keenly anxious to meet her. She kindly called and invited me to the Canton Hospital, the largest in China. There is room for about three hundred patients and no charge is made for those too poor to pay. Over 20,000 outpatients were treated in 1884 and 2,000 operations performed."[47]

Dr. Fulton was a woman of unusual bravery and strength of mind when she started dispensary work at Guiping in Guangxi Province, where there was not a single missionary at the time of her appearance. She rented two rooms in a mud house for the dispensary and hospital; the medical work developed favorably and splendidly. She had a most valuable assistant, Mrs. Mei Yagui, who had trained at the hospital under Dr. Kerr and was able to talk to the Chinese women directly, while Dr. Fulton, still unfamiliar with the Chinese language, had to talk through her interpretation. A new hospital building was erected and almost ready for occupancy at the beginning of May 1886, but a gang, which was incited by the Confucius scholars, burned it to the ground. Luckily, Dr. Fulton managed to run away uninjured, but she never returned to Guiping.[48]

Convinced that there ought to be a hospital for women in Canton, Dr. Fulton opened a dispensary near the Canton Hospital in 1888, so that the women had a place to come. One hopeful feature was that an increasing number of women visited her dispensary, although many of them were too late. In 1891, she opened another one with the help of Dr. Niles, who took charge of the dispensaries when Dr. Fulton was away on trips to rural areas. Dr. Fulton became so famous in Canton that in November 1889, she answered an imperative call from a high-ranking Chinese official in Canton to treat his 82-year-old mother. A bodyguard was sent with her from Canton, and Dr. Niles was treated very well on the way and traveled for several days to Shantou, a city 300 miles east of Canton. After the patient was successfully treated, Dr. Fulton obtained most admiring tributes to her competence and thankful appreciation of the value of her medical work.[49]

Dr. Mary Fulton assumed responsibility for the women's work of the Canton Hospital in 1897, assisted by faithful Miss Mei who remained there until her resignation in September 1900. Fulton had established herself as the hospital and medical school's most important woman physician while the mission's first woman doctor Mary Niles dedicated herself more to caring for the blind. During Dr. Niles's last absence, Dr. Fulton was in charge of the women's wards again, which made it possible for the medical work to continue without disruption.[50] Within the American mission community, both in Canton and back at home, Fulton had great support from both the Canton Hospital and her strongly evangelical family, which included her brother, the Reverend Mr. A. A. Fulton of the Canton mission.

The Hackett Medical College for Women, 1899–1933

The work at Canton Hospital's medical school was making good headway, and by 1898 the school had thirty-seven pupils. The expansion of the medical education at the Canton Hospital helped promote recruitment of women medical students, the number of whom steadily increased. There were only three women medical students in the class of twelve in 1882, four in 1886, and the number of women had grown to nine by 1890. Under Kerr's supervision, female students were trained regularly in the Canton Hospital medical classes from 1879 to 1899. The female students, like their counterparts, provided assistance in the hospital during their study years, beginning hospital work immediately and making house calls to upper-class women. As the reputation of the Canton Hospital extended to other provinces and the female students' professional care of female patients was improved considerably, the number of women patients increased considerably: six gynecological-related calls in 1884, thirteen in 1885, and 162 in 1894.[51]

The Hackett College, 1899–1915

The medical apprenticeship arrangement worked well for many years, but it ended abruptly in 1899 when Kerr retired from the Canton Hospital to devote his entire time to the care of the insane. He took with him the boys in the medical class and left the girls without an opportunity to complete their courses. Dr. Kerr's leaving provided a chance for which the Hospital's women's physician had been waiting, however. Resigning from the Canton Hospital staff, but not withdrawing from the support of the Presbyterian missions, Dr. Fulton announced her plan to organize a specifically female medical school and hospital compound as part of the mission's work in Canton. These five female students and two Chinese women doctors became the nucleus of the new medical college for women; it was the first attempt in China to teach medicine at a formal school for women.

The school was at first housed on the ground floor of the Theodore Cuyler (First Presbyterian) Church in the western suburbs of Canton, but this accommodation was not sufficient because the students were forced to have their meals in the outpatient room. Endeavors were made to provide a special hospital for women and children in association with the school.[52]

When returning to America, Mr. Fulton was able to raise $3,000 from the Lafayette Avenue Presbyterian Church in Brooklyn, and subscriptions amounting to $3,000 were soon raised from Chinese donors, too. Dr. Fulton and her brother then found an open space where two hundred pigs were lying in the mud and put all their money on this poor land, laying down the foundation of a college. A church with rooms for a dispensary was the first building erected in 1900 through the charity of Mr. E. A. Hackett of Indiana for the use of the medical school, which assumed the name of the Hackett Medical College for Women in honor of the donor. As a result of the second well-timed endowment from Mr. Hackett, a second college building to house lecture theaters and laboratories was erected, named the David Gregg Hospital for Women and Children. The first large three-story building for typical college use held lecture theaters and reception rooms on the second floor and bedrooms on the third. The students with pleasure relocated to the third floor. By 1902, the College had two fine buildings.[53]

Just after Chinese New Year in 1901, nine students were admitted. The original staff, in addition to Fulton, consisted of John Kerr, J. J. Boggs, Chas. C. Selden, Mary Niles, Su Daoming, He Zijin, Yu Meide, and Shi Meixing, and the students were instructed in the Cantonese dialect. Dr. Fulton made this clear from the inception, instructing potential medical students in 1901 that they would "learn that while medicine is a beautiful fruit of Christianity, the practice of it is not the sole aim of a Christian physician. It is to be a means in aiding suffering ones to look to the life beyond."[54] Dr. Fulton repeated this theme later, as she wrote:

> The purpose of the college is to train Christian women physicians to go out amongst their own countrywomen. Our graduates do excellent skilled work, and in a year save scores of lives, besides bringing a knowledge of common sanitation into homes, as well as making known the simplest rules for the common-sense treatment of the sick.
>
> Since this is at present the only college in the empire distinctively for women, its usefulness and needs should appeal to every heart that desires to mitigate human agony, elevate women, and bring knowledge of a Savior to heathen homes.[55]

To Dr. Fulton, the distribution of Christianity and modern medicine and the elevation of Chinese women's social status were the objectives of the College. Dr. Fulton offered in 1902 a training course, and eleven young women were "brave enough to present themselves as students." It was an astounding inauguration at a time when there were few professional opportunities for women in China.[56]

In January 1903, diplomas showing the new college seal were given to two students who were the products of a three-year set of courses, enhanced by participation in Dr. Fulton's large dispensaries and her many house calls. In 1904, four students received diplomas, and they were instantly employed at mission hospitals and several government institutions.[57] The curriculum was extended from three to four years in 1904. The women students attended clinics, helped lance boils, and delivered babies, but, when they graduated, they had never seen a major operation.[58] In 1907, thirty-five students were enrolled in the College, of whom seven students received diplomas. The viceroy of Guangdong and Guangxi provinces stamped the diplomas, with the seal of the U. S. Consulate in Canton, the only diplomas in the province thus stamped with the highest official recognition.[59]

The Hackett School was really an institution for women's education, and application numbers without difficulty exceeded the number the college could admit. Since the Hackett students were considered fine, educated women, they were highly demanded as wives of the upper class. As a result, the College lost so many women physicians to marriage that Dr. Fulton finally made a strict regulation: anyone to be married was prohibited from studying at the Hackett College. In 1908, six students graduated, including the first students from a distant province. The former Chinese ambassador to the United States addressed the ceremony, and the viceroy attended the commencement ceremony personally, awarded the graduates with their diplomas, and gave his address in Mandarin. It was the first time in missionary history in this part of China that women's medical education was very well respected by a prominent official.[60]

The reputation of the school and the foundation for women's education was boosted by the attendance of the mayor of Canton and Dr. Amos Wilder, American consul general in Hong Kong and Dr. J. C. McCracken of the Canton Christian College at the commencement in 1909. Dr. Fulton went over the main points in her historical outline of the College that by 1909 over thirty students had graduated, some of whom had secured desirable status in Canton and elsewhere as physicians as well as surgeons. Seven young women received medical degrees among thirty-one graduates, with students coming from Fuzhou, Xiamen, Hainan in South China as well as Honolulu.[61] The staff then consisted of fifteen teachers, most of whom were Chinese.[62]

In 1912, the Hackett Medical College was honored by the attendance of Dr. Sun Yat-sen, the first president of the Republic of China, at its commencement ceremony. In 1913, American Consul General F. D. Cheshire presided over the opening ceremony of the Hackett College in June.[63] In 1914, two new faculty members were hired at Hackett, bringing with them the hope to raise training benchmarks. Martha Hackett, the founding donor's daughter, received her M.D. from the Rush Medical College in Chicago in 1913, and Harriet Allyn received her Ph.D. in biology and scientific education from the University of Chicago in 1912. Drs. Hackett and Allyn graduated from the latest medical schools, but they were shocked by what pretended to be modern scientific training at Hackett. In 1915, there were more than sixty students, nearly all of them living on the campus. The Hackett Medical College was officially recognized and registered as it satisfied official standards, and its diplomas were marked with the official stamp of the Guangdong government.[64]

Referring to her illness and her desire to work full-time in Shanghai to translate medical texts, Dr. Fulton resigned as head of the Hackett medical complex—hospital, medical college, and nursing school—in 1915 after serving as dean of the school for sixteen years. Before Dr. Fulton went to Shanghai, more than sixty young women had finished the four-year courses and about fifty students then were taking the regular courses. Dr. Fulton's personality and religious faith were so forceful that almost all the nurses and physicians she educated were alleged Christians except for three.[65]

As a result of the small number of medical schools at that time in China, it was very hard to get good medical textbooks in Chinese. Dr. Fulton left Canton for Shanghai, at the request of the Chinese Medical Missionary

Association, because she intended to devote herself to the translation of medical books. Afterward, Dr. Fulton kindly presented the Publication Committee of the Chinese Medical Society with a supply of her translation, one of which was Dr. Anna M. Fullerton's *Nursing in Abdominal Surgery and Disease of Women*, a book of thirty-six pages in seven chapters printed in Chinese style, the last chapter focusing on formulas for sanitarium food. This was a very valuable gift because at that time there was only one book on nursing—*The Manual of Nursing*.[66] Dr. Fulton translated other two books, the *Diseases of Children* and *Nursing in Abdominal Surgery*. Thereafter, many Chinese general practitioners and medical teachers allegedly adopted her Cantonese translations of very important English-language textbooks on surgery, gynecology, diseases of infants and children, and both general and surgical nursing.[67]

A gifted surgeon, administrator, and educator, Dr. Fulton was recognized for the most part as the initiator of the Hackett Medical College for Women. She lived to see the enterprise that she had launched expand into an excellent institution providing plentiful openings for mission medical assistance to Chinese women.[68]

The Hackett College, 1915–33

In 1915, Dr. Martha Hackett was appointed as president of the whole compound of three medical institutions, Dr. Hariet Allyn as dean of the Medical College, and Hellen Stockton, who arrived in China in October 1912, as the superintendent of the Nurses' Training School and matron of the Gregg Hospital. The Hackett College, remaining for the most part female, was brought up to date and thus kept efficiently running, at any rate by the benchmarks of Western medical education in China. Before long, the College required difficult entrance examinations, one year of mandatory, premedical preparation, and one year of internship.[69] Both physicians and nurses, foreign and Chinese women, were employed at the College. Major fund drives started to pay for the on-going costs. In 1919, Hackett became a coalition establishment, which was sponsored by a number of mission boards.[70]

The Chinese students studied hard at the college. American doctors presented favorable comments on their female students, as Mary Fulton was quoted by a prominent Chinese:

> After many years' experience I can testify that the Chinese girls become almost ideal doctors. They learn quickly and have good memories. They are calm, dignified and self-possessed, clean in their personal habits, and dainty in their dress. Their small hands are finely adapted for delicate surgical work. They are seldom elated or cast down. They seem steadily year by year to grow in grace and knowledge. They bear heavy and important responsibility readily and cheerfully. I do not remember in all these years to have heard

one murmur or complaint, although they are busy all day and often all night in homes anything but sanitary. They are instant in season and out of season.[71]

All four of the women physicians working at Hackett between 1915 and 1922 had left by the end of 1922, either to wed or to look after the rich families. Three-fourths of the medical students were Christians and were enthusiastically involved in Christian witness and service in rural areas. By 1922, the College had graduated a total of 112 women.[72] The Hackett compound, although still lagging in the wake of medicine in the United States, was in any case within the lowest criteria of that time, a continued success in terms of its students.

In 1923, both Drs. Allyn and Hackett resigned from Hackett. When its two leading women departed, the Hackett Board, in looking for its next president, turned to Dr. John Allen Hofmann, a qualified male physician who was not only enthusiastic, but willing to go to make a position for himself within a women's medical institution. Dr. Hofmann, with special training in medical education, was appointed the president of the College and the superintendent of the Hospital. He managed an international staff of twenty-nine, half of whom were Chinese, including the dean and the nursing school director. The Hackett compound was expanded. Some of the aged houses were destroyed and a new dormitory, named Mary Fulton Hall, modern and well equipped, was constructed in 1923, in which forty-nine medical and seventeen pre-medical students were accommodated.[73]

A report published in August 1929 stated that ten students were graduated after the fourth year of medical study of Hackett and had begun to serve as interns at the David Gregg or other hospitals while the M.D. degree was granted to ten women who had completed their internship. In the fall semester of 1929, the admission examinations were raised so that only the graduates of recognized senior middle schools or their like might be admitted to the pre-medical course, which all at once was extended to two years instead of one. The set of courses had slowly but surely become extended to six years, including a two-year pre-medical course as well as a year of internship in a standard hospital.[74]

Hackett's faculty and staff changes began in the 1920s. One very important factor for the speed of this change was the increasing competence of the Chinese-trained physicians. Locally-trained Chinese general practitioners then could continue for more medical training without high expenses because they did not have to leave China to study in other countries and could do so at several advanced Western-style medical centers in China, the best of which at that time was the Rockefeller-funded Beijing Union Medical College.[75] Additionally, more and more Chinese were given administrative positions in preparation for the registration work and in the atmosphere of growing Chinese equality because the Chinese staff was doing very good work, as Dr. Hofmann commented in 1928: "We foreigners must decrease while the Chinese increase."[76]

In July 1931, Dr. Ross Huang, a male professor of surgery and anatomy, was selected by ballot to be the president of the whole Hackett compound to follow Dr. J. Allen Hofmann, who was due leave of absence. Dr. J. Franklin Karcher was elected to be superintendent of the David Gregg Hospital after the death of Dr. Hofmann on April 11, 1933.[77] Respected by many Cantonese, Dr. Hofmann was regarded as "one of the busiest and most popular doctors in the hospital and in the city."[78] By the end of 1932, Hackett, like other missionary institutions, was entirely managed and enrolled by the Chinese, and all the top administrative positions were occupied by men, except for only several women accountable for nurses and nurses' education.

The David Gregg Hospital

Since its conception, the David Gregg Hospital (Yuji Hospital) had provided significant medical services to the women in Canton and made medical knowledge available to pregnant women. The Cantonese women, who were going to produce babies, could stay at the hospital and give birth with the help of gynecologists. In 1927, maternity clinics were started and a Home Visiting Department was opened. The number of visitors to the maternity clinics increased, although they did not make good progress in the beginning.

New momentum was coming in 1928 when the Young Women's Christian Association inaugurated a public health campaign and worked together with the David Gregg Hospital. Since then the Hackett Medical College always had supplied many of doctors and nurses needed for those annual health campaigns. A Mothers' Club was organized, and instruction on health topics was offered at several schools.[79] In 1932, the Maternity Clinic of the Gregg Hospital organized a baby contest, the first time in Canton.[80]

The Gregg Hospital also provided outpatient service for child health. Mothers of infants from one to five years old were encouraged to participate in the health program, and they were taught how to raise children and were given basic health information. When children were diagnosed with physical or health problems, their parents were urged to correct the problems so that their children would continue healthy and grow well without illness. Every year about 3,000 patients visited the Yuji Hospital for consultation, and by 1934, 500,000 patients had stayed at the David Gregg Hospital wards. In 1934, 1,857 inpatients and 18,192 outpatients received medical treatments at the David Gregg Hospital for Women and Children, which had twenty-seven doctors, one hundred beds, 22,523 outpatients and inpatients annually.[81]

The Yanzai Pharmacy School

The Hackett Medical College was making good progress and began to train pharmacists when the Yanzai Pharmacy School was opened in 1926, the only school of its kind in south China. It was with Dr. Hofmann that the idea of the school of pharmacy originated. Since Dr. Hofmann's special medical field was internal medicine and therapeutics, he had the full understanding of the problems in pharmacy. He recognized the importance and value of well-trained pharmacists and helped in every way to set the school on its feet. The School soon received an unanticipated number of applicants. In 1930, three students were graduated as qualified pharmacists. In 1931, nine students were enrolled, according to the report of G. F. Sauer, the dean of the Yanzai School in 1931.[82] In June 1932, four students were graduated.[83]

The Hackett Medical School, the Gregg Hospital, and the Yanzai School continued their impressive activities in the early 1930s. The Institutions showed steady growth in material equipment, the number of their students, the standard of work, and in the quality and enthusiasm of their students. These three institutions developed into the largest medical complex for women in China at that time.[84]

The Sun Yat-sen Medical College of the Lingnan University

Medical education was another field, into which the Canton Christian College (later Lingnan University) expanded. Established by a group of American missionaries in 1888, this private institution was relocated a couple of times, moving to Macau in 1900 to escape the repressive policies executed by the Qing Dynasty, then back to Canton in 1904. In 1906, the University Medical School (UMS) founded in Canton was sponsored by the Christian Association of the University of Pennsylvania in the United States, an organization to encourage Pennsylvania medical graduates to practice medicine in China.[85] In 1910, the UMS had five students, four male and one female, in its own house on its own land neighboring the College campus, and the faculty consisted of two American physicians and one nurse, Miss Mary C. Soles.[86] Lack of unanimity caused tension among the faculty members, and efforts to work together with the Canton Christian College were unsuccessful for various reasons. As a result, the UMS pulled out officially from Canton in April 1914 after much disappointment and was relocated to Shanghai at the invitation of St. John's University there. Thus the Canton Christian College was allowed to use the medical school property, whose campus adjoined the premises of the College.[87]

In January 1915, the staff of the Canton Christian College offered ward classes for the students of several medical schools in Canton and tried to embark on public clinics. A legacy of $25,000 was put down by General Horace W. Carpentier of New York to the Trustees of Canton Christian College for medical work under the competent leadership of Andrew H. Woods.

This made it possible in 1919 to purchase the land and the buildings of the University Medical School, which was closed in 1914. The hospital building was thereafter called the Carpentier Hall.[88]

At that time, the founding of a united medical college in Canton was discussed among the medical missionaries and the Chinese medical professionals. Beginning in 1921, the students from the three medical colleges, Gongyi, Guanghua, and Hackett attended to the patients at the Canton Hospital, and the staff of the Canton Hospital gave lectures daily to those medical students. In 1929, the Lingnan University regents and the governing board of the Hackett Medial College reached an agreement to make Lingnan one of the largest co-educational schools in China. This program was firmly initiated in September when the Canton Hospital, which was to form the third link of this union, was officially re-opened with the support of the Lingnan University. Negotiations then began for the creation, with the Canton Hospital as a foundation, of a medical college, a cooperative venture of both the Lingnan University and the Hackett Medical College. In the middle of these negotiations, Zhong Rongguang, the president of Lingnan University, persuaded the new Nanjing government to construct a building on a site adjacent the Canton Hospital.[89]

On account of President Zhong's enthusiasm and vigorous endeavors, the Nationalist government in Nanjing assured the amount of half a million Mexican dollars and the support of yearly grants for the erection and establishment of the Sun Yat-sen Medical College, a suitable name for Lingnan's Medical College. After its registration with the Nationalist government in 1932, the Hackett Medical College adopted the standard six-year program, which was a requirement of all medical colleges in China, and required its students to have their internships at the hundred-bed David Gregg Hospital. In 1933, the Hackett and Canton Hospital complexes, in company with several smaller, mostly missionary ventures, were relocated by their boards to Lingnan University. The Hackett Medical College for Women was shut down and incorporated into Lingnan University as its medical department; the Canton Hospital became the teaching hospital for the medical students. Both Hackett and Lingnan University offered premedical courses, Hackett in Chinese and Lingnan in English. Consequently, the academic standard was raised steadily, the tuition and fees escalated, and the move to bilingual teaching with emphasis on English started. The students took introductory medical classes on the Lingnan campus and later did clinical work at both the Hackett and the Canton Hospital facilities, which were then put under Lingnan control. All those medical institutions were combined into the new Sun Yat-sen Medical College, registered with the Nanjing government in the 1930s.[90] These medical colleges and hospitals are still the most important medical and health institutions in Canton in the present day.[91]

The Effects of Medical Education for Women on Chinese Society

The establishment of the Hackett Medical College for Women had a great impact on China. With regard to the role the Hackett College would play in the Chinese society, the viceroy of Guangdong asserted at Hackett's 1907 commencement ceremony, "Money invested in such institutions as this college will bring vast relief, dissipate prejudice, and open the way for other needed reforms that will enable China to take a high place among other nations."[92] The formation of medical education for women in Canton played a role in modern transformation in China in four major areas.

First, the medical education for women in Canton and the American doctors' determination and encouragement, helped change many lower-class women's lives and elevate their social status. Luo Xiuyun was one of them. She was married at fourteen years old to a man she had not seen after the man paid her relatives 125 dollars for her. Some months after they were married, he went to New York where for ten years he was a laundryman. Occasionally, he sent some money, but, indeed, she was one of "such helpless girls being sold to men and becoming so much property to be used and disposed of as the men choose," according to Dr. Fulton.[93] Her aunt was a fine teacher of Chinese and had systematically trained her niece in the reading and writing of that language. At nearly sixteen years old, she applied to study medicine, and Dr. Fulton admitted her as a student. Dr. Luo described how Dr. Fulton had won her over during her years at a nearby Presbyterian girl school:

> I was selected by Dr. Fulton to study medicine. I was not fond of medicine, though I lived with Dr. Shi Mooi Hung. Whenever she came into the room from the hospital, I went out because I did not like the smell of iodoform. Dr. Fulton often asked me to study medicine. I did not agree to it at all. She wanted me to become interested in medicine so she took me to see students, interesting cases and operations. Within half a year, it melted my heart so I decided to study medicine.[94]

In 1904, Luo graduated from the Hackett Medical College. After graduating, she continued her work at Hackett for twelve years. Since there were only four members of staff without a single nurse in 1906, the staff had to perform many kinds of work. They sterilized utensils, kept the operating room clean, wrote diet lists, and counted the patients' clothes before and after washing. Even when they did have nurses later, they still had to teach them how to work and give lectures to them every day. Dr. Fulton later hired Luo as one of the instructors and as one of her assistants in the operating theater. In just several years, Luo became a competent surgeon, performing forty-five successive severe abdominal operations without the loss of a patient. She conducted 200 cases of caesarean section and took a big tumor of 105 pounds from a woman patient, which later was sent to Nanjing for display. She never weighed a hundred pounds and was pretty, delicately neat, quick and accurate. Dr. Fulton saw neither any lack of confidence even in cases of the severest risk, nor her hands shake in the most dangerous and complicated surgeries. She was excellent in surgery.[95]

When the nurse training school was opened, no students applied for the school at the commencement. As a determined recruiter, Dr. Fulton was always looking for smart, bright young girls interested in Christian medical services. Consequently, six or more clever, young women submitted applications and were accepted. They had never witnessed a qualified nurse before and were wary about a white set of clothes, white cap, and white socks because white was the Chinese symbol of grief. They, however, wanted to be "like American nurses," and appeared clean and pretty in the new uniforms.[96] Luo took up position as the head of the nursing school after helping Dr. Fulton open the Hackett College and the David Hospital. She once became the superintendent of the David Hospital and the president of the Hackett Medical College. The case of Dr. Luo indicated how the Hackett College turned a slave girl into a very successful and professional woman. American doctors in Hackett helped change many poor Chinese women's lives, as Luo Xiuyun wrote, "She [Dr. Fulton] gave more blessings to Chinese women than can be expressed in words. She elevated the position of Chinese women and gave them a good occupation. She trusted her students, gave them work to do, and helped them do their best. She loved God and mankind. She not only treated sickness but also gave comfort of soul."[97]

Mei Yagui was another example. She was born six hundred miles from Canton, a third child. When she was eight years old, her father had several wives but had lost all from gambling. Wives and sons were abandoned to take care of themselves, and the daughters were put up for sale. A man purchased her for twenty-eight dollars, and two years later, she was resold for fifty. She never again had any information about her family and was later taken to Canton. At the age of eighteen, she was paid eight dollars to marry a man, but two years later, he died in California. She was sent to a girls' school and became a Christian later. At the missionary school, she asked Dr. Kerr to teach her medicine, although at that time she had never seen a woman doctor. After finishing her medical studies, she became Dr. Kerr's assistant in the women's department.[98]

Returning to Canton, her former mother-in-law found herself in great poverty, losing her belongings without any money because her husband's uncle, an opium smoker, had sold everything. When Mei visited her mother-in-law and her uncle, they beat her and ordered her to worship the tablets and to light the incense stick. When she refused, her uncle bargained to sell her, and she escaped to her pastor, who advised her to marry a Christian man, just returning from Honolulu. When her mother-in-law heard that

Miss Mei attempted to get away from her, she mobilized her clan members, took a chain, and started forcibly to enter Dr. Fulton's dispensary to carry her back. As a result, urged by Dr. Fulton, the American consul in Canton asked the Cantonese official to send soldiers to protect the medical premises and disperse the mob. Miss Mei later became Dr. Fulton's assistant and was very helpful during their Guiping adventure in Guangxi Province in 1889. One of Mei Yagui's two daughters, after studying medicine, became one of the hospital directors and an instructor at the Hackett College. Miss Mei's case was typical of many poor girls in China at that time and the American doctors' effort to change their lives.[99]

Second, medical education for women in Canton helped promote women's medical education and new careers for women in China. Medical missionaries were pioneers in the education of Chinese women in medicine. The medical education for women attributed its foundation to the endeavors of American medical missionaries. The admission of two Chinese women to the South China Medical School in 1879 was the beginning of medical educational opportunities offered to Chinese women. Later, more medical schools in Canton as well as in other cities in China began to admit women students to study medicine. In the 1930s, medical missionaries supported only two women's medical colleges in China, the Hackett Medical College in Canton and the Women's Christian Medical College in Shanghai, but more female students graduated from other medical colleges. In 1933, 463 female medical students graduated from all ten medical colleges in China, not just the women's colleges, and ninety-six women students came back to China after finishing their medical studies in the U.S., Canada, Japan, and Great Britain.[100]

When the Nanjing government initiated comprehensive medical and public fitness programs in the 1930s, the request for women doctors increased considerably because most Chinese women had a preference to seek advice from female physicians.[101] Beginning in 1929, registration of physicians became compulsory, and in 1937, the number of registered Chinese male doctors was 8,191 exceeding that of 907 female doctors by the ratio of 9 to 1, as stated by the statistics of the Nanjing government.[102] Without a doubt, the number of female medical students looked small, and most of them by and large came from prosperous families. Medical missionaries, however, not only opened the door of medical education to women but also provided a new professional alternative for women. Medicine was becoming one of the best-paid professions open to women in China at that time.

Third, medical education for women in Canton marked the beginning of coeducation in colleges in China. Since the Hackett College opened up higher education to women, Chinese women could go to colleges for the first time. Influenced by the Canton Hospital's medical school and later the Hackett College, the Canton Christian College bravely led in this remarkable direction and conducted the most progressive, coeducational experiments in Canton. The Canton Christian College became the first college in China to admit women when it opened its Preparatory Department to four girls in 1906, who attended classes with the boys. President Oscar F. Wisner was careful to state that the College was not committed to coeducation but had made such an arrangement since at that time there was no other condition in Canton for the higher education of women. The experiment was making good progress, and the girls performed so well that the practice was later extended to the Collegiate Department. Under the influence of the Canton Hospital and Hackett to some extent, the Guanghua Medical School also put co-education into practice in 1908 to recruit not only male but also female students. In 1910, a medical school for women was opened, and in 1911 male and female students were combined into one school.[103]

The Gongyi Medical School followed. In 1911, Gongyi opened the Zanyu Medical School for Women on the opposite bank of the Pearl River with only six students, originally and principally, to take care of maternity and children's cases. In 1912, Gongyi took charge of a hospital situated in the heart of Henan Island and turned it into a clinic for outpatients, and its activities were extended to include the Zanyu school.[104] In 1921, women students were re-admitted to be educated together with the men in combined classes at Gongyi. Thus, Canton became China's first city where colleges were made coeducational. The regular colleges in China did not become coeducational until 1919 when coeducation first began at the government university in Beijing. Other Christian colleges followed more slowly: Shandong Christian Medical College in 1921, West China Union University in 1924, Shandong Christian College in 1926, Suzhou University in 1928, and Hangzhou University in 1929.[105]

Finally, the Hackett College helped promote nursing programs in China. China's traditional health therapy was usually provided by a variety of para-medical and medical persons with family members taking care of their ailing relatives every day. The profession of nursing did not actually appear until the late nineteenth century, and modern Chinese nursing developed as a result of the inspiration of the medical missionaries. In 1902, the Julia M. Turner (Rouji Duanna) Training School for Nurses was organized in connection with the David Gregg Hospital at Canton, offering a curriculum of two years.[106] Six female students were admitted to the school, but only one student Li Fengzhen graduated in 1906, who thereafter became China's first nurse-in-chief. By 1909, when the second graduation was held, four pupils had successfully passed while eleven were in training.[107] In late 1928 when the Hackett's chief American missionary nurse departed to care for her sick mother, a Chinese woman was for the first time appointed both superintendent of nurses and acting principal of the nursing school.[108] A total of 180 nurses had graduated by 1934, and most of the graduates were working in Canton and in other provinces as well as Honolulu.[109]

The Rouji School generated public health nurse, the first one of such kind in China. To solve such problems as maternal and child health, tuberculosis, venereal disease, or nutrition, it was necessary to use health workers who could teach and work with those people in a manner personalized to their practical needs. Endeavors to provide home nursing on an organized basis for the sick poor were made in Canton in the 1920s. Since public health work was becoming important for the Cantonese, the Rouji Hospital sent Turner Nursing School's graduates to the Beijing United Hospital to study the nursing work. After completing their studies and returning to Canton, the Hackett Medical College was able to send public health nurses to the patients' homes for recovery. Those public health nurses visited those patients at their homes after they had visited the hospital or produced babies at the hospital but still needed nursing services. Those nurses took care of the patients and charged them according to patients' economic conditions; sometimes they did not charge any money.[110] In 1931, the Turner Training School for Nurses put greater emphasis on its public health work. The School's prenatal and postnatal clinic and child welfare clinic were making gratifying progress and the nurses of the School gave valuable help at the two health campaigns held in Canton in March and November in 1931, according to the School's 1931 report.[111]

The founding of the Hackett nursing school led to the increasing number of the nursing schools in Canton. The Canton Hospital started training of female nurses in the late nineteenth century, but systematic training of nurses did not start until a nursing school for both men and women was organized in 1912 with the help of Mr. and Mrs. Louis Schwa of New York, who started to provide the annual support. Consequently, the services of Miss Evelyn M. Manful were secured. The training school for nurses was completely reorganized when the American Baptist Missionary Society transferred Miss Luciele A. Whithers in 1915 from Shantou, 300 miles east of Canton, to the Canton Hospital. When the Canton Hospital was reopened in 1933, Miss Lillian Xu, a Cantonese nurse accepted the position of superintendent.[112] In 1913, only three students were studying at the Nursing School and twenty-six in 1921, half of whom were female. From 1916 to 1926, sixty-seven students graduated from the three-year program of the School, thirty of whom were female. When the Nursing School was reopened in 1933, all of the students were female, and this school had trained a great number of nurses, both men and women, for the care of patients.[113]

The Gongyi Hospital at Canton made endeavors to open a nursing school under Mrs. Margaret S. Todd, R. N., in 1911 not long after its commencement. It was later registered with the Nurses' Association of China in 1918. By 1925, thirty-seven students had graduated from the school, seventeen of whom had obtained the official diplomas. In 1912, the Guanghua Medical College opened a nursing school with a three-year program to solve the problem of lack of nurses in Canton and did not charge students tuition. In 1934, 167 midwifes graduated from Guanghua, and by 1935, eighty nurses graduated. The Two Guang Baptist Hospital also opened an advanced nursing school in 1924. Thus, by the 1930s, Canton had about ten nursing schools, taking the lead in training nurses in China.[114]

The first school for Chinese nurses was opened by American Ella Johnson in 1888 in Fuzhou, the capital of Fujian Province. The training of nurses began in 1909 in Changsha, the capital of Hunan Province. In 1935, China had about thirty formal nursing schools.[115] Canton did not train formally the first nurses in China, but produced many well-trained nurses between the 1920s and 1930s, which had an effect on the medical and health work not only in Canton, but also in other cities.

Medical and Health Work of Hackett's Alumnae

Dr. Fulton asserted that the best program to satisfy the increasing request for competent physicians was to instruct the Chinese to serve their own people and that her students did "enter to learn, go forth to serve."[116] American doctors' encouragement helped their students assume new and difficult tasks in Chinese society. Many doctors and nurses whom American doctors had instructed were responding to requests and were taking on demanding tasks in Chinese society. Some of the alumnae were working at the government or missionary hospitals and dispensaries established by philanthropic people for the poor, some were practicing medicine at their own private clinics, and some were teaching at medical schools.

Since Hackett's founding, its many students had gained good reputations in Canton and elsewhere to meet the shortage of women doctors and nurses. This small group of women doctors, together with the female nurses, not only provided modern medical services to the Chinese women but also promoted health care and child welfare and organized health campaigns, contributing considerably to the improvement of many women's physical condition in the 1920s and 1930s. The women doctors and nurses also became involved in the introduction of new conceptions of women's bodies and Western systems of health care and instructed the masses in social hygiene. Their endeavors to introduce scientific knowledge about female biology and physiology destroyed the myths and restrictions in connection with menstruation, pregnancy, and childbirth.[117]

Medical and Health Work in Canton

Xia Aiqiong contributed significantly to women's and children's health in Canton in the 1920s and 1930s. After graduating from Hackett, she worked as a gynecologist at the Canton Hospital. At the beginning of the early twentieth century, the infant mortality rate was high because most Cantonese women, like other Chinese women, assisted by their midwives, delivered their children at home under unsanitary conditions. Thus, some Cantonese businessmen and merchants helped build modern hospitals and encouraged pregnant women to produce their babies in the sanitary environment of a hospital. Most women, however, still preferred staying at home rather than going to modern hospitals because of some male midwives at such hospitals or the high cost of medical expense. After witnessing traditional, backward methods used by midwives to deliver babies, Xia resigned from the Canton Hospital in 1907 and opened a seventeen-bed hospital for women and children (maternity home) in western Canton. She also opened obstetric workshops so as to train midwives, which later became the obstetric medical school. The Women and Child Hospital opened a maternal school of a two-year term later. In 1912, she expanded the women's and children's hospital by opening another branch in central Canton, where a maternity home was housed. In the late 1920s, she transformed the maternity home into a midwifery school, which consequently recruited 200 students, including ninety boarding students.[118]

In 1932, the midwifery school became the center of the hospital while the original hospital became a branch. At that time, four physicians were working at the ninety-ward-bed hospital, and about 250 babies were delivered at the hospital each month. The delivery and medical costs were free for poor women while the hospital often donated funds in support of social welfare and charity. By 1934, more than 1,000 students graduated from the school. The two dispensaries had four doctors, eleven nurses, ninety-eight ward beds, and yearly treated 827 inpatients and 1,681 outpatients.[119]

Xia's maternity clinic and school, without doubt, helped many Cantonese women change their attitudes toward Western professional midwives, who had modern medical knowledge and arts as well as efficient tools of delivery. By the 1930s, many Cantonese women had accepted Western medicine, producing their babies either at hospitals or at home with the help of the modern-trained midwives, and there was a significant reduction of maternal death rate. Dr. Xia contributed considerably to the improvement of many Cantonese women's physical condition in the 1920s and 1930s.[120]

Liang Yiwen, born in Guangzhou in 1903, studied medicine at Hackett Medical College for Women from 1917 to 1923. After her graduation, she became resident physician at Shanghai Hospital for Women and Children. In 1925, she returned to Canton, working at the David Gregg Hospital and the Canton Hospital. In 1926 she studied maternity and pediatrics at Beijing Union Medical College, and in 1927 she was a physician in the Department of Obstetrics and Gynecology at the David Gregg Hospital and later the chair of the Department in 1928. In 1929 she was studying obstetrics and gynecology at the Medical College in Philadelphia in the United States, gaining her doctorate degree in medicine. After studying obstetrics, anatomy, and pathology at the medical center in Vienna, Austria for a while, she returned home and assumed again the position of director of the Department of Obstetrics and Gynecology at David Gregg Hospital in Canton in 1931, according to the 1931 Report of Jessie A. MacBean, the superintendent of the Hospital.[121]

Dr. Liang contributed considerably to women's medicine. In the 1930s, many Cantonese women died when delivering babies. Dr. Liang was the first in Canton to transfuse the patients' own blood in cases of ectopic pregnancy (a complication of pregnancy in which the pregnancy implants outside the uterine cavity) and to use new technologies for the diagnosis of ectopic pregnancy bleeding. She also pioneered the use of Western medical treatment of dysmenorrhea (a gynecological medical condition characterized by severe uterine pain during menstruation), using chromosomes in the inspection of uteritis (inflammation of the womb) and conducting screening of the cervix of the womb so as to diagnose early cancer of uterus.[122] Many Cantonese boatwomen, who lived on boats along the banks of the Pearl River, had frequent difficult births in the 1930s. Dr. Liang, while trying to seek medical treatments of dystocias (abnormal or difficult childbirth or labor) for those boatwomen, carried out research in detail on their lives on boats. She finally came to a conclusion that those boatwomen living on boats tilted forward while they were working. Their workload was so heavy that their pelvises changed, which led to difficulties in childbirth. As a result, while attending her patients, Dr. Liang always asked those young women of reproductive age to be very careful, especially to sleep supine so as to avoid changes of the position of their pelvises. Her suggestions helped greatly reduce the mortality rate of both babies and their mothers attended by her. By 1933, she had assumed the deanship of the Hackett College.[123]

Dr. Liang also committed herself to the treatment of infertility in Canton in the 1930s. During that time, infertile women had to endure tremendous mental pressure, some of whom were forced out of their husbands' homes. Dr. Laing was the first in China to adopt the method of cervical dilation, in proportion to women's physical characteristics. It was said that when women sought Dr. Liang's treatment, approximately 60 percent of them would become pregnant. For this reason, she became well known in China in the 1930s.[124]

Zhang Zhujun also contributed significantly to the Cantonese women's health. She was born to a wealthy family in Canton. Early in her childhood, Zhang suffered from polio, stricken with a semi-paralyzing illness. Since the local famous physicians of Chinese medicine did not know how to cure the disease, her prosperous family sent her to the Canton Hospital for healing. After being treated for a long time, she was finally restored to health. She then converted to Christianity and was determined to study Western medicine. She was admitted in 1897 to the medical school of the Canton Hospital but graduated with honor in 1900 from the Hackett Medical College for Women, which was affiliated with the Canton Hospital at that time. She began practicing Western medicine and established her Difu Dispensary and Nanfu Dispensary in Canton in 1901, becoming the first Chinese to open a dispensary and the first female head of a dispensary in China. In 1902, she was appointed as the president assistant of the China Hospital in Singapore while visiting there.[125]

When a cholera epidemic occurred in Canton in 1904, nine charity associations held a meeting to discuss methods to control the disease. During the conference, Zhang suggested that perishable melons and vegetables be banned from being sold, and that the patients' excrement be burned instead of being dumped in rivers. She also pointed out that both the patients' excrement and water pollution in river contributed to the spread of the disease, discouraging inhabitants from drinking contaminated water from river and wells. She even urged the county magistrates to use big ships to transport clean water from the outskirts of Canton to the Cantonese residents. As a result, the magistrates of both Nanhai and Panyu counties adopted her suggestions to take preventive measures and requested the military authorities to send four warships to tow forty ships to transport clean water for Canton residents. The epidemic was eventually under control. Because of her outstanding medical experience and friendly personality, she won immense admiration, recognition, and friendship from local people irrespective of age or sex. Her medical activities, which aimed to help the poor as well as the rich, kept her treatment center crowded with patients night and day.[126]

Liang Huanzhen was an alumna of the Hackett College, too. Impressed by the image of doctors of Western medicine, she had a dream to become a physician when she was young. At the age of fifteen, she was admitted to study medicine at the Hackett College for Women. After her graduation in 1905, Liang was working at the Canton Hospital as a resident doctor. In 1910, Liang and other Cantonese medical elite organized the Guanghua Medical Society and opened a medical school for women. Given that many hospitals in Canton focused only on diagnosis and surgery without teaching the patients how to maintain their health at that time, Liang Huanzhen, together with Liang Peiji, Luo Xiuyun, and others, established in the late 1910s a convalescent hospital in eastern Canton in order to help the people learn how to keep their health. In 1921, the Canton Municipal Health Department established a medical advisory committee in order to seek the medical experts' suggestions in connection with the development of Canton health program. Ten famous medical professionals in Canton served on the committee, including Liang, an expert in public health.[127]

Huang Dexin, after graduating from the Hackett Medical College in 1918, worked at the Rouji Hospital as resident doctor and later assumed the chair of the Department of Obstetrics and Gynecology. Afterward she left Rouji and worked at the Baoyu Shanhui, a charitable organization, for several years.

In the 1927, Dr. Huang and opened the Baosheng Hospital and an obstetric nursing school where she was teaching women medicine.[128]

Medical and Health Work outside Canton

The Hackett College trained China's first women medical professionals, who played a significant role in medical modernization not only in Canton but also in many provinces in China as well as in other countries. By the 1930s, all Chinese women physicians in southern China had been educated either by Dr. Fulton or by her students. Their influence extended wherever Cantonese-speaking people were found, as Dr. A. A. Fulton wrote: "Out of the unfavorable environment of those early days has grown the splendid institution whose beneficent influence saves life and spreads light on thousands of home in many provinces of old China."[129]

Gao Xinrong was one of the examples. Gao was born to a middle-class family in Hubei Province in 1905. In 1921, Gao's mother was so severely sick that she was in danger of dying, and later her life was saved after a operation performed by a surgeon. Gao was so grateful to the surgeon that she decided to study Western medicine to become a doctor. She enrolled in the Hackett Medical College and graduated in 1929. After graduation, she practiced women's medicine in the city of Qingdao in Shandong Province. In 1935 she moved to the city of Tianjin, about 100 miles east of Beijing, to continue practicing of medicine at a hospital. Some young men wanted to be engaged with her when she was studying at the college and was practicing medicine after graduation, but she refused because she kept in mind the admonitions of Dr. Guan Xianhe, then the dean of the Hackett College for Women. Dr. Guan once stated that it would take at least thirty years to become a famous doctor and that the most important period was the first five years immediately after graduation from the medical college. Guan also claimed that a doctor would not have a lot of successful achievements if he or she was too much engaged in routine family business. As a result, Gao remained unmarried and dedicated herself to treating women patients. She soon became an eminent doctor of women's medicine in China in the 1930s.[130]

Huang Xuezhen was another case. After graduation in 1902 from Hackett, she was assisting Dr. Nile and was teaching at the college. Later she served as the director of the Zanyu Xueshe in Canton, a philanthropic institute helping the poor women deliver their babies without any charges. As the only one female doctor to assist with delivery, she worked very hard because too many poor women came to visit her for medical treatments and consultations. Later, she moved to Zhongshan County in Guangdong and served as the director of both the foundling hospital and the Baoyu shanhui, a charitable institution. In 1913, she returned to Canton and served as the director of the Guangzhou Yuyingyuan (Guangzhou Foundling Hospital). In the 1920s, she moved to Changsha, the capital of Hunan Province, and served as the president of the Xinyi Hospital there. Practicing medicine for more than twenty years, she took care of many cases, most of which were gynecology, obstetrics, and pediatrics.[131]

Zhang Zhujun also significantly contributed to the improvement of women's health in Shanghai. In 1904, Zhang moved to Shanghai and founded a Sino-Western Medical College for Women as a joint project between a professional merchant and herself. Her male colleague was responsible for the traditional sector of the program, and she taught medical courses. She was the president of the College, where forty students were enrolled. The College was to train women in obstetrics and gynecology, the first medical college for women in Shanghai.[132] In July 1909, the Shanghai Hospital was opened, the first modern hospital run by the Chinese in Shanghai, and Dr. Zhang was appointed as the superintendent.[133]

After 1912, Zhang continued her medical practice in Shanghai, but lived quietly and never asserted herself above others. She remained unmarried and dedicated herself to curing patients in the 1920s. In 1926, when cholera erupted in Shanghai, she transformed her Jianhua yiji yuan (Convalescent Hospital) into to a Huxi shiyi yiyuan (Hospital for Infectious Disease) provisionally to accommodate an increasing number of patients assaulted by the disease. Zhang made great endeavors to set up more beds, urge very sick patients to stay at the hospital, and do away immediately with all remains of the patients so as to control the spread of the plague.[134] Later, with the financial assistance from her friends, she founded several Western-style hospitals and schools in different provinces.[135]

It was said that 90 percent of the Hackett College alumnae were confirmed practicing medicine energetically in fourteen provinces in China and in other countries.[136] A new historical outline of the Hackett Medical College appeared in 1926 when the *China Medical Journal* issued an educational edition. In this article, Dr. Hofmann wrote,

> Hackett has graduated 155 students during its twenty-seven years. This includes the students who came to it from Dr. Kerr's class. The graduates have scattered to at least ten of the provinces of China, to Hong Kong, Macao, Singapore, Java, and Borneo. About 60% are in private practice, 20% are in the employ of Missions, and the rest are with government or other native charities, are doing post-graduate study, or are not practicing.[137]

The Hackett College alumnae played an imperative part in promoting Western medicine, providing medical services to Chinese women, and carrying out health work, especially women's health work, in China in the first three decades of the twentieth century.

The Cantonese Women Doctors and Social Reform in China

The medical missionaries went to China initially to promote Christianity, rather than as a deliberate driving force of social change, but they advocated a bigger role for women both in their own missionary communities and in Chinese society. The changes that were brought about by that were significant, but were not their objective. Medical missionaries wanted to renovate Chinese society along Christian notions without revolutionizing its basis. With the introduction of Western medicine into China, social restrictions on Chinese women were broken by two phenomena in Canton in the late Qing and early Republic periods. The first phenomenon consisted of American male and female doctors who broke with the Chinese custom of taking care of Chinese women in public places, and the women patients who were willing to be attended to at the modern hospitals.

The second phenomenon consisted of the Chinese women medical students and the Chinese women doctors. American doctors gave their students useful tools with which they could begin to become independent from the traditionally subordinate role of women in China. In addition, American doctors trained the Chinese women not only to make their way in a still very male world, but also emphasized the ideas of women's rights to some degree, while teaching their students. Most female medical students could not have graduated without learning at least some parts of Western culture or some core Western values from their teachers who had wide-ranging influence in them. It is a little difficult to assess how the Cantonese female medical elite absorbed American culture, but they, while carrying out medical and health work, did challenge Chinese traditions. Some of them promoted social reform and took the lead in the modern women's rights movement in China, especially in Canton.[138]

Women's Social Role

The Cantonese women doctors began to play a role in Cantonese society. They became pioneers of what it meant to be a new woman in Canton. They opened new businesses or established new organizations, helped women learn equality of the sexes, and promoted women's social involvement. Dr. Harriet M. Allyn, the dean of the Hackett College in the 1920s, believed that the Hackett College not only trained China's first female medical professionals, but also China's new women. She wrote:

> Not only does their training in college fit them for leadership, but also the practice of their profession itself.... They develop courage and initiatives. Such women are resourceful, serious thinkers, full of determinations.[139]

Zhang Zhujun was one of the examples. After graduation, for instance, Zhang Zhujun opened a philanthropic clinic of her own in Canton. She apparently cut a striking figure when making her house calls, usually dressing in Western clothing, putting on leather shoes, reading an English-language book, and riding a specially designed sedan chair held by four men. To avoid the summer high temperatures, she stayed in a vessel along the Pearl River. She was very active in Cantonese society, traveling freely everywhere and frequently giving public speeches.[140]

As a devoted Christian, Zhang organized Bible study classes for her friends and disbelievers and preached the Gospel in a temporary chapel beside her clinic. She delivered speeches every night on Christianity and sometimes talked about the wrong restrictions of St. Paul against women speaking in church. As a feminist, by way of her lectures and writings, Zhang encouraged equality between men and women, in accordance with Christian doctrines, and advocated women's education and independence. She claimed that if all the Chinese, men and women, performed their obligations as citizens, China could keep pace with Western countries. Her energetic, radical activities led to her being admired as a new woman, acclaimed as the Female Liang Qichao (the famous Cantonese reformer).[141] Several Hackett alumnae became the community leaders in Cantonese society in the 1920s. As Dr. J. Allen Hofmann wrote, "There is also a growing helpfulness among the alumnae, many of whom have become influential members of society."[142]

Women's Educational Rights

Education rights were an important part of women's rights. In 1902, Zhang Zhujun and several others established in Canton the first private girls' school, named Gongyi nuxue, run by the Chinese, and later opened another one, Yuxian nuxue.[143] While practicing medicine, Zhang taught her students science as well as medicine. In her class of about ten students, she always discussed current affairs and criticized the national crisis in China. She talked about the disadvantages of the low social status of Chinese women, her opinions of self-conduct, and her own stories.[144] The main purpose of her project in Canton was to train the Cantonese girls to learn skills so that they could earn their own living when necessary. Influenced partly by Zhang's schools for girls, more private girls' schools were established by the Cantonese at the beginning of the twentieth century. In 1904, the Kunwei School was founded in Canton, and by 1907, there were seven private girls' schools in Canton. In the meantime, more private girls' schools began to appear in other cities in China, eleven schools in Shanghai, three in Nanjing, and two in Tianjin. By the late Qing period, Canton's education for women took the lead in China in terms of the number of girls' schools, particularly the number of Christian students, but in terms of the number of the women's schools run by the Chinese, Canton was behind Beijing, Shanghai, and other cities because the political situation was not stable in Canton.

Canton, however, took the lead in women professional education. In China, professional education for women started with medical education, and missionary medical training of women physicians remained virtually the only possible source of modern professional education for Chinese women at the end of the nineteenth century. Canton became the first city to develop women medical education. At the beginning of the twentieth century, other professional education for women, in addition to medical schools, began to appear in Canton, such as nursing schools. In 1917, the Guangdong Professional Institute for Women was established, which had such departments as embroidery and Western tailoring, the first professional school for women in Canton.[145]

Women's Working Rights

Women's working rights were a significant part of women's rights. The Cantonese female doctors began to appear in Canton in the 1880s, the first female professionals in imperial China; Afterward, female nurses and teachers began to emerge, becoming new female professionals. At the beginning of the twentieth century, the most popular profession among the modern educated women was as doctors and nurses, apart from teachers; the medical profession perhaps remained new women's most popular lifework. By 1935, Hackett had graduated approximately 240 women doctors, Guanghua Medical School 146 female physicians, and Gongyi Medical School sixty-two.[146] Most of those female medical doctors as well as nurses and pharmacists worked at hospitals, dispensaries, and medical institutions in Canton; some worked in other provinces in China, even abroad in such countries as England, the United States, France, and Australia.

The medical training of women played a role in changing women's lives in the journey towards women's equal participation in a larger world, which, to some extent, contributed to the rise of women manufacturers, technicians, office clerks, and workers in Canton. Women manufacturers began to appear in Canton in the 1910s, where no less than forty factories, making socks, shirts and the like, were owned and operated entirely by the women. Nine or ten factories employed from forty to fifty women each while the rest had from eight to ten. The Yuhung Knitting Company of Canton, run by the women, employed more than fifty persons, making annual profits of US$100,000.[147]

More professional jobs were open to the women in Canton in the 1920s. On January 27, 1921, the Guangshan Railroad Bureau held open examinations in Canton to recruit female trainee ticket sellers and ticket inspectors. Forty women, thereafter, were employed as accounting clerks and office secretaries as well as ticket sellers. Thus female office clerks began to be acceptable for the first time in China, which opened more office jobs to women employment.[148] The Telephone Bureau also adopted such measures as the Railroad

Bureau and hired new female employees. By the beginning of 1924, 157 female telephone operators were employed, and most Cantonese were satisfied with their excellent service. Female telephone operators began to be appealing in Canton, an important step to open a new career for Cantonese women.[149]

Zhang's Thinking on Women's Rights and Her Practice in Shanghai

Zhang Zhujun, a vigorous Cantonese feminist, not only promoted the women's rights movement in Canton, but also in Shanghai. In 1904, Dr. Zhang moved her practice to Shanghai. Once in Shanghai, she was warmly accepted by the local people as a public figure because her fame was widespread, due to a laudatory biography of her, which appeared in the April 1902 issue of *Xingmin congbao* (Journal of New Citizen).[150] During that time Dr. Zhang began to develop her thinking on women's rights and played a role in the modern women's rights movement in Shanghai.

First, Zhang believed that Chinese women needed education to combat ignorance and gain independence economically. In an article published in 1907 in the journal, *Alarm Bell*, Zhang described a number of settings, in which the upper class women found themselves economically helpless. Zhang claimed that such circumstances could be avoided or rectified through education making them self-sufficient. Taking her own case as an example, Zhang stated, "I study hygiene and am involved in manufacturing in order to attain women's self-strengthening and self-support." She maintained that ignorance had confined the women to a dependent existence and forced families to rely simply on their own endurance, and that male subjugation was only a part of the problem. Zhang contended that the women were accountable for their tolerance of this miserable situation as a result of their lack of the knowledge, the same inspirations as those advocated by Liang Qichao before. She also told the prosperous Chinese women once more that "wealth and honor are inconstant," and that the Chinese women should regard both Harriet Beecher Stowe and Florence Nightingale as models. Finally, Zhang claimed that women's ignorance, as well as the low level of maternal education, produced a weak Chinese race, which would struggle to survive in the modern world. As a solution to the women's education issue, supported by the Aiguo nuxuexiao (Patriot Girls' School), Zhang opened a girls' school in Shanghai in 1904.[151] She also founded Nuzi xinxue baoxian hui (The Women's Association for Security through Learning) in the same year to promote women's education, open new schools, and provide some financial assistance, as the objectives of the society set forth in her announcement stated.[152]

Second, Zhang criticized women's bad habits and advocated improvement of women's ill health. In 1904, she founded the Society for the Promotion of Hygiene, an organization to offer a three-month course in basic medical information and practice and a preliminary step towards a medical school for women.[153] During its first meeting, Zhang connected the Chinese's backwardness to their weak bodies. She explained the damage done by make-up from a hygienic point of view because the lead-based make-up was harmful and sometimes deadly. She claimed that women had to keep these harmful practices, because their dependence meant they needed to attract men to support themselves. Zhang argued that a key solution to this was to combine bodily culture with the knowledge of trade, so that women could be in good physical shape and economically independent. Later, Zhang offered lectures on hygiene and provided free medical consultation and treatment, which helped the women understand the significant role of modern sanitation in the preservation of the Chinese race. Zhang also condemned the evil of footbinding, claiming that during the Song dynasty, Confucianism had a stronger bias against women than ever before, and that since then many rich Chinese men regarded little feet as beautiful and forced their daughters to bind their feet in order to satisfy the men's perspective of beauty. The Chinese had to eliminate such evil in Chinese society, Dr. Zhang wrote in 1907.[154]

Third, Dr. Zhang thought that Chinese women needed to establish their own organizations and institutions to gain their independence and rights, joining together in effective groups to work toward their goals. Grieving over the miserable position of Chinese women and listing the difficulties and dangers which Chinese women had to face, Zhang proposed her programs for organizing women into a large association so that the position of women in society would be improved through mutual help and learning. Zhang did soon organize several enterprises to encourage the social and economic independence of women. In 1914, Zhang founded Nuzi shougong chuanxi suo (Handicraft Institute for Women) at the Girls' Patriotic School, which had a three-month program in hand and machine sewing. The Institute thereafter became an independent workshop where the students studied music, English, and composition. Zhang's Institute helped the women learn their skills to acquire the means of self-support and to use their power in the public interest. Under Zhang's influence to some degree, more women associations were founded in Shanghai. By 1914, a women's bank and several women-run shops, such as the Women's Encouragement of Enterprise Company, the National Women's Products Company, and the Women's Love of China Association, had been founded in Shanghai to promote the use of native products.[155]

Finally, Zhang pushed the Chinese women, like Chinese men, to fight for national survival and to play a role in the nation-building movement. Zhang, after examining the current condition of Chinese men, said "Chinese men today are exposed to outside pressure to less extent than women, but like women, they put up with a dark, backward country under Western subjugation as well as tyrannical rule." As said by Dr. Zhang, the situation of Chinese men was not much better than that of the women, and the men, like the women, did not have any political powers so the women could not press hard upon the men and could not expect them to make efforts to improve women's social status and to promote their rights. Dr. Zhang claimed that China was in a critical situation, and that Chinese men had to take half of the blame while the humble women took the rest. As a result, Zhang alleged that the Chinese women's rights movement should not become a women's rebellion against men's domination, as in Western countries. Both the Chinese men and women had to answer the national call to participate in the national salvation and the self-strengthening movement. Zhang, however, believed that the women had a different role in nation-building, urging the women to look beyond the armies. She expressed her disapproval of women's fighting role because the women, not physically up to the men, would be an obstruction on the battlefield, and that there were many other ways women could make themselves useful for the nation. She stated in 1912, "The new Republic has just been founded, and countless businesses were lying ahead for us to do. Those women, who have the ambitions to help our nation and society, have the greatest value, and their tasks are numerous. I discourage women, however, from serving in the army."[156] At that time, Zhang was critical of the contemporary call for women's participation in bloody battles, albeit for the sake of a very noble goal—the Chinese nation. Zhang strongly opposed the establishment of women armies because, as a general practitioner, she believed that practicing medicine or saving lives could serve the Chinese nation better than a noble death in fighting.[157]

In brief, Zhang addressed the issue of the women question and the question of women's education, and the link between women and the national question, taking on the problems of national rejuvenation and female liberation. These questions and issues were first discussed and theorized in reform journals of the late 1890; several justifications for women's education as a key component of national strengthening had been put forward by the enlightening Cantonese reformers, such as Liang Qichao. Zhang, however, not only upheld and promoted those ideas but also carried out social reform in Shanghai by establishing the girls' schools, the women's institute, and the women's association. She was a promoter of women's education and professionalization, playing an imperative role in the modern women's rights movement in China.

The Cantonese Women Doctors' Political Role and Influence

The Hackett's alumnae and students not only raised women's social and economic status in the women's rights movement, but also played a political role in Chinese society. They began to cultivate their national consciousness, became involved in the revolutionary movement, and were vigorous in the anti-Western campaigns. Their political role and influence in part inspired the Cantonese women to fight for their voting and political rights.

The Revolutionary Movement

The Hackett alumnae took part in the revolutionary movement. Liang Huan-zhen was one of them. When Liang was studying at the Hackett Medical College, Professor Xu Ganlai was interested in revolutionary ideas and often discussed with her about China's destiny and the reasons for a revolution to overthrow the Qing dynasty, sometimes conversing until midnight. Deeply impressed by his talk, Liang became interested in the anti-Manchu movement and tried to devote herself to the revolutionary cause. During that time, both Shi Meiqing, alumna of the Hackett Medical College, and Liang, sharing the same political ideology, became good friends and often discussed the issues of reform and revolution.[158]

After graduation, Liang was working at the hospital as a resident doctor. In 1905, Liang was depressed because Professor Shi, her good friend, died of a disease. Liang left the Canton Hospital in 1906 after one-year service there and practiced medicine at the Zanyu xueshe, a charitable institution taking care of the poor and the sick. In 1907, Liang joined Tongmeng hui (Revolutionary Alliance) founded by Sun Yat-sen in Tokyo in 1905 in an attempt to overthrow the Manchu regime. Thereafter Liang established an office for the Guangdong revolutionaries at her clinic, together with such well-known revolutionaries as Zhu Zhixin, Hu Yisheng, and others. Liang secretly promoted revolutionary ideas and encouraged the medical students and the Christians to participate in the Revolutionary Alliance. In 1909, Sun sent Liang and others to Canton to establish the Canton branch of the Revolutionary Alliance, and soon the Canton branch had recruited more than 2,000 members, most of whom were soldiers in Canton. Impressed by Liang's activities, Wang Jingwei, one of the leaders of the Revolutionary Alliance, visited her clinic and discussed revolution strategies with Liang. Both of them agreed that it was urgently needed to promote revolutionary ideas among the lower classes. For this reason, Liang decided to establish a hospital and an obstetrics school for the ordinary people. While teaching medicine and giving lectures on diagnosis at the Hackett Medical College and other schools, she tried to promote revolutionary ideas among students to overthrow the Manchu government.[159] The revolutionary doctor Liang Huanzhen played a role in the revolutionary movement in Canton before the 1911 Revolution because the Hackett College, like the Canton Hospital, provided a new public sphere to the Cantonese women. With this advantage, the medical students had the opportunity and freedom to discuss their ideas of reform and revolution, which helped turn them into reformers and revolutionaries.

Liang was not an isolated case; the revolutionary doctor Zhang Zhujun was another example. Prior to the 1911 revolution, Zhang was practicing medicine and running her several hospitals in Shanghai. Many of her close associates, such as Hu Hanmin and Shi Jianru, later were prominent Republican politicians. In October of 1911, the revolution began with small-scale fighting at the city of Wuchang and then spread swiftly. Many Chinese women supported the revolution. The women street orators in Shanghai pushed the masses to help the revolution with money and volunteer service. The women in the force, sent by the Revolutionary Alliance to free Guangdong from the Qing government, worked as barbers to cut the pigtails of those people denying the Manchu regime. The women began to organize volunteer corps. Some doctors in Wuhan seemed to have started a Red Cross relief undertaking at an earlier time.[160]

Zhang wanted to take the advantage of her practical competence as a medical doctor by organizing a Red Cross Society when writing a strong letter to the director of the Red Cross Association, attacking its indifference and the confidentiality of its accounting. Zhang's own volunteer Red Cross Society then launched a campaign for the relief work, and her activities were closely related to the Shanghai Girls' Volunteer Corps Daring to Die. She united several local hospitals to establish a medical corps consisting of sixty-nine men and fifty-four women to help the wounded in Hankou. They formed two teams, leaving Shanghai separately for Hankou on September 3 and September 29. They put on quasi-military dress, rode small horses, and led the medical unit to the battle zones.[161]

Zhang and her teams cared for over one thousand injured solders in the two-month period in which she was stationed in Hankou and Hanyang, and she consequently took care of another thousand or more wounded troop when the revolutionary armies marched from Zhengjiang to Nanjing. Zhang also alone performed over a hundred amputations in three days. Not one of her nurses left under attack, performing well in relief activities in aid of the wounded. A women's team was effective in preparing clothing and blankets for the wounded soldiers.[162]

In the meantime, Dr. Zhang was asked by her sponsor, a very intimate friend who previously put money into her hospital building, to safeguard some revolutionaries traversing the Yangzi River so as to get to Hankou and to organize the revolt. As a result, the leaders of the Wuhan Uprising, including Huang Xin, disguised as member of the Red Cross, were able to arrive at their destination unharmed with the assistance of Zhang's medical team.[163]

On December 25, 1911, Zhang gave a speech during a meeting. She was so saddened by the high number of causalities among the revolutionaries that she would like to surrender the Red Cross relief work and enroll in the revolutionary armies against the Qing military. Her appearance in military dress drew the attention of the listeners.[164] Zhang and her medical team played a role in the Wuhan rebellion of the 1911 Revolution.

Nationalistic Women Doctors

Ironically, Western medicine helped cultivate anti-Western nationalism among the female medical elite. The Hackett students began to build up national consciousness at the beginning of the twentieth century. They started to realize that Western medicine was unusually important not only to individual health, but also to the Chinese nation and that if China's modern medical institution was dominated by Western countries, Chinese lives would be controlled by the Westerners. As a result, after their graduation, they were active during the campaign for the restoration of medical education rights to the Chinese. Nationalistic Liang Huanzhen was one of the examples. After graduation from Hackett, while practicing medicine, she and several other Cantonese medical doctors organized the Guanghua (Revive China) Medical School in Canton in 1908 so as to win medical sovereignty and the rights to medical education by the Chinese.[165]

Revolutionary Zhang Zhujun was not only a feminist, but essentially a nationalist. As expected, Zhang aggressively took part in the 1905 anti-American boycott campaign, a nationwide protest against America's Chinese Exclusion Act, which prohibited Chinese immigrants. The Chinese women in Shanghai played a vital role in this anti-imperialist mass movement, in which the Chinese merchants, industrialists, intellectuals, students, and workers cooperated. The women organized their own protest gatherings and adopted such resolutions as "promotion of Chinese handicraft industry." Zhang delivered a speech at one of such meetings on July 19, 1905, stating that the Chinese women had chosen to reject American manufactured goods, even though they were using the most. She wrote a letter on the issue, and her antagonism towards the imperialist countries was apparent.[166] Zhang often warned that China was in grave circumstances and that if the Chinese accepted this development and did not change it, China would be discarded in the process of natural selection before it was divided up by the major powers. It was clear that Zhang's claim manifested her perception of the dangerous situation of China in an impending threat of division by the Western powers after the Boxer Rebellion.[167] In 1910, when the black plague spread in Shanghai, Dr. Zhang made an objection to the policies of the Municipal Council of the Shanghai Settlement controlled by the Westerners. She claimed that the government had abused its power in carrying out such policies against the plague as entering private houses for examination without permission, compulsorily taking away the suspected victim from the dwelling, etc.[168]

Guan Xianghe was another nationalist. After graduating from Hackett, Guan served as resident physician at the Canton Hospital. Later, she was employed as assistant at the Hackett College in 1913. She took a year of study at Mount Holyoke College and another year at Columbia University in the United States. Upon returning to Canton, she was appointed as the assistant dean of academic affairs of the Hackett Medical College from

1915 to 1922 and the dean from 1923 to 1927.[169] During the anti-imperialist revolutionary campaign in Canton in the 1920s, Guan Xiahe, together with several Christian principals of high school and Zhong Rongguang, president of Lingnan University, published a declaration on October 5, 1926, strongly condemning and protesting against Britain's aggressive policy. British gunboats boarded other ships forcibly and bombed inhabitants in Wan County in Sichuan Province, which contributed to the death of many Chinese during the bombings on September 4.[170]

The Cantonese women doctors also participated in the fighting against Japanese imperialism. When the Japanese armies attacked Shanghai in January 1932, Xia Aiqiong of the Hackett alumni voluntarily organized a rescue team to go to the city of Suzhou, eighty miles west of Shanghai, to take care of the wounded Chinese soldiers at a military hospital, an effort to help resist Japanese invasion.[171]

Nationalism at Hackett

The Chinese control of the Hackett College was an indication of the rising nationalism at Hackett. In 1927, waves of Chinese national sentiment were rising very high in Canton, having great effect on both Hackett's students and Chinese faculty. Since the missionary schools were a symbol of imperialism in Chinese nationalist ideology and education was regarded as a means of political propaganda, the new Nanjing regime tried to impose tight government control of education in China. The new unified Nationalist government demanded that all foreign schools register with the Chinese government in 1927, a piece of legislation putting them formally under the control of non-Christian organizations. At the Hackett, Dr. J. Allen Hofmann, like many of his American colleagues, resisted the registration when the issue first was discussed in the spring of 1927. In reply, many students and Chinese professors and staff wanted the registration because they understood clearly that the medical college in China had to be subject to Chinese management and guidance. They made it clear that their future relationship to the institution depended on its dominantly Western nature bowing to Chinese control and leadership.[172]

During the registration crisis, the reactions of the Hackett's Chinese women, professors, staff, students, and alumnae astonished Dr. Hofmann and other American doctors. Eventually, the conflict receded because the students did not want their school suspended and the members of the Hackett Alumnae Association played a significant part in solving this problem, acting as the arbitrator between the several parties concerned. The consequence was that the Board of the Trustees of the Hackett, with the authorization of the Presbyterian Board of Foreign Missions, transferred the management of the Hackett College to a board of trustees selected by the Chinese-run Church of Christ in Canton. In response, the new board assumed main monetary liability for the Hackett compound and assured the enduring Christian spirit of the institution. The Presbyterians, on the other hand, carried on providing medical missionaries.

The most vital ingredient in this registration crisis was Chinese nationalism. Western medicine played a role in the rise of the anti-Western nationalism at Hackett in some measure, although many factors were responsible for this anti-Western campaign, such as the Communists' propaganda and the mass mobilization strategy of the Nationalists.

The First Women to the Assembly and to the Government

The rise of women medical professionals in Canton and their social activities helped awaken not only Cantonese women's social consciousness but also their political consciousness in some way.[173] It was not surprising that the Cantonese women started to demand political rights. After the 1911 Revolution, the Cantonese women organized a study group on women's rights and continued their movement for the legal enactment of gender equality in the government.[174] This campaign won the endorsement of Sun Yat-sen who supported women's participation in the government. As a consequence, ten women supported by the male progressive politicians were elected to the Guangdong provincial assembly of 165 representatives in December 1911. For the first time in the Chinese history, the women delegates attended a provincial assembly, and, needless to say, this was the first instance of elected women delegates in Asia.[175] The franchise for Guangdong women, however, existed for only several months. When the provincial assembly election law was published on September 2, 1912, the women delegates were kept out of the provincial assembly of Guangdong.[176]

The Cantonese women were not only the first to win the women's franchise, but also were the first to serve in the government in China. Zheng Yuxiu (1891–1959) was an example.[177] In 1919, the minister of foreign affairs of the Canton Military Government under the leadership of Sun Yat-sen appointed Zheng as the honorary member of the Society of the Foreign Investigation. She became the first Chinese woman to participate in political affairs and serve in the government. During the conference in Versailles in 1919, Zheng, a member of the delegation of the Republic of China, was in charge of translation work and communication with other countries' delegations, serving as a correspondent for the Chinese newspapers in Canton. She later served as the Chinese ambassador to France and the chief justice of the Court of Shanghai in the 1920s.[178]

Conclusion

The formation of the Hackett Medical College for Women had noteworthy effects on Chinese society in three major areas. First, Hackett's American doctors, students, and alumnae played a significant role in the introduction of modern medicine, especially women's medicine, into Chinese society. American missionaries founded the Hackett Medical College for Women, the first women's medical college in China. The Hackett College trained nearly five hundred Chinese women doctors from 1899 to 1935. American medical missionaries were the pioneers in women's medical education in China. During that time, American doctors and the Chinese women doctors saved many women's lives and healed many women and children in the modern medical way, introduced modern methods of aiding childbirth, and improved conditions and the care of women's health and child welfare in China, particularly in Canton. American doctors and the Chinese women doctors also introduced scientific knowledge about female biology and physiology and modern conceptions of women's bodies, instructed Chinese women in social hygiene, and changed their traditional medical ideas. The Hackett College brought in and advanced modern women's medicine in China.

Second, Hackett's American doctors, students, and alumnae played a role in modern women's rights movement in China generally and in Canton particularly. American doctors challenged Confucianism's bias against the women when removing obstacles to the treatment of Chinese women in the medical sphere. The Canton Hospital and the Hackett College treated the women patients in a public space, challenging the traditional practice that the women could not been treated by male doctors outside the women's quarters. For the first time the Chinese women were able to enjoy the same rights as the Chinese men did, to some degree, to medical attention and treatments. Hackett equipped the women to make their way in a still very male world, giving their students useful tools, with which they could begin to break away from the old, subordinate role of women in China. American medical missionaries' determination and encouragement helped change many lower-class women's lives and elevate their social status when the Chinese women practiced medicine after graduation from the Hackett College.

Medical missionaries' attention remained focused steadfastly on the much more traditional task of arming women to serve the cause of established Christianity, but they asserted the ideas of women's rights, such as women's rights to medical attention, women's educational rights, women's working rights, while teaching their students. Most female medical students certainly could not have graduated without at least absorbing, in some way, some of these ideas. Thus, the Cantonese women doctors, China's first women professionals, not only carried out medical and health work in China but also took the lead in the modern women's rights movement in China, especially in Canton. They opened their hospitals and dispensaries for women and children, started professional schools for women to learn skills to make a living, taught women the ideology of women's rights, and encouraged women, like themselves, to play an active role in their communities and their society.

They contributed to an awareness of women's rights among the Chinese and helped promote women's status.

The Hackett College opened higher education for women, and the Chinese women for the first time could go to colleges, an imperative education reform in China. Influenced by the Canton Hospital's medical school and later the Hackett College, the Canton Christian College bravely led in this remarkable direction, conducted the most progressive, coeducational experiments in Canton, and became the first college in China to admit women. Hence the Hackett College marked the beginning of coeducation in colleges in China.

Finally, Hackett's students and alumnae not only played a role in medical and social transformation of China but also played a part in the political movement. They took part in the revolutionary movement to overthrow the Manchu regime before and during the 1911 Revolution. Ironically, they also participated in the anti-Western nationalist crusades and in the campaign of the restoration of medical rights to the Chinese in the nation-building movement at the beginning the twentieth century, although they were trained by American doctors. The rise of nationalism in Hackett was so powerful that the administrative authority of the Hackett College was forced to be transferred from the missionaries to the Chinese. Many factors were responsible for the growth of Chinese nationalism among the Cantonese medical elite, but Western medicine was one of the factors. By that time, the Hackett's alumnae and students, even the Chinese faculty members, had realized that Western medicine was extraordinarily critical not only to individual health but also to the Chinese nation and that China's modern medical institutions had to be controlled by the Chinese, rather than by foreigners.

American doctors played a role in the modern women's right movement in China generally and in Canton particularly, but they were the promoters of this movement only when providing a new public sphere—hospitals—for Chinese female patients, a new opportunity—medical education—for Chinese girls, and a new concept—women's rights and role in society—for the Cantonese elite. It was the poor female patients who first bravely escaped momentarily the binds of Confucian morality and decorum to enter the Canton Hospital to seek a foreign male physician. It was the Cantonese girls who first approached the Canton Hospital to express their interest in studying medicine. It was the Canton female medical students and alumnae themselves who initiated the modern women's rights movement in Canton as well as in China. It was the enlightened Cantonese male elite who campaigned for the women's educational and working rights.

American medical missionaries' contributions to women's education in Canton should not be denied, but it was clear that many diverse, sometimes conflicting interests and ideas at play in the history of Cantonese women's education. Equation of medical missionary involvement in female education with Chinese feminism or a nascent Chinese women's right movement should not be too easy, as American women missionaries, through supportive of women's education and opposed the seclusion of women, were not necessarily acting against or voicing criticism of patriarchy or the distinctly male prerogative embodied by church hierarchy. Women like Mary Niles and Mary Fulton are probably best recognized for their exceptionalness, rather than their adherence to social convention.

Notes

1. See, for example, Sara Tucker, "A Mission for Change in China: The Hackett Women's Medical Center of Canton, China, 1900-1930, in Leslie A. Flemming, ed., *Women's Work for Women: Missionaries and Social Change in Asia.* (Boulder: Westview, 1989), and Pang Suk Man, "To Save Life and Spread the True Light: The Hackett Medical College for Women in China (1899-1936)," MA Thesis, Hong Kong Baptist University, 1998.

2. S. M. Tao, "Medical Education of Chinese Women," *Chinese Medical Journal* 47 (1933). 1010-28.

3. In 1890, Mary Niles, one of the early women missionary doctors, worked with Kerr and taught obstetrics at Canton. In 1890 she wrote an account of her seven years experience of observing native midwifery. See Mary W. Niles, "Native Midwifery in Canton," *China Medical Missionary Journal* 4, no. 2 (1890): 52.

4. R. H. Graves, *Forty Years in China or China in Transition* (Baltimore: Woodward, 1895. Reprint, Scholarly Resource at Wilmington, Delaware, 1972), 236-37.

5. John Stoddard, *China*, (Chicago: Belford, Middlebrook & Company, 1897), 76-77.

6. G. H. Choa, *"Heal the Sick" was Their Motto: The Protestant Medical Missionaries in China* (Hong Kong: Chinese University Press, 1990), 81.

7. Pui-Lan Kwok, "Chinese Women and Protestant Christianity at the Turn of the Twentieth Century," in Daniel H Bays, ed., *Christianity in China from the Eighteenth Century to the Present* (Stanford: Stanford University Press, 1996), 196.

8. George B. Stevens and W. Fisher Markwick, *The Life, Letters, and Journals of the Rev. and Hon. Peter Parker, M.D., Missionary, Physician, and Diplomatist, the Father of Medical Missions and Founder of the Ophthalmic Hospital in Canton* (Boston: Congregational Sunday School and Publishing Society, 1896), 127-8.

9. Edward Gulick, *Peter Parker and the Opening of China*, 51, 57.

10. Cadbury, *At the Point of a Lancet*, 49.

11. *The Twentieth Annual Report of the Board of Foreign Missions of the Presbyterian Church in the United States* of America (New York, 1857), 72-3.

12. Medical Missionary Society, *Report of the Medical Missionary Society in China for the year 1866* (Canton, China: The Medical Missionary Society, 1867), 9.

13. Medical Missionary Society, *Report of the Medical Missionary Society in China for the Year 1860* (Canton, Friend of China Press, 1861), 12.

14. John Swan, "Caesarean Section," *The China Medical Journal* VII, 3 (September 1893), 173-77.
15. Born in Pennsylvania, Happer received his education at Jefferson College and Western Theological Seminary and his medical doctor degree at the University of Pennsylvania in 1844. As the son of pious parents who led him early on to the ministry, Happer accomplished an enduring dream to become a missionary when being ordained to the Presbyterian ministry on April 23, 1844. To answer the appeal of the Presbyterian Board for Foreign Missions, right away after his graduation, Happer, in company with several other missionaries, boarded a ship for Macao in the same year. After arriving in Macao, Happer opened a school for boys and then moved to Hong Kong to become an associate leader of the Morrison Education Society. See Loren W. Craftree, "Andrew P. Happer and Presbyterian Mission in China, 1844-1891," *Journal of Presbyterian History* 62, 1 (Spring 1984): 19-35.
16. *Annual Report of the Board of Foreign Missions of the Presbyterian Church in the United States of America, 1854* (New York: Published for the Board, 1854), 48.
17. *Annual Report of the Board of Foreign Missions of the Presbyterian Church in the United States of America, 1884* (New York: Published for the Board, 1884), 100.
18. Loren W. Craftree, "Andrew P. Happer and Presbyterian Mission in China, 1844-1891," *Journal of Presbyterian History* 62, 1 (Spring 1984): 19-35.
19. *Dictionary of American Biography*, 8: 234 and Charles H. Corbett, *Lingnan University* (New York: Trustees of Lingnan University, 1963), 7.
20. *History of the South China Mission of the American Presbyterian Church, 1845-1920* (Shanghai: The Presbyterian Mission Press, 1927), 10-12
21. *Annual Report of the Board of Foreign Missions of the Presbyterian Church in the United States of America, 1854* (New York: Published for the Board, 1854), 47f.
22. Presbyterian Board of Foreign Missions, Missions Correspondence and Reports (1833-1911), Hong Kong Baptist University Library.
23. *The Twentieth Annual Report of the Board of Foreign Missions of the Presbyterian Church in the United States of America* (New York, 1857), 69.
24. Harriet Noyes, *A Light in the Land of Sinim-Forty-Five Years in the True Light Seminar, 1872-1917* (New York: Fleming Revell, 1919), 13.
25. Harriet Noyes, "Fifty Years in the Foreign Field," *The Continent*, May 13, 1920, 650-651.
26. Liu Xinchi, *Zhengguang guangron jianshi* (A brief history of True Ling Seminar) (Hong Kong: Heyintang Press, 1972), 2.
27. Letters of South China Mission, Presbyterian Church in the United States, Group Number 92, File 4, Document 4, Archives of Guangdong Province, Guangzhou.
28. *Records of the General Conference of the Protestant Missionaries of China* (Shanghai, Presbyterian Mission Press, 1878).
29. R. H. Graves, *Forty Years in China or China in Transition* (Baltimore: Woodward, 1895. Reprint,Scholarly Resource at Wilmington, Delaware, 1972), 237.
30. Ibid., 249.

31. Harriet Noyes, *A Light in the Land of Sinim-Forty-Five Years in the True Light Seminar, 1872-1917* (New York: Fleming Revell, 1919), 85.

32. Letter of Kerr to Ellinwood, August 26, 1884, vol. 18: 326, Presbyterian Church Board of Foreign Missions, *China Letters, 1837-1900,* microfilm, Presbyterian Historical Society, Philadelphia, Pennsylvania; Letter of Board to Canton Station, Nov. 21, 1881, vol. 32: 56, Ibid.

33. Ibid.

34. John Kerr, "The Bubonic Plague," *The China Medical Missionary Journal* 3 (1894): 178-80.

35. Letter Ellinwood to Happer, Jan. 21, 1881, vol. 31: 24, Presbyterian Church Board of Foreign Missions, *China Letters, 1837-1900,* microfilm, Presbyterian Historical Society, Philadelphia, Pennsylvania.

36. For a study of the history of American women doctors, see Gloria Moldow, *Women Doctors in Gilded–Age Washington: Race, Gender, and Professionalization* (Illinois: University of Illinois Press, 1987) and Judith Lorber, *Women Physicians: Careers, Status, and Power* (New York: Tavistock, 1984).

37. Niles, the first female missionary doctor in Canton, was born on January 20, 1854 in Wisconsin, where her father was a pioneer missionary. She graduated from Elmira College in 1875 at the age of twenty-one and spent the next three years in New York City, where she taught at some of the public schools. In 1878, she began the study of medicine at the Women's Medical College and received her M.D. degree in 1882 as well as her M.A. degree from Elmira College at the same time. In 1917, her alma mater conferred upon Dr. Niles the degree of LL.D. in recognition of her work in China. See Dr. Mary W. Niles' Home Letters, Group 92, File 4, Document 10, 84, Guangdong Provincial Archives, Guangzhou, China.

38. Ibid.

39. Letter of White to Ellinwood, Feb. 9, 1885, vol. 18: 135, Presbyterian Church Board of Foreign Missions, *China Letters, 1837-190,* microfilm, Presbyterian Historical Society, Philadelphia, Pennsylvania. See also Mary Niles: Dr. Niles' Home Letters, Group 92, File 4, Document 10, 84, Guangdong Provincial Archives.

40. Cadbury, *At the Point of a Lancet,* 145-46.

41. The new dispensary was open for five afternoons during the week, and one room was used entirely as a chapel or waiting room where a Bible woman had a word with and read to the waiting women. See Cadbury, *At the Point of a Lancet,* 147-48.

42. *History of the South China Mission of the American Presbyterian Church, 1845-1920,* 68.

43. *Annual Report of the Presbyterian Board of Foreign Missions* (New York: The Board of Foreign Missions, Presbyterian Church in the U.S.A., 1890), 43.

44. Dr. Mary W. Niles' Home Letters, Group 92, File 4, Document 10, 84, Guangdong Provincial Archives, Guangzhou, China.

45. G. Thompson Brown, *Earthen Vessels and Transcendent Power: American Presbyterians in China, 1837-1952* (Maryknoll, N.Y.: Orbis Books, 1997), 88. Some historians of mission studies believe that Brown's

book is riddled with errors, but I believe that this piece of information is accurate.

46. See David James Evans, *Obstetrics: A Manual for Students and Practitioners* (New York: Lea, 1900). Dr. Mary W. Niles' Home Letters, Group 92, File 4, Document 10, 84, Guangdong Provincial Archives, Guangzhou, China.

47. Mary Fulton, *"Inasmuch": Extracts from Letters, Journals, Papers, Etc* (West Medford, Mass.: The Central Committee of the United Study of Foreign Missions, n. d.), 13.

48. For more information on Mary Fulton, see the Mary Hannah Fulton entry of *Notable American Women 1607-1950: A Biographical Dictionary*, vol. 1 (A–F), (Cambridge, Mass.: The Belknap Press of Harvard University Press, 1971), 685-86.

49. *History of the South China Mission of the American Presbyterian Church, 1845-1920*, 67-8.

50. Mary H. Fulton, *"Inasmuch": Extracts from Letters, Journals, Papers, Etc*, 97.

51. Cadbury, *At the Point of a Lancet*, 147-48.

52. "Hackett Medical College," *China Medial Missionary Journal* XV, 3 (July 1901), 243-44.

53. Mary H. Fulton, "Hackett Medical College for Women, Canton," *China Medical Missionary Journal* 13, 5 (1909): 324-29.

54. Mary H. Fulton, *The Woman's Medical College—Announcement: Session 1901-1902*, 9. Accession 69, Folder 46, The Medical College of Pennsylvania Archives and Special Collections, Philadelphia, Pennsylvania.

55. Mary H. Fulton, "Hackett Medical College for Women, Canton," *China Medical Missionary Journal* XXIII, 5 (1909): 324-29.

56 . *Annual Report of the Presbyterian Board of Foreign Missions* (New York: The Board of Foreign Missions, Presbyterian Church in the U.S.A., 1902), 46.

57. J. Allen Hofmann, "A Short History and Sketch of Hackett Medical College and Affiliated Institution, August, 1926, Group Number 65, File Number 42, Guangdong Provincial Archives, Guangzhou, China.

58. *History of the South China Mission of the American Presbyterian Church, 1845-1920* (Shanghai: The Presbyterian Mission Press, 1927), 116-17.

59. Wu Tingfang, formerly minister to the United States, compassionately presented an address, saying that "he was warmly in sympathy with this medical college and that it was desirable that a woman should fit herself for a work so eminently suitable to her abilities and so peculiarly adapted to the needs of her own sex." As an additional symbol of his admiration, the viceroy sent three gold watches to three graduates who passed the highest in the final examination. See Mary H. Fulton, *"Inasmuch": Extracts from Letters, Journals, Papers, Etc*, 97.

60. Ibid., 98.

61. Ibid.

62. The faculty members were:

Mary H. Fulton	Dean, Clinical Surgery
Harry W. Boyd	Ophthalmology and Bacteriology
Edward Machle	Neuropathology
Charles Selden	Neuropathology
Mary W. Niles	Emeritus Professor of Obstetrics
Luo Xiuyun	Obstetrics and Diseases of Women and Children
Su Daoming	Surgery
Liang Ganchuo	Practice
Wong Sin Shang	Chemistry
H. A. Cheng	Physiology
Chen Ruihua	Dermatology and Physical Diagnosis
Liu Ziwai	Dentistry

See *Annual Report of the Presbyterian Board of Foreign Missions* (New York: The Board of Foreign Missions, Presbyterian Church In the U.S.A., 1909), 157.

63. "Hackett Medical College: The Opening Ceremony," *The China Mail*, June 26, 1913.

64. Drs. Hackett and Allyn received much more current scientific trainings than did Mary Fulton. When Mary Fulton received her M.D. degree in 1884, the germ theory was not yet extensively recognized, only simple operations could be performed, hospital buildings were still quite small, and pharmacy of drugs accessible was extremely restricted. All of this was changing almost daily in 1913. See J. Allen Hofmann, "A Short History and Sketch of Hackett Medical College and Affiliated Institution, August, 1926, Group Number 65, File 42, Guangdong Provincial Archives, Guangzhou, China.

65. Mary H. Fulton, *"Inasmuch": Extracts from Letters, Journals, Papers, Etc*, 120-2.

66. Lucy A. Gaynor, "A Nurses Association," *China Medical Journal* XXIII, 2 (March 1909), 118-20.

67. In 1897, Mrs. J. J. Boggs, M.D., of the Hackett College, completed a version of Hampton Robb's *Principles and Practice of Nursing*, too. See Anna Fullerton, *Nursing in Abdominal Surgery and Diseases of Women* (Philadelphia: P. Blakiston, 1891) and "Book Review: Manual of Nursing," *China Medical Missionary Journal* XX, 2 (March 1906), 86.

68. Fulton was compelled to return to America on account of ill health and died at her home at Pasadena on January 8, 1927.

69. *Xiage nu yi xue xiao zhang cheng* (The regulations of xiage medical school for women) (Guangzhou: Xiage nuyi xue xiao, 1919), 2-3.

70. *History of the South China Mission of the American Presbyterian Church, 1845-1920*, 131-32.

71. Harriet Noyes, *A Light in the Land of Sinim-Forty-Five Years in the True Light Seminar, 1872-1917* (New York: Fleming Revell, 1919), 90. See also Min-Ch'ien T. Z. Tyau, *China Awakened* (New York: The Macmillan, 1922), 59.

72. Harriet M. Allyn, "The Hackett Medical College: The Healing of His Seamless Dress by Chinese Beds of Pain," *The Presbyterian Magazine* (April, 1922): 218.

73. "Hackett Medical College, Canton," *China Medical Journal* XLI, 7 (July 1927): 667-68; "Hackett Medical College and Affiliated Institution," Ibid. XLIV (September 1930): 961-62.

74. *Hackett Medical Center Report of the Director, 1936-1937* (Board of Foreign Missions, Presbyterian Church, USA Papers), Archival Records, Presbyterian Historical Society, Philadelphia, PA.

75. *Bulletin of the David Gregg Hospital for Women and Children, Hackett Medical College for Women, Julia Turner School of Nursing* (Canton, 1929), 14.

76. J. Allen Hofmann to Miss Mary T. Bankes, May 17, 1928, Folder 21, Box 28, Record Group 82, Presbyterian Church in the U.S.A. Board of Foreign Missions. Secretaries Files: China Missions, 1891-1955, Presbyterian Historical Society, Philadelphia, Pennsylvania.

77. J. Franklin Karcher, "Report of the Superintendent," December 1, 1933, Folder 4, Box 5, ibid.

78. Lereine Ballantyne, *Dr. Jessie MacBean and the Work at Hackett Medical College, Canton, China* (Toronto, Canada: Women's Missionary Society of the Presbyterian Church in Canada, 1934), 27-28.

79. Taylor Ross, "A Child Welfare Clinic," *China Medical Journal* 41 (1927): 250-4.

80. Lereine Ballantyne, *Dr. Jessie MacBean and the Work at Hackett Medical College, Canton, China* (Toronto, Canada: Women's Missionary Society of the Presbyterian Church in Canada, 1934), 35, 57.

81. The numbers of inpatients who stayed at the hospital every year were as follows:

Department of Surgery:	400
Department of Internal Medicine:	600
Department of Gynecology:	400
Department of Obstetrics:	600
Department of Pediatrics:	600

. See, Brief History of the Hackett Women College, November 29, 1934, Group Number 18, File Number 43, Guangzhou Municipal Archives, Guangzhou, China.

82. *Annual Report of the David Gregg Hospital for Women and Children, Hackett Medical College for Women, Turner Training School for Nurses, Yau Tsai School of Pharmacy* (Canton: Shameen Printing Press, 1931), 18.

83. G. F. Sauer, "Report of the Principal, Yau Tsai School of Pharmacy," December 1933, Folder 4, Box 5, Record Group 82, Presbyterian Church in the U.S.A. Board of Foreign Missions. Secretaries Files: China Missions, 1891-1955, Presbyterian Historical Society, Philadelphia, Pennsylvania.

84. *Guangzhou shi dierrenmin yiyuan shi, 1899-1999* (The History of the Second Municipal Hospital of Guangzhou, 1899-1999)(The Committee of the History of the Second Municipal Hospital of Guangzhou, 1999), 4-23.

85. In 1907, the UMS assumed the support of Dr. Andrew H. Woods of the Canton Christian College, who was a medical graduate of the University of Pennsylvania and was appointed to the staff to deal with the medical requirements of the Canton Christian College. See William W. Cadbury, "History of the Medical Work of Lingnan University," Group 8, Box 107, Yale Divinity School Library.

86. "University Medical School, Canton," *The China Medical Missionary Journal* 23, 6 (1909): 406-07.

87. Barron H. Lerner, "The University of Pennsylvania in China: Medical Missionary Work, 1905-1914" (BA Thesis, University of Pennsylvania, 1982), 52-59, 94-95.

88. Charles Hodge Corbett, *Lingnan University* (New York: The Trustees of Lingnan University, 1963), 61.

89. On January 24-30, 1917, eighty–two members of the China Medial Missionary Association and eighty-eight of the National Medical Association attended a joint conference held in Canton and enjoyed the most energetic collaboration of Governor Zhu Qinglan. After reviewing the medical educational situation in Canton, the attendants stated that the Gongyi Medical and Guanghua Colleges should unite together and form a Guangdong Union Medical College. In February 1920, the Board of the Directors of the Canton Hospital sent Dr. John Kirk, a surgeon of the Canton Hospital and a member of the Council of the New Zealand Presbyterian Mission, and Dr. J. Oscar Thomson, the president of South China Branch of the CMMA, to the CMMA conference in Beijing. Drs. Kirk and Thomson presented to the conference the Resolutions adopted by the Board of Directors of the Canton Medical Missionary Union with regard to the establishment of a school of medicine at the Canton Christian University. See Memorandum of Delegation Representing the Canton Hospital, China, Presented to the Canton Christian College and Other Missionary Boards Working in South China, Folder 22, Box 11, Record Group 82, Presbyterian Church in the U.S.A. Board of Foreign Missions. Secretaries Files: China Missions, 1891-1955, Presbyterian Historical Society, Philadelphia, Pennsylvania.

90. William Warder Cadbury, "Mission Hospital and Medical Educational Work in Canton," *China Medical Journal* No vol. (October 1933): 1-2 and Mary Anderson, *A Cycle in the Celestial Kingdom* (Mobile, Alabama: Press of Heiter-Starke, 1943), 227.

91. The David Gregg Hospital of Hackett becomes the Second Municipal Hospital of Guangzhou today, a chief hospital in Canton, which has more than 1,000 doctors and staff as well as 700 beds. See http://www.fm120.com/zt/hospital/html/0024/0024-1.html. In the 1950s, Sun Yat-sen Medical College of Lingnan University, Guanghua Medical College, Gongyi Medical College were combined into the Sun Yat-sen Medical University. It has more than 10,000 medical students and eight teaching hospitals now, a leading medical institution in China. See http://www.gzsums.edu.cn/2008/index.php.

92. Mary H. Fulton, *"Inasmuch": Extracts from Letters, Journals, Papers, Etc*, 93.

93. Ibid., 85-6.

94. J. Allen Hofmann, "A Short History and Sketch of Hackett Medical College and Affiliated Institution," August, 1926, Group Number 65, File Number 42, Guangdong Provincial Archives, Guangzhou, China.
95. Ibid.
96. Mary H. Fulton, *"Inasmuch": Extracts from Letters, Journals, Papers, Etc*, 82-5.
97. J. Allen Hofmann, "A Short History and Sketch of Hackett Medical College and Affiliated Institution, August, 1926, Group Number 65, File 42, Guangdong Provincial Archives, Guangzhou, China.
98. Ibid., 54-5.
99. *Guangzhoushi ge yiyuan yange* (History of the Hospitals in Canton) (Guangzhou, 1934).
100. Tao Shan Ming, "Zhongguo zi yixue jiaoyu," *Zhonghua yixue zazhi* 19, no. 6 (1933): 849-64.
101. Tao S. M, "Medical Education of Chinese Women," *Chinese Medical Journal* 47 (1933): 1010-28.
102. *Weisheng tongji* (Health Statistics) (Chongqing: Neizhengbu, 1938).
103. See *Guanghua biye tongxuehui tekan* (Special issue of Guanghua medial alumni), Guangzhou, 1935.
104. O. J. Todd, "Cooperation with the Chinese in Medical Education Work," *China Medical Journal* XXVII, 3 (May 1913): 143-47.
105. Gael Graham, *Gender, Culture, and Christianity: American Protestant Mission Schools in China, 1880-1930* (New York: Peter Lang, 1995), 85.
106. *Annual Report of the Presbyterian Board of Foreign Missions* (New York: The Board of Foreign Missions, Presbyterian Church in the U.S.A., 1903), 55.
107. Lucy A. Gaynor, "A Nurses Association," *China Medical Journal* XXIII, 2 (March 1909): 118-20; Mary Fulton, "Hackett Medical College for Women, Canton, ibid. XXIII, 5 (September 1909): 324-29; J. Allen Hofmann, "A Short Historical Sketch of Hackett Medical College and Affiliated Institutions," ibid. XL, 8 (August 1926), 776-79.
108. 1932 Hackett Report, Folder 4, Box 5, RG 82, and J. Allen Hofmann letter to Scott, received October 29, 1928 Folder 4, Box 5, RG 82, the Presbyterian Historical Society, Philadelphia, Pennsylvania.
109. *Guangzhou wenshi ziliao* (History and literature of Guangzhou) (Guangzhou shi wenshi ziliao weiyuan hui) 45 (1993): 151.
110. Zhu Qinglan, *Guangdong tongzhi gao* (The first draft of Guangdong history), vol. 3 (Beijing, Special Collection Department, 2001, reprint): 1110-3.
111. *Annual Report of the David Gregg Hospital for Women and Children, Hackett Medical College for Women, Turner Training School for Nurses, Yau Tsai School of Pharmacy* (Canton: Shameen Printing Press, 1931), 21.
112. *Rouji duanna hushi xuexiao zhang cheng, 1934-1935* (The catalog of the Rouji Hospital and the Turner Nursing School, 1934-1935) (Canton, 1935), 25-36.
113. Canton Hospital, *Annual Report of the Canton Hospital for the Year 1914* (Canton: Too Leung Printing Press, 1915), 17-19; Canton Hospital, *Annual Report of the Canton Hospital for the Year 1916* (Canton: Too Leung

Printing Press, 1917), 17-18; Canton Hospital, *Annual Report of the Canton Hospital for the Year 1920* (Canton: Too Leung Printing Press, 1921), 69-70; Canton Hospital, *Annual Report of the Canton Hospital for the Year 1922* (Canton: Too Leung Printing Press, 1923), 71-72; and Canton Hospital, *Annual Report for the 99th Year of the Sun Yat-sen Memorial of the Canton Hospital* (Canton: Too Leung Printing Press, 1934), 21-24.

114. *Sili Guangdong Guanghua yixue yuan gai kuang* (The outline of the private Guangdong Guanghua Medical College) (Guangzhou: Guanghua yixue yuan, 1936), 1-10 and *Guangzhou zhinan* (Guide to Canton) (Guangzhou: Guangzhou Municipal Government, 1934).

115. Wu Lien–teh, "A Hundred Years of the Modern Medicine in China," *The China Medical Journal* 50, 2 (February 1936).

116. J. Allen Hofmann Letter to Scott, Wooster, Ohio, September 15, 1924, Folder 14, Box 17, RG 82, Presbyterian Historical Society, Philadelphia, Pennsylvania.

117. "Hackett Medical College, Canton," *China Medical Journal* XLI, 7 (July 1927): 667-68; "Hackett Medical College and Affiliated Institutions, Canton, 1929," Ibid. XLIV, 9 (September 1930): 960-61; "Announcement," XLV, 7 (July 1931), 680. See also "Universities and Colleges," *National Medical Journal* 15, 4 (August 1929), 505.

118. "Students of Midwifery School Demanded for Improvement of Treatment," *Guangzhou minguo ribao*, March 27, 1927, 10.

119. Zhu Qinglan, *Guangdong tongzhi gao*, vol. 3, (Beijing, Special Collection Department, 2001), 1113.

120. Dr. Xia's Women and Children Hospital was taken over by the Chinese government in 1949 and is under the control of the Guangzhou municipal government today.

121. Jessie A. MacBean, "Report of Superintendent of David Gregg Hospital, 1931," Folder 4, Box 5, Record Group 82, Presbyterian Church in the U.S.A. Board of Foreign Missions. Secretaries Files: China Missions, 1891-1955, Presbyterian Historical Society, Philadelphia, Pennsylvania.

122. Interview with Dr. Wang Xiaoping, physician of the Second Municipal Hospital of Guangzhou on June 21, 2007.

123. Hackett Medical College: Report of the Dean, November 1933, Folder 4, Box 5, Record Group 82, Presbyterian Church in the U.S.A. Board of Foreign Missions. Secretaries Files: China Missions, 1891-1955, Presbyterian Historical Society, Philadelphia, Pennsylvania.

124. In 1937 when the Japanese air force bombed Canton, a lot of people died or were wounded. Dr. Liang tried her best to rescue and take care of the wounded at her own risk. After the Japanese occupied Canton, she remained at the hospital to provide medical service to the people. In 1944 she successfully extracted an ovarian tumor of 90 pounds from a woman, a piece of news widely disseminated all over the city. She went to study medicine at the Medical Center in New York in 1949 and came back to Canton after the Chinese Communists took over Canton in 1950. She served at the David Gregg Hospital (later renamed the Second People's Municipal Hospital of Canton) as chair of the Department of Gynecology and Obstetrics, vice president, and president of the hospital until 1991. See Liang Yiwen, "Recollections of Xiage Medical College for Women,"

Guangzhou wenshi ziliao (History and literature of Guangzhou) 35 (1986): 147-151 and "Liang Yiwen: An Expert on Obstetrics and Gynecology," Ibid. 45 (March 1993): 81-87.

125. Feng Ziyou, "Nu yishi Zhang Zhujun" (Female doctor Zhang Zhujun), in Feng Ziyou, *Geming yishi* (Unofficial history of the [1911] revolution (reprint, Taibei: Taiwan shangwu yinshuguan, 1965), vol. 2, 41-45.

126. T. Kobayashi, "Chang Chu-chün for Women's Rights," *Journal of the Oriental Society of Australia* II (1976), 62-80.

127. Shen Yanshen, "Recollections of Rouji Hospital," *Guangzhou wenshi ziliao* (History and literature of Guangzhou) 45 (1993): 144-158.

128. *Xiage yike da xue sanshi zhounian jinian lu* (The thirtieth anniversary of the Hackett Medical College for Women) (Guangzhou: xiage yike daxue, 1929).

129. J. Allen Hofmann, "A Short History and Sketch of Hackett Medical College and Affiliated Institution, August, 1926, Group Number 65, File 42, Guangdong Provincial Archives, Guangzhou, China.

130. Gao went to study at the Johns Hopkins Medical School in Baltimore in the United States in 1936 and later became a famous physician in Hubei Province after her study. When the Sino-Japanese War erupted in 1937, Dr. Gao stopped her study and returned home in 1939. She served as associate chair of the Department of Gynecology and Obstetrics at the Central Hospital in Chongqing, the temporary capital of the Nationalist government during the war. After the war, Dr. Gao, returning home town opened a hospital in the city of Wuchang in Hubei province until 1952. After the Chinese Communists took over China in 1949, Dr. Gao donated all equipments of her hospital and a lot of medications to the government. She was the chair of the Department of Gynecology and Obstetrics at the Second Hospital of Wuhan, and later the vice president of the hospital until she retired in 1988. She was so dedicated to her medical duty that she won great appreciation from her colleagues and patients at the hospital. She held several important positions at the Medical Association of China. See *Wuhan shizhi: Weishen zhi* (Annuals of Wuhan: Annals of health) Wuhan: Wuhan difang shi weihuan hui, 1993), 304-306; *Wuhan wenshi ziliao* (History and literature of Wuhan). Wuhan wenshi ziliao weiyuan hui, 2002), 152-24. Interview with Gao Xinrong's colleagues on December 1, 2009 at the Second Hospital of Wuhan in Wuhan, Hubei Province.

131. *Xiage yike da xue sanshi zhounian jinian lu* (The thirtieth Anniversary of the Hackett Medical College for Women (Guangzhou: xiage yike daxue, 1929).

132. *Zhongguo jindai xueji shiliao* (Sources of the educational system of modern China), vol. 2 (Shanghai: Huadong shifan daxue chubanshe 1989): 642-48.

133. *Minli bao* (People's daily), July 19, 1909, 2

134. *Guangzhou shizhi: Minzheng zhi* (Annuals of Guangzhou: Annals of civil administration), vol. 19 (Guangzhou: Guangzhou shizhi weiyuan hui, 1996): 190.

135. Li Yuning and Zhang Yufa, eds., *Jindai zhong guo nuquan yundong shiliao 1842-1911* (Documents on the women's rights movement in modern China, 1842-1911) (Taipei, 1975), 1: 1088.

136. Harriet M. Allyn, "The Hackett Medical College: The Healing of His Seam-less Dress by Chinese Beds of Pain," *The Presbyterian Magazine* (April, 1922): 218.

137. J. Allen Hofmann, "A Short Historical Sketch of Hackett Medical College and Affiliated Institutions," *The China Medical Journal* 8 (August 1926): 776-79.

138. Lately, a great deal of work has been published on the role of women in the construction of Chinese modernity in the late Qing and early Republic. The most significant contribution to the scholarship is Joan Judge, *The Precious Raft of History: The Past, the West, and the Woman Question in China* (Stanford, California: Stanford University Press, 2008). Judge emphasizes the role of Japan in modern women's rights movement in China.

139. Harriet M. Allyn, "Is a Woman's Medical College Worth While in China?" *Post Jubilee News* 5 January 1921.

140. Feng Ziyou, "Nu yishi Zhang Zhujun" (Female Doctor Zhang Zhujun), in Feng Ziyou, *Geming yishi* (Unofficial history of the revolution) (Shanghai: The Commercial Press, 1981), 2: 40-44.

141. Charlotte L. Beahan, "In the Public eye: Women In Early Twentieth Century China," in *Women in China: Current Directions in Historical Scholarship*, ed. Richard W. Guisso and Stanley Johannesen (New York: Philo Press, 1981), 217-18; Esther Lee Yao, *Chinese Women, Past and Present* (Mesquite, TX: Ide House, 1983), 149-50.

142. J. Allen Hofmann, "A Short History and Sketch of Hackett Medical College and Affiliated Institution, August, 1926, Group Number 65, File 42, Guangdong Provincial Archives, Guangzhou, China.

143. "Biography of Miss Zhang Zhujun," *Dagong bao*, October 19, 1902; "Biography of Miss Zhang Zhujun, Part 2," *Daggong bao*, October 21, 1902.

144. Ma Junwu, "Zhang Zhujun zhuan," *Xinmin cong bao* (Renovation of the people journal) 7 (May 1902).

145. *Guangzhou jibainien jiaoyu shiliao* (Guangzhou: Wenshi ziliao weiyun hui, 1983), 74.

146. See *China Year Book, 1935, 1936* (Tianjin and Shanghai: Tianjin Press and the North China Daily News); *Guanghua biye tongxuehui tekan* (Special issue of Guanghua medial alumni) (Guangzhou, 1935); and *Guangdong Gongyi Yixue Zhuanmen Xuexiao, Guoli Guangdong daxue yike ,zhongshan daxue yixueyuan biyeshen mingce* (1909-1955) (the Graduate Register of Guangdong Medical School, Medical Department of National Guangdong University, and Medical College of Zhongshan University) (Canton, 1962).

147. Min–Ch'ien T. Z. Tyau, *China Awakened* (New York, The Macmillian Company, 1922), 59-60.

148. Editorial, "Chinese Women, to Demand Social Status!," *Shanghai minguo ribao* (Shanghai republican daily), February 18, 1921.

149. "Disturbance of Employment of Women Telephone Operators," *Guangzhou minguo ribao* (Guangzhou Republican daily), May 11, 1924.

150. *Xinmin congbao* (Journal of New Citizen) 7 (April 1902): 116-19.

151. *Jingzhong ribao* (Alarm bell daily) (Shanghai), September 28, 1904 (Taiwan reprint, 1968), 7-8.

152. Zhang Zhujun, "Announcement of the Women's Association for Security through Learning," *Jingzhong ribao* (Alarm bell daily). April 1904.
153. Zhang Zhujun, "Zai weisheng jiangxi hui chengli hui shang de yanshuo," *Jingzhong ribao* (Alarm bell daily), May 24 and 25, 1904.
154. Zhang Zhujun, "Nuzi xinxue baoxian hui xu" (Introduction to Women Society of Learning and Security), *Zhongguo xinnüjie* (New Chinese women's world) (Tokyo) 4 (May 1907): 7-11, in *Xinhai geming jianshinianjianshi lun chunji* (A collection of the essays on the 1911 Revolution for ten years), vol. 2 (Shanghai: Shanlian, 1977), 898.
155. Li Yuning and Zhang Yufa, eds., *Jindai zhong guo nuquan yundong shiliao 1842-1911* (Documents on the women's rights movement in modern China, 1842-1911), vol. 1 (Taipei, 1975), 1088. See also Mary Rankin, *Early Chinese Revolutionaries: Radical Intellectuals in Shanghai and Chekiang, 1902-1911* (The Cambridge University Press, 1971), 97.
156. Zhang Zhujun, "Lun Chuzhi Nuzi Jundui (On organizing women's army)," *Dongfang zazhi* 8,10 (1912), 6.
157. Hu Ying, *Tales of Translation: Composing the New Woman in China, 1899-1918* (Stanford: Stanford University Press, 2000), 111.
158. *Xiage yike da xue sanshi zhounian jinian lu* (The thirtieth anniversary of the Hackett Medical College for Women (Guangzhou: Xiage yike daxue, 1929), 4-5.
159. Ibid., 6-8.
160. Feng ziyou, "Nu yishi Zhang Zhujun" (Female doctor Zhang Zhujun), in his *Geming yishi* (Unofficial history of the [1911] revolution (Taibei reprint: Taiwan shangwu yinshuguan, 1965), vol. 2, 41-45.
161. Chun-tu Hsueh, *Hunag Hsing and the Chinese Revolution* (Stanford University Press, 1961), 110.
162. Gardner L. Harding, *Present-Day China: A Narrative of a Nation's Advance* (New York, 1916), 40-43.
163. Shixue, "Nuzi hongsshizi hui zi kejing," *Minli bao* (People's daily), October 10, 1911. See also "The Red Cross' Meeting, Ibid., October 20, 1911, 5; Ibid., October 25, 1911, 5.
164. "Zhang Zhuqun's Speech, President of the Red Cross Society," *Shen bao*, December 27, 1911 and "Zhang Zhuqun's Speech, President of the Red Cross Society," *Sheng bao*, December 30, 1911.
165. *Xiage yike da xue sanshiz zhounian jinian lu* (The thirtieth anniversary of the Hackett Medical College for Women (Guangzhou: Xiage yike daxue, 1929), 9-11.
166. "Yijiu ninwu nian fanmei aiguo yundong "(The 1905 anti-American patriotic movement), in *Jindaishi ziliao* (Sources of modern history), vol. 1 (Beijing, 1954).
167. *Zhongguo xinnüjie* (New Chinese women's world) (Tokyo) 4 (May 1907): 7-11.
168. *Minli pao*, November 11, 1910.
169. Guan was the head of the Board of Hackett College and Affiliated Institutions. See the Record of Hackett Medical College in Foreign Language, Folder 29, Record Group 65, Guangdong Provincial Archives, Guangzhou.
170. "Canton Christians Opposing British Gunboat Policy," *Renmin zhou kan* (People's weekly) 25 (1926).

171. *Guangzhoushi ge yiyuan yange* (History of the Hospitals in Canton) (Guangzhou, 1934).
172. *Xiage yike da xue sanshi zhounian jinian lu* (The thirtieth Anniversary of the Hackett Medical College for Women (Guangzhou: xiage yike daxue, 1929), 12-15.
173. Liu Zhiqin, ed. *Jindai zhongguo shehuiw wenhua bianqianlu* (History of modern social and cultural changes in China), vol. 3 (Hanzhou: Zhejiang chubanshe, 1998), 447; "Diyici guonei geming zhangzheng shiqi de Guangdong funu yundong" (The women's movement in Guangdong during the first revolutionary civil war) in *Guangdong dangshi ziliao* (Source materials on party history in Guangdong), vol. 8 (Guangzhou, 1986): 152-91.
174. Wang Hongjin, "Qingmo Minchu de de Guangdong yihui zhengzhi" (Guangdon parliamentary politics at the end of the Qing and beginning of the Republic), in *Guangdong Xinhai geming ziliao* (Historical sources of Guangdong in the 1911 Revolution) (Guangdong: Guangdong renmin chubanshe, 1981), 426-36.
175. Sun Yat-sen praised this new change. He stated, "After the founding of the Republic of China, the Chinese women had enjoyed some political rights as the men. Women, for example, were elected to the Guangdong Provincial Congress. Those congresswomen, like congressmen, were able to discuss state affairs, significantly splendid and glorious!" See *Sun Zhongshan xuanji* (Selected works of Sun Yat-sen), vol. 2, 566.
176. Liu Zhiqin, ed. *Jindai zhongguo shehuiw wenhua bianqianlu* (History of modern social and cultural changes in China), vol. 3 (Hangzhou: Zhejiang chubanshe, 1998), 447.
177. Born to a high-ranking official's family in Guangdong Province, Zheng Yuxiu became a revolutionary of Sun Yat-sen's Revolutionary Alliance while studying in Japan in 1908. She returned home and participated in revolutionary revolts in an attempt to overthrow the Manchu regime from 1908 to 1911. After the Republic of China was established, Zheng decided to go to Paris to study laws and later received a master's degree in law in 1917 from University of Paris. Zheng later received a doctoral degree in law in 1925 from the same university, the first oriental woman upon whom this recompense had been conferred. See Van Vorst, *A Girl from China* (Soumay Tcheng) (New York: Frederick A Stokes Company, 1926), 239-40.
178. "Zhongguo nüzi yaojiu canzheng de xianshen" (The first cry for Chinese women's participation in government), *Jiefan hua bao* (Liberation pictorial journal) 5 (Shanghai, May 1920).

4

American Doctors and the Modern Philanthropic Movement in Canton, 1835-1935

Medical Missionaries transplanted Western medical institutions into China. This not only contributed significantly to the development of modern medicine in China, but also promoted the modern philanthropic movement in China. This chapter examines how the missionary hospitals provided free medical service to the Cantonese, and how American medical missionaries extended their philanthropic services to the blind and to the insane, opening China's first mental hospital and south China's first school for the blind. The chapter also studies how American medical missionaries influenced the Cantonese reformers and elites in their attitude towards traditional philanthropic concepts and inspired them to launch a modern philanthropic movement in Canton in late Qing and early Republican China. Finally, this chapter examines why and how the Canton government took over Kerr's Refuge for the Insane and became involved in the Mingxin School for the Blind.

Traditional Chinese Charitable Institutions

Emphasizing amity and generosity without entitlements, traditional Chinese charity meant compassion, kindness, mutual help, and personal relationships. These concepts reflected Confucian and Buddhist beliefs in benevolence, righteousness, rite, order, and loyalty, and a rigid social hierarchy that defined love and loyalty. Charitable behavior had continued for centuries in China within the communities, clans, and kinships. Many philanthropic institutions founded by local officials or merchants provided relief to the poor and the needy. The objectives of such institutions were to maintain peace and stability in society, promote Confucianism's benevolence, and obtain rewards after death.[1]

China's pre-modern benevolent ventures were divided into two categories: official and civic. The Qing government, understanding the importance of the philanthropic institutions, decreed the foundation of benevolent institutions in local communities in the empire. Government-sponsored public relief homes existed for centuries, but they did not function continuously. Many were destroyed during the peasants' rebellions. For this reason and others, both local elites and officials organized and managed the united welfare institutions to carry out a variety of welfare functions. These institutions stored grain, distributed gruel to the hungry, cared for the ill, aged, widows, and foundlings, corrected disobedient youths, handed out money to the poor, saved the abandoned, and buried the dead. Thus, government agencies and private benevolent societies provided for aid when needed, even though discriminatingly, temporarily, and limitedly.

In late Qing China, official charitable ventures had declined, many of which were shut down. The number of the poor and needy exceptionally exceeded that of those who were cared for by the government, and China lacked a central, specific, and wide-ranging organization for the relief of misery. On regional levels, the government's noble objectives fell noticeably behind its endowments, and the official emergency supply allocated to the disaster areas was badly insufficient. Since the government was not determined to make available comprehensive social welfare assistance to the poor all the time, families and clans took the main responsibility for philanthropic work. Thus, the formation of community relief societies made up for the lack of adequate government aid to destitute commoners. Official relief funds for the poor continued, but the commune's mutual support was more helpful during a short-term crisis. The rural community heads or spiritual leaders played a more important role than the government in providing assistance to the poor because they owned and managed lands, schools, and shrines.

Private charity was very deep-rooted in Chinese society. Traditional charitable enterprises were clan-kin-oriented. In China, the donors anticipated and accepted public acknowledgment of the funding, which was one of the primary incentives for generosity. Under this system, the concentration of benevolence in general was limited to a local area, for which the benefactors had sympathy. The philanthropists donated their lands or wealth to support the poor, orphans, the blind and others of their kith and kin only, and the kinfolk would take advantage of such charitable help and aid. Thus clan-kin loyalty, rather than state loyalty, was emphasized in traditional China. In terms of medical philanthropic institutions, such institutions as Shiyi ju (Medicine House for the People) and Huiming ju (House Benefiting People) existed in the Qing society, but they had a limited role because these temporary institutes functioned only in time of plague, not serving the poor sick regularly. Even so, those medical philanthropic institutions were declining in the late Qing dynasty.[2]

The Canton Hospital's Charitable Service and Fund-Raising Drives, 1835-1935

Founded in Europe in the nineteenth century, the charitable hospital was an agency of poverty relief, as well as a religious institution. Such hospitals, not governmental undertakings, had primarily social rather than medical functions, intending to serve the sick whose deficient homes could not provide the accommodation their pain needed. Such private institutions tended to take care of the acute cases and short-stay patients while the chronic cases, the incurable, the mentally ill, and those suffering from communicable diseases had to visit public institutions.

The Western missionaries transplanted such hospitals to China once they were there at that time. The purpose of these missionary hospitals was to provide free medical care and healing to the Chinese in an attempt to promote Christianity. The Canton Hospital was one of the examples, the first medical charitable institution in China.

Medical Charitable Services

The Canton Hospital was founded on the basis of brotherly love to promote God's benevolence among the Chinese. American medical missionaries tried to change the Chinese attitude toward the Westerners through the hospital so that they were able to teach the Chinese Christianity, as Dr. Peter Parker, as well as Drs. T. R. Colledge and E. C. Bridgman, announced in their statement of the Medical Missionary Society on April 14, 1838:

> Their patients will not only hear, but feel that the people from the West are good men. The effect of such influences will be silent, but powerful, for there is something irresistibly impressive in a benevolent action, especially when it appears to be exempt from the imputation of interested motives.[3]

From the beginning, the Canton Hospital provided free medical service to its patients. During Parker's times, the Canton Hospital did not accept any fees of any kind from either rich or poor. Many patients were aware of the hospital's benevolent purpose.

After Dr. Kerr took charge of the Canton Hospital, in 1859, he opened a vaccine department offering free service of vaccination against smallpox to the Cantonese children. During Kerr's times, the poor patients did not pay medical service fees, but the inpatients at the Canton Hospital had to supply their own food, which was cooked for them by their relatives or friends. The patients kept their supplies under their beds. Their untrained relatives and friends did the nursing work, except in rare and serious cases when the doctor would sit up all night with them. Even so, many patients were forced to leave the hospital before they were restored to health because either their relatives would not stay any longer or their money ran out. To solve this problem, the Canton Hospital established new funds in 1861 to supply food to some of the poor patients. In 1873, the Canton Hospital made an effort to encourage rich patients to pay a small amount of rent if they would like to stay in separate rooms and to pay for medical services they received so that the Hospital had more funds to support the work of healing the poor.[4]

John Kerr endeavored to encourage his medical colleagues to understand the significance of free medical services for Chinese patients. He wrote,

> It needs no argument to show that practicing for money, or fixing a price for serves rendered, must of necessity present to the Chinese mercenary and selfish motives, thus taking away from the healing of the sick that which gives the missionary physician his power as a co-worker in Christian missions.[5]

It is clear that John Kerr tried to make an impact on the Cantonese of the noble and benevolent spirit of Christianity; acceptance of service fees could hurt missionaries' standing. Dr. Mary Fulton also offered her services without charge to the poor women and children by means of both home visits and neighborhood hospitals in the 1880s and 1890s.

The Canton Hospital began to charge some service fee at the beginning of the twentieth century. In 1914, each patient was charged only fifteen cents a day and a private room only from ten yuan to twenty-five yuan per month. This, in Canton money, was less than half the amount in American currency. The Canton Hospital remained a charitable institution at that time, however. The philanthropic accomplishments of the Canton Hospital was noteworthy, as Dr. J. O. Thomson, the superintendent of the Canton Hospital, later wrote in a summary of the hospital report in 1941:

> Many things have impressed me most when I looked back the history of this institution during the past thirty years: the great influence for good that it has exerted in the city of Canton and throughout south China, in medicine, education, religion, and philanthropy; the large number of persons, of all classes of society but particularly the poor, who have been efficiently cared for; during the past thirty years, more than 30,000 people have been operated upon; more than two thirds of these were poor people.[6]

The Canton Hospital established a model of a modern medical philanthropic institution in China, which contributed to the modern philanthropic movement in Guangdong Province in general and in Canton in particular in the following years.

Fund-Raising Campaigns

Fund-raising was a very important activity for the survival of charitable institutions. When the undertakings of the Canton Hospital increased and expanded, the requirement for healthy finances became increasingly important. American medical missionaries were aggressive in fund-raising campaigns, which to some degree inspired the Cantonese to support the Canton Hospital and found more philanthropic institutions.

Dr. E. C. Bridgman made clear in a report to the American Board in May 1836 that financial endowments for the hospital were generously obtained from both the Chinese and foreign inhabitants of Canton, and the lack of a managerial association to deal with this business suggested that "the hand to prescribe and administer what is requisite, cannot be so readily supplied." As a matter of fact, the funds needed to maintain the hospital's functions were in excess of the donations contributed by both the British and American traders in Macao and Canton when Parker gave an account to the American Board only several months after the commencement of the Hospital. He wrote, "The hospital has received liberal, voluntary patronage from benevolent residents here and at Macao—$1,050 has already been subscribed. These donations are uniformly accompanied with kindest wishes for the success of the undertaking."[7]

The need for money was a real and pressing problem to the Canton Hospital, and a wider basis of support was vital if the Medical Missionary Society was to continue its benevolent work. American doctors had to be energetically engaged in the fund-raising campaigns. Due to the closing of the Canton Hospital in 1839, caused by the First Opium War (1839-1842), Dr. Parker left China in 1840 to spend two years in the United States and Europe. To win Congress's support for his Hospital, Dr. Parker, the best-informed man on China in the United States, was given the privilege of speaking before U.S. Congress on January 31, 1841. He spoke of his medical work among the Chinese, the establishing of hospitals at Canton and Macao, and the importance of his medical work in overcoming the Chinese's prejudices and laying the basis for good Chinese-American relations.[8] After delivering his speech before Congress, Dr. Parker gave his lectures to various religious groups in Washington and New York and addressed a group of doctors and the Boston Medical Association, asking their support for his work in China. At the end of the meeting with Dr. Parker, according to the report of James Jackson, the chairman of the Committee of the Boston Medical Association, the Association resolved to "invite the attention of men of property to the medical establishments in China, and earnestly to recommend that they should furnish such assistance as shall give a permanent maintenance to these establishments."[9] The Boston physicians endorsed Parker's aims and commended his efforts, agreeing to publicize his work in the hope of securing more funds for the Medical Missionary Society in China. The Americans,

191

impressed by Dr. Parker's achievements, showed their support for his benevolent work.[10]

As the war in China continued, Parker had to cancel his original plan to return to China immediately and planed a trip to Europe to raise more funds to support his work. After arriving in London, Parker spent six weeks there, writing the pamphlet, *Statements Respecting Hospital in China*, published in Glasgow in 1842, which had a wide circulation and became one of the chief aids in his work. In London, Dr. Parker spent his time visiting doctors and ministers, trying to arouse their interest in his work in China, and many famous people, such as the Duke of Sussex and the Bishop of London, did show an interest in his mission. Parker visited several major cities in England and Scotland. After a meeting with Parker, many prominent citizens in Edinburgh set up a committee, which later turned into the Edinburgh Medical Missionary Society, to raise money for Parker's work. Citizens in Liverpool also appointed a committee to raise funds for Parker. In May 1842, Dr. Parker decided to return to China, even though the war was still in progress. By the time he reached Canton, a peace treaty had been signed, ending the war between Britain and China. Parker took with him a collection of new books, instruments, and medicines as well as a sum of $6,030.62 to be delivered to his Medical Missionary Society. Dr. Parker, a good fund-raiser, helped promote medical charitable work in Canton.[11]

Beginning in 1862, inspired and encouraged by American doctors in some way, the viceroys, merchants, professional people, civil and military officials of the Guangdong Province donated their money to the Canton Hospital and contributed annually towards the expenses of the Hospital and its many dispensaries, including the special funds for new buildings. In 1863 came the first plea from Dr. John Kerr, the superintendent of the Canton Hospital, for a new site for the hospital. His plan was to renovate the old hospital in Jinlifan to receive outpatients routinely and to build a new one, Boji Hospital, to accommodate inpatients. After the Medical Missionary Society spent a good deal of time in discussing Dr. Kerr's suggestion for the enlargement of the hospital, it was resolved that in view of the deficiency of the building occupied, a new hospital should be constructed and that a committee of management would be appointed to devise the best means of accomplishing this object. As a result, a committee composed of Dr. Huang Kuan and two others was founded and began to function, examining the buildings. In the meantime, Dr. Kerr made a great effort to raise money for the hospital; his method was to enlist the Chinese who were really interested in the success of Boji. Consequently, the cost of the new buildings constructed in 1865 mostly came from the Chinese donors. On October 1, 1866, the new hospital was ready for occupancy, complying with all expectation as an appropriate house for the treatment of patients. In 1867, the new complex was built, a chapel, a supply room, and a temporary ward for the use of patients. In 1869, the residence for the physicians was erected. Between 1860 and 1870, the Cantonese contributed over $4,000 to Dr. Kerr's hospital.[12]

In the 1880s, when the Canton Hospital was in financial crisis, Dr. Kerr appealed to the Cantonese again for donations, distributing copies of the brochure to the Cantonese residents. Kerr wrote in the pamphlet:

> The Canton Hospital, a charitable institution, provides modern Western medicine to the Chinese, and since its establishment, the Hospital has seen countless patients and helped numerous patients be restored to health. I am not Chinese and live in a country thousands of miles from China, but I volunteer to offer medical assistance to the Cantonese in order to show God's compassion. Thus, prosperous and wealthy merchants and well-to-do families, please contribute money to help your brothers and sisters.[13]

Dr. Kerr's fund-raising was very successful, collecting sufficient funds from many Chinese and foreign merchants and the Manchu officials, including Governor Zhang Shushen's donation of 200 yuan and Viceroy Zhang Zhidong's 200 yuan, the largest payment of that time.[14]

By means of the kindness of the Cantonese who raised the money for purchase of hospital equipment, an X-ray machine was added to the hospital, which was greatly wanted, and the ownership of this machine not only pleased the doctors but also the patients. A fine gift of surgical instruments for litholopaxy (the crushing of a stone in the bladder and washing out of the fragments) was received in 1896, presented by Dr. W. S. Forbes, who had designed them, and eleven other Philadelphia physicians. In 1916, the eightieth anniversary of the founding of the Canton Hospital, even Li Yuanhong, the president of the Republic of China, contributed five thousand dollars to the Canton Hospital.[15]

A letter written in 1918 by Su Daoming, Dr. Kerr's pupil and later a doctor on the staff of the Canton Hospital for thirty years, showed that the Canton Hospital was the pioneer in Canton in work for the poor and needy with the support of many donors. He wrote:

> Relative to the Canton Hospital of the Canton Medical Missionary Society, I have the privilege to state that as of 1867, there was no charitable institution to provide for the relief of the sick and suffering in Canton, except the Canton Hospital, founded some ten years before my returning from America forty-nine years ago....
> Therefore, I respectfully join in soliciting for whatever funds are available from all loving persons to enable the Canton Hospital to continue to relieve the needy and suffering of their pain and misery through its modern medical and surgical service.[16]

According to the financial report of W. Russell Augur, the business manager of the Canton Hospital, the Canton Hospital received $9,674 from the Chinese and $29,865 from the foreigners in 1923.[17] Encouraged and inspired by Americans to some extent, the Cantonese became more energetically involved in the charitable institution. Charitable giving was becoming a new trend in Canton, and the Chinese donations became one of the financial sources of the Canton Hospital, which had been a missionary charitable institution since its start. More importantly, the Canton Hospital provided a model of a modern philanthropic medical institution for the Chinese.

American Medical Missionaries' Philanthropic Thinking

American medical missionaries not only founded charitable medical institutions and acted very vigorously in the fund-raising drives, but also enthusiastically promoted the establishment of modern philanthropic institutions in China. First, American doctors criticized traditional Chinese welfare institutions. After his watching and coming into contact with the poor in Canton, Dr. Kerr published in 1873 in the journal *China Review* a report based on his assessment of the Chinese charitable institutions. Kerr's motivation to study the Cantonese welfare institutions was to "find something worthy of imitation in their modus operandi...to point out where reforms are needed and improvements are to be made." Kerr confessed that the Chinese had many welfare institutions that were supposed to offer aid to the poor and the needy, but these welfare institutes were not run in the spirit of genuine compassion because "the officials rob the poor and defraud the states."[18] As a result, China's traditional welfare institutions had to be reformed, according to Kerr.

Second, the American doctor encouraged the missionaries to help the Chinese establish modern philanthropic institutions because the Chinese did not have genuine benevolent institutions. He claimed that "truly benevolent institutions are found only in Christian countries and not others" and that the Chinese should be given "the knowledge of those truths which are revealed to us in the Bible," a course of action that would bring about the development of "truly benevolent institutions." Kerr believed that "There is urgent need of reform in the management of these institutions.... Let us, however, teach them by example."[19] Kerr's comments on China's traditional benevolent institutions of that time are controversial, but it is very clear that Kerr was urging the missionaries to help the Chinese found Western-style charitable institutions in accordance with Christian principles.

Finally, American doctors believed that medicine and its practitioners played a significant charitable role in society and that more hospitals should be founded in order to promote Christianity. In 1877, in discussion of relations between medicine and miracles, Kerr asserted that Western medical advantage over Chinese medicine was completely by reason of "means and institutions which modern science and philanthropy have devised."[20] Kerr claimed that the supreme "means of elevating our race" were "schemes of benevolence which depended on the medical profession" and that medicine was "above all others except the clerical, a profession of benevolence." Kerr underlined that this generosity was anchored in a physician's science, not his donations, and that benevolence was rooted in a doctor's knowledge of "the laws of hygiene and their application to the prevention of disease."[21] When developing the relationship between science and benevolence, Kerr believed that medicine was a profession of benevolence, and physicians curing patients and healing the sick were engaged in charitable work.

Dr. R. H. Graves, who practiced medicine in south China for more than thirty years, echoed Dr. Kerr's points of view and advocated opening more dispensaries and hospitals in China to promote Christian benevolence. He wrote in 1895:

> Like the Day School in the education scheme, the dispensary has the advantage of spreading the benefits of Christian benevolence over a wide sphere. It is especially valuable in opening new stations, and thus medical missions do the preliminary work for which they are specially adapted.[22]

To Dr. Graves, the more missionary dispensaries, the more Chinese would benefit from Christian benevolence, which would help make more Chinese to convert to Christianity.

The Progressive Cantonese Reformers' Promotion of Modern Charity

American doctors' thinking on relations between charity and physicians as well as their charitable hospitals in Canton had an effect on the Cantonese reformers and elites to some extent, urging them to promote a modern charitable movement in Canton, although numerous forces had inspired them. Progressive Cantonese reformer Zheng Guanying was one of them.

Cantonese reformer Zheng Gunying's modern charitable thinking was seen in his essay *"Shanju"* (Charity) in his famous book, *Shenshi weiyan* (Words of Warnings to a Prosperous Age), published in 1892. Zheng inherited Buddhism's teaching of causality in Chinese traditional charitable enterprise to encourage rich people to do charitable works so that they would be rewarded after their death. In an article on both hospitals and doctors, he cited an example of a traditional Cantonese physician, who was doing a lot of good works, e.g., free drugs, free coffins, and free medical care to the poor. As a result, Zheng wrote, the physician's family gained good fortune before long because of his beneficent activities.[23]

Zheng was in favor of studying the Western charitable system, a perfect model for the Chinese, accepting as true that Westerners were actively engaged in charitable business due to such factors as Western values, traditions, and Christianity. He also believed that the laws on charitable activities were important in development of benevolent actions in Western countries, and that, because of the laws, many rich Westerners were happy to donate millions of dollars after their death, instead of giving to their children, to such charitable institutions as schools, hospitals, orphan houses, refuges for mental illness, and others. He condemned many rich Chinese merchants and businessmen of wasting money to do a lot of useless things. Zheng, praising the Western welfare system, wrote that the workers paid their medical care and aid as well as their retirement plans from their wages every month, and, under this welfare system, if the workers felt sick, lost jobs, or retired, the government would help and support them. Zheng was the first Chinese to introduce the Western welfare system.[24]

Zheng stressed the multiple functions of modern charitable institutions. He claimed that in Western countries social relief, reducing the number of baggers and thieves in societies, helped maintain a stable social order, and that social relief was not only to provide economic assistance to those needy persons but also to help them learn skills to earn their own living. He underscored the government's role in developing the charitable system, asserting that government and merchants should work together to afford social relief in time of natural disaster and offer assistance in time of tranquility. Zheng advocated that social relief funds should be established, social relief offices should be opened, and social relief workers should be hired in China, as those in Western countries, and that the Chinese government, like Western governments, should establish workshops, training centers, and others to teach people how to cultivate land, make clothing, and produce tools, etc.[25]

Zheng not only advocated Western charitable enterprises but also got involved in charitable campaigns. In 1878, there was a great natural disaster in northern China, and many peasants died of hunger. Zheng, together with several rich merchants and businessmen, established a relief office in Shanghai to launch a campaign for donations and to provide relief to the desperate peasants in northern China. Zheng himself even donated 1,000 taels of silver (1 tael = US$1.40) that his mother left to him after her death. To praise Zheng's great philanthropic endeavor, the Qing government honored him, permitting his hometown to erect a memorial archway, on which "Great Generous" in Chinese characters were engraved. His hometown officials recorded his charitable activities in the annals of the county, too.[26]

Great Cantonese reformer Kang Youwei was another case. Kang's philanthropic ideology took shape in the late twentieth century. First, Kang encouraged the Chinese to abandon traditional Chinese philanthropic institutions based on the clan relationship and to adopt modern charitable institutes. To Kang, the Chinese were willing to help only their clan members or their relatives, as opposed to anyone who needed help. After comparing Western philanthropic institutions with China's counterparts, Kang stated that Western charitable ventures had played a significant part in societies because all kinds of people, regardless of clan and kin, benefited greatly from the benevolent endeavors. Underlining nation-state loyalty, rather than kin-clan loyalty inherited in Chinese society, Westerners were happy to donate a lot of money to the public charitable institutions to help their citizens.[27] Kang advocated founding of such modern official philanthropic institutions in China as hospitals, schools, home for the elderly, orphanages, and others, to provide relief to anyone who was in urgent need of help, regardless of kin or clan connections. Such charitable institutions sponsored by the government would help weaken kinship loyalty and strengthen national patriotism, as indicated by Kang.[28]

Second, Kang was in favor of multiplying functions of the philanthropic institutions. He divided the poor into two categories, lazy people and disabled people including the blind, the deaf, and the dumb. To the first group, Kang stressed teaching them the skills to support themselves; to the second group, he supported the founding of charitable institutions to adopt them.[29] To Kang, Shantang (Benevolent Society) had functions of not only giving aid to the poor and the needy but also teaching Confucianism and introducing Western leanings, carrying out political and cultural missions. He pointed out, "Shantang has been established for some years to promote Confucianism's benevolence by giving aid to the poor, the needy, the sick, and widows and orphans. Now we have to promote studying Confucianism at this institution as well as learning Western science and technology. As a result, like the Western charitable institutions, Shantang is of educational function."[30] Kang was the first Chinese to raise the modern charitable concepts, such as public support, public education, public relief in his book, *Datong shu* (Great Harmony). Published in 1902, this book outlined Kang's perfect society, underscoring government's role, instead of clan-kin's, in helping the poor, the sick, the old, the disabled, and the weak.[31] In Kang's utopian society, the people would have freedom to marry, children would be raised by the state, free education would be for all the people, and the government would take care of those people who were in need of help.

Finally, Kang stressed the relationship between the assistance to the distressed and the liberation of a nation from subjugation. He believed that government should be responsible for giving relief to the poor and funding a welfare system. The relief to the poor was a part of his reform program in the reform movement. In his 1895 petition to the emperor, Kang encouraged the Qing government to found different types of charitable institutions, like the Western charitable ones, to provide relief to the poor, the needy, the disabled, the handicapped, the sick, and others; otherwise, many Chinese would be still very poor and weak, and a rich China would not come into being, according to Kang.[32] Kang was the first Chinese to connect charity with the revitalization of China.

Sun Yat-sen was very involved in medical charitable work. In February 1894, Sun was forced to leave Macao because his medical license was not recognized by the colonial government of Macao, although he had been practicing medicine in the city for a couple of years after his graduation from the medical college in Hong Kong. Sun then opened a dispensary in western Canton. He attended to patients at his clinic and provided free medical services in the morning every day, and in the afternoon, he went out to see patients, receiving service fees only when patients were willing to give. In time of emergency, such as difficult labor or poisoning, Sun lost no time in rushing to their homes no matter whether they were rich or poor.[33] In 1895, Sun put his charitable thinking in the constitution of the Revive China Society, pointing out that this organization was to gain the benefit for the 400 million Chinese people, and that no one would be suffering in the new Republic of China. In 1924, he claimed that the government should carry out relief to improve the suffering of the workers and peasants and that the old should be supported and the young should be educated. Sun also designed a system, under which agricultural, mineral, lumber, and other economic resources would be controlled by the state so that the government would have enough funds to organize and to run the charitable enterprises.[34]

Liang Qichiao was in support of the charitable institutions, especially the charitable work of medicine. He and other reformers established Yixue Shanhui (Charitable Medical Society) in Shanghai in 1897. The objective of the medical organization was to promote medical science in China, but this organization was a charitable association with educational function.[35] Liang also stressed setting up more Shantang (Charitable Society) to give assistance to the homeless, the poor, the sick, the weak, and the aged, providing them with books to read and study and helping them learn skills. Liang even suggested making *Shantang* a place like Western parliaments to discuss politics.[36]

Tang Shiyi, John Kerr's student, was a philanthropist. After graduation from Canton Hospital, for example, Tang provided free services to 7,546 patients from January to September in 1909 at the China Reform Association, a charitable organization in Canton.[37] Later, after making profits from his pharmacy business, Tang began to donate money to build a primary school and purchased a lot of equipment for the boarding school in his hometown in the 1920s. This school, free to all students, became the largest and most well-equipped school in the county; he contributed significantly to education in his hometown.[38]

Partially exposed to American medical missionaries' Christian benevolent philosophy and impressed by American-run charitable institutions in Canton to some degree, the Cantonese elites began to develop modern charitable thought and advocated modernization of Chinese traditional practice of clan-oriented philanthropy in China, especially in Canton.

The Early Modern Charitable Enterprises in Canton, 1871-1912

The influence of the Canton Hospital had been extensive on the setting up of modern charitable institution in Canton; a new form of philanthropic institution began to appear, combining the charitable institutions of traditional China with the modern medical administration and treatment of Western hospitals. The first one of this type of the so-called charity hospital was opened in Hong Kong under the name of Donghua Hospital in 1871, and another one was the emergence of Aiyu shantang (Hall of Sustaining Love) in Canton in the same year. Both Donghua and Aiyu were not merely hospitals and dispensaries, but included other channels of benevolent work, such as opening free schools, preaching ethics, supporting the aged and orphans, giving coffins to the poor, supplying food and clothing to the impoverished, and helping widows and others. Aiyu shantang's objectives were all admirable, beyond hospital and dispensary work. It offered aid to the needy without requiring that they belonged to or be identified with a particular group of tradesmen, or a particular clan, or fit into any category except that of the impoverished. Those people were not expected to give in return for the assistance given to them.[39]

Westerners in part inspired the Cantonese to establish the modern charitable institution. As Dr. Kerr commented in 1874, "The Chinese merchants and compradors who were the originators of the scheme, had been for many years connected with foreigners, and had learned from them much of foreign ideas, philanthropy and something of religion."[40] Aiyu shantang was modeled on the Canton Hospital, when Kerr claimed, "Taking Oi Yuk Tong [Aiyu tang] as a specimen of these institutions, a sketch of its administration and of its work will show how far they are copied from the foreign models and how far native ideas have developed them on new lines."[41]

As a matter of fact, at the beginning, Aiyu shantang received American doctors' support. Many Chinese doctors of the old type, for example, were asked by Dr. Kerr through Aiyu shantang to receive instruction in vaccination at the Canton Hospital.[42] In his report Dr. Kerr described Aiyu shantang as a highly commendable benevolent society with these remarks, "We recognize the institution under consideration...as a step in the right direction, to place the Chinese on a level with Western nations."[43]

The founding of Aiyu shantang paved the way for the formation of more Shangtang (Benevolent societies) in Canton in the following years. In 1873, a new medical welfare institution, Fanbian suo, was established to "provide a place in which to receive the homeless and friendless persons who are hopelessly ill."[44] By the end of the nineteenth century, there were nearly twenty non-government charitable institutions of such kind in Canton as Guangren shantang established in 1884, Renji Hospital in 1889, Chongzhen shantang in 1896, Fangbian Hospital (Place of Charity) in 1899, Lesan Hospital and Huixing sanyuan in 1900, and so on, nine of which were very famous at that time in Canton.[45] Institutions of this kind later were quite numerous in south China. The gazetteer of Nanhai county in Guangdong wrote, "This was the very beginning of benevolent societies in Guangdong province."[46]

The motivations for local prominent leaders to become engaged in voluntary organizations of modern times were several. The privileged members of the benevolent societies for the most part had the identical moral value as the Chinese nation had. Their benevolent activities would earn them the empathy of important persons with Confucian integrity, enhance their influence and social status, show their social sense of right and wrong, give them some authority in the community, provide them with extra incomes, compensate them with individual value, and others.

The Characteristics of Shantang

Shantang was a new form of charitable society in Canton, combing traditional charitable organizations with Western institutions. Such Chinese-style associations had several characteristics. The first common feature of Shantang was its multiple duties. Traditional widows' departments, orphan houses, and old men centers provided for only a single category of the destitute correspondingly. The new benevolent societies presented assistance and advice to all kinds of the needy; they were diverse in classifying different kinds of the poor. The benevolent societies afforded food, clothing, and housing to the poor young and the aged; bestowed free medicine; taught the poor children, offered coffins and free burials, instructed on ethical principles, salvaged the stranded, provided street lights, and did a broad variety of other charitable works.

The second feature of such benevolent societies was that their benefactors and administrators generally included both the gentry and merchants. Theoretically, the social position of merchants still trailed behind that of scholars and officials and did not play a significant role in the charitable enterprises. In the late nineteenth century, the Cantonese merchants were becoming a driving force in the modern charitable movement in Canton because the benevolent associations required a large amount of funds for their operations, and merchants possessed sufficient financial resources to support them. The founding of the Fangbian Hospital was an example. In the summer of 1899, many inhabitants died of the plague. The dead bodies were not buried immediately, and some patients in danger of dying were lying in the streets, a horrible scene encouraging some Cantonese merchants to open a hospital to help those dying people and to collect and bury those corpses. Under the leadership of Chen Huipu, twenty-four merchants launched a campaign for donations and contributions throughout the city of Canton. As a result, a philanthropic medical institution was opened.[47]

The third feature was not clan-kin oriented. Shantang in Canton not only served the residents of the city of Canton but also the people in Guangdong and other provinces, as well as other countries. These new, modern charitable institutions were distinguished from the traditional charitable institutes that provided relief only to the kin or clan members. In 1907, when the pandemic transpired in Saigon, Vietnam, and Phnom Penh, Cambodia, Fangbian Hospital dispatched doctors of Chinese medicine to relieve the people in suffering countries. In 1908, when the epidemic erupted again, Fangbian Hospital provided free treatment of Hong Kong patients, except transportation fees, and free medical care and free transportation to the poor residents in Hong Kong as well as other poor Chinese overseas.[48]

The fourth was the modern management skills adopted by the local elite to manage their benevolent societies. To be able to provide services on a continual basis, the benevolent society needed a steady source of funds. The administration of the shops and houses owned and rented out by Aiyu shantang required modern management skills and knowledge. Dr. Kerr praised the stable financial sources of Aiyu shantang with such observations, Shantang "becomes, therefore, a large business establishment, requiring time, talent, and skill for its administration. This arrangement for a permanent income is an evidence of the fact that voluntary contributions cannot be relied on to sustain the institution."[49] He stated in another report that this business talent would "fill this land [China] with institutions for the relief of human suffering in all its forms, as well as for the elevation of the people intellectually, morally, and spiritually."[50] Shantang also learned how to make a united effort—a modern management skill. During the 1894 plague, all nine Shantang were united together and primarily conducted medical relief efforts in Canton beyond those officially mandated measures. These Cantonese civil leaders worked together to take charge of plague relief effort among the Cantonese residents. In 1896, when the plague occurred in Hong Kong, several Shantang cooperatively sent hospital ships to take care of patients there, and some of them were brought back to Canton for further treatment. Shantang made a united effort to provide food and medicine to the people of Guangxi province in natural calamities in 1896 and mailed 500 silver taels of donation in 1900 to alleviate the people in Guizhou Province.

The fifth was to educate the masses with Confucian teachings. Lectures were delivered at Shantang open to the community, based on the content of *Shengyu guangxun* (Confucian Teachings), a book published by the Qing government in 1670, which emphasized Confucian thought on topics such as morality, good and evil, filial piety, family value, benevolence, loyalty, learning, and others. In addition to teaching at Shantang, the lecturers hired by Shantang traveled to the countryside to deliver their lectures and to loan to peasants the books on Confucianism. The aim of the teachings was to edify the masses with the intention of the establishment of a stable and peaceful society.[51] Dr. Kerr, noting that Aiyu tang paid 285 taels to five lectures in 1871, unhappily remarked that "the amount of money spent...does not indicate any great enthusiasm either for the education of the masses or the propagation of morality or religion."[52] In 1872, twenty Confucian teachers taught 564 students in nineteen schools, and in 1873, sixteen teachers taught 391 students in fifteen schools. Kerr claimed that the exercise of community teachings of this type had declined but was revitalized in 1874 so as to offset the preaching of Christianity.[53]

The last one was to carry out professional education—free schools for the poor. Shantang not only provided relief but also helped train the poor to earn their living by themselves. They set up free public schools to help the poor children learn how to read and write and the skills to make their living. According to Dr. Kerr's account, the Aiyou shantang hired twenty teachers and opened nineteen schools in 1872 and employed sixteen teachers and opened fifteen schools in 1873.[54] In 1913, Shantang opened a medical school, Hongzhong Medical School, to teach predominantly Chinese medicine and partially Western medicine with a six-year term in order to train more medical professionals to meet the demand of the Cantonese. Chen Huipu, the president of the Fangbian Hospital, was appointed as the principal of the medical school. The first semester successfully recruited 300 students in three classes.[55]

American medical missionaries were one of the forces that inspired the Cantonese to found this new form of philanthropic institutions to some extent, although many forces motivated the Chinese to launch a modern charitable movement in Canton, such as the model of the charitable associations in other cities in China. More significantly, the Cantonese combined the traditional Chinese benevolent institution with the Western counterpart, rather than only copying totally Western charitable institutions.

The Role of Shantang

The new modern charitable institutions in Canton played a momentous role in the philanthropic movement. First, the new charitable institutions provided social relief to the poor and medical services to the sick. Shantang distributed free food and clothing and collected and resettled homeless persons, vagrants, and prostitutes. As indicated by Dr. Kerr's statistics, Aiyu tang played a significant part in the modern charitable movement in Canton.[56] In addition to social relief, voluntary doctors of Chinese medicine established dispensaries at Shantang to provide medical treatments for poor outpatients and accommodate beds for the poor inpatients. The Aiyu Benevolent Society maintained a dispensary as part of its regular charitable activities, and patients could select doctors who were working for the dispensary. Unlike traditional dispensaries, this dispensary in daily operation was open throughout the year.[57] Furthermore, Shantang dispatched physicians to provide medical attention to poor patients at homes, such as free smallpox vaccination and free medications.[58] For example, the China Reform Society founded in western Canton in 1908 was a charitable institution providing relief in time of natural disaster and free Western medical services to the poor. Each month the volunteer doctors of Western medicine served approximately 900 patients without any charges. The famous woman doctor Chen Lunhun, an expert at gynecology, obstetrics, and pediatrics, served at this Society and played an important role in providing medical services to residents in western Canton.[59]

Second, the institutions alleviated the people in stricken areas in time of natural disaster. In 1902, due to a crop failure in Guangdong Province, many peasants were on the edge of starvation; Shantang lost no time delivering grain to famine-stricken areas. These charitable institutions worked together to carry out relief works due to the limit of one institution's financial and human resources. In the spring of 1907, because of great inflation, the hungry people were plotting a revolt in Dongguan, sixty miles east of Canton. Under such momentous circumstances, each Shantang in Canton donated funds or loaned money sufficient to purchase rice from Vietnam, and they immediately delivered grain to the hungry peasants in April.[60] Shantang played an imperative part in dissemination of relief to the victims of natural calamities.

Finally, they played a crucial function in preventing the spread of epidemics. During the 1894 plague, for example, Tungshan tang in eastern Canton employed a doctor to be in charge of a quantity of medicines and to distribute them along the streets of the suburbs, so that those people who lived too far away from the city center or were unable to seek the doctor for advice were able and to receive preventive medicines. Renji tang, because of its location in the city's business districts, which were full of plague patients, used a very large boat as a floating hospital to take care of the patients. An article in the journal of *North China Herald* wrote, "Placards also had been posted calling upon skilful physicians to apply to the charity institutions for regular engagements.... Moreover, such doctors as stayed at home were called upon to give aid, gratis, at their office, and then apply to the institutions for remuneration if so desired."[61] Shantang also operated as a sanatorium for the dying and offered interment for the departed during the plague. Dr. Mary Niles gave an account that at the end of the third month of the epidemic Aiyu shantang had given out over three hundred free coffins, much more than the regular monthly number of twenty or thirty, and that at the Fangbian suo "there was a mortality of 296 of the epidemic on their grounds in the third month, whereas last year 108 died of the spring epidemic."[62] Besides, charitable elites launched a campaign to collect and dispose of rats so as to stop the epidemic. Shantang played a momentous part in control of the transmission of the plague.

Modern charitable institutions gained their strength in Canton at the beginning of the twentieth century. Both the Canton Hospital and the Cantonese generous institutions coexisted well. The Canton Hospital continued receiving Chinese contributions. Shantang was carrying out good works in its own traditional way but emulated the Canton Hospital's objective and approaches in some degree. As Dr. Su Daoming summarized the philanthropic institutions in Canton in a letter of 1918, he wrote such observations, "Since then Oi Yuk [Aiyu] and other Chinese charitable organizations have been established, all imitating the purpose and methods of the Canton Hospital to remove pain and distress especially from the poor."[63]

American Doctors' New Charitable Institutions in Canton, 1889-1935

When China's charitable institutions were providing relief, medical service, and moral education to the Chinese so as to maintain social order and stability in the late nineteenth century, Western philanthropists were extending their philanthropic service. They not only established hospitals and employed doctors to treat patients, but also opened new charitable institutions, such as refuges for the mentally ill, orphanages, schools for the blind, deaf, or dumb, and others. They not only offered relief to the poor, the sick and the needy but also helped those unfortunate people learn their skills to make their living. American medical missionaries transplanted such institutions into Canton, opening the Mingxin School for the Blind in 1889 and Kerr's Refuge for the Insane in 1899.

The Mingxin School, 1889-1932

The blind in China, together with the deaf, and the dumb, normally were not cared for as a separate class of the destitute. Those who could not care for themselves or be looked after by their relatives, family members, or friends were eligible for the same relief as provided to other destitute. Few special institutions existed for their care in China generally, and official effort to encourage or teach the poor blind to earn a living was lacking at that time.

The local governments, generous societies, and charitable individuals did not have any education or remedy programs for the physically or mentally handicapped, but Canton did have a home for the blind, maintained and supported by the Nanhai and Panyu county magistrate. The Qing court at the beginning provided some support for the sightless persons in Canton. The total number was increased to 1,476 in 1846. The resources provided for the blind were put in the local government and were given to the sightless every three months. The blind were enrolled by name, age, and appearance. The unsighted kept money they were given, but they were not offered with any lodging, provisions, or medicines, not including medical care accessible from the benevolent hospitals. In 1875, John Henry Gray, a British consular chaplain at Canton, published his observations in Canton in his book, *Walk in the City of Canton,* recording observations about the blind in some detail. He claimed that in Canton the blind lived in the asylum and might receive medical attention, and that the number of residents was about 300 in 1875.[64] The situation of the blind girls in Canton was very miserable. Called "sing-song girls," they were led through the streets at night with their musical instruments, singing while begging. The money they collected sometimes was stolen by thieves. They lived as slaves in the singing houses, which were dirty with filth and rats and infected with illness.[65]

The miserable situation of the blind in Canton was identified by American medical missionaries. When Dr. Mary Niles was working at the Canton Hospital, Dr. Kerr's interest in Chinese charitable institutions no doubt influenced her, and she began to take an active role in relief for the blind. Her interest in the blind apparently began in 1889 when a little waif of three years was picked up from an ash heap and brought to the hospital for healing. The rescuer later identified that the child was hopelessly blind. Shocked by a singing blind girl's miserable stories, Dr. Niles decided to keep the girl with her. Soon after, four little blind girls were rescued and were taught to memorize at the Canton Hospital's school run by Mrs. Martha Noyes Kerr, Dr. Kerr's wife.[66] The School for the Blind was begun, as Dr. Mary Niles wrote:

> They had been brought as patients, but when found incurable and their friends were proposing to commit them to worse than useless lives, we rescued them from this fate…. Friends in America, moved to compassion by my mother's recital of their woes, furnished their support.[67]

When Dr. Niles returned to America in 1890, Mrs. Kerr took charge of these little girls. As soon as their friends in America were told of the troubles, money was sent for their maintenance. A native home in Henan in southern Canton was rented at first and later a house in Macao. A blind teacher was employed to teach the students Braille and knitting, and a lady was engaged to take charge of them soon after Dr. Niles returned to Canton. After four years, ill health compelled the lady to return to America, and the school for the blind came back to Canton where the True Light Seminary generously gave them a room in the fourth story of one of their buildings.[68]

Dr. Niles, determined to provide a place to care for these blind girls, wrote in 1892 to the secretary of the Presbyterian Board of Foreign Missions to apply for assistance. Rev. Dr. William Speer's reply was unenthusiastic. As a result, Niles contributed an article, "The Blind Girls of Canton," to the journal, *Woman's Work for Woman,* which touched the minds of many sponsors in America. The appeals of many in the home church were made aware, and the Board finally approved Mary Niles's school for blind girls in 1894. The School for the Blind was formally founded in 1896, and later the School had its own house when a new building capable of housing thirty pupils was erected. Dr. Niles and her father, who had come to visit his daughter, moved from the Canton Hospital to the new building for the blind school. In 1897, Niles renamed the school as Mingxin School (School of Clear Heart or Understanding Heart). The objectives of the school were to adopt blind children and to teach them life skills so that they would earn their living by themselves and become useful persons in society.[69] Thus, American missionary doctors initiated a new form of philanthropic institution in Canton, extending beneficent service to the blind.

In 1899 when Dr. Niles came back to Canton after her second furlough, she severed her connection with the Canton Hospital in order to devote her entire time to the needs of the expansion of her school, resigning as a doctor and assuming a position as an administrator of the Mingxin School. In 1906, the School for the Blind was relocated to Fangcun in southwestern Canton where a piece of land of three acres was purchased along the river at low price through the generosity of the missionary medical doctor, Chas. C. Selden. With the support of the Canton government, wealthy people, and foreigners in Canton, the School collected more than US$3,200, sufficient for a new building. A new three-story dormitory was constructed for student and faculty. The sale of knitted goods made by the girls helped provide support. In a couple of years, when the new buildings were completed, the School became a picturesque place with adored old banyans and many other trees, bricked and winding trails, and neat and bright classrooms.[70]

Inspired by the administration system of other philanthropic organizations, the Board of Trustees of the School was established in 1908. The Board of Trustees had meetings regularly, three or up to six times annually, discussing fund-raising activities, expenditures and incomes, employment, appointments, lay-offs, and so forth.

In 1908, the School started to charge students tuition as well as fees for their room and board, but most helpless pupils did not pay any fees. The curriculum was offered from kindergarten through junior high. Music was an important section of the program with classes in piano, organ, and singing. Twenty-nine students were at the School. During the opening ceremony held on October 25, 1910 for the new building of the School, the prominent officials, such as Tartar general, the minister of education, the salt commissioner, and the provincial judge, sent their representatives to attend, showing their interest in the educational work carried out for the sightless.[71]

The Canton government began to realize the significance of the School for the Blind after the new Republic of China was founded. On August 8, 1912, the Department of Police of Canton sent to the School sixty-six blind singing girls and seven blind boys, unclean, tattered, scared, and weeping. For that reason, the school soon expanded so greatly that the enrollment of the school multiplied three-fold, and boy and girl departments were established separately. In 1913, a building was erected for the accommodation of 140 pupils.[72]

At the beginning, the chief of the Police Department promised that the Canton government would pay to the School the room and tuition of the blind students it sent every month and would pay for a school building, but several months later the chief suddenly died, and the Police Department again and again failed to honor the promise the chief had made. Since the building program was in progress, the debts had to be paid, and the Chinese recognized an obligation to pay off old debts on the last day of the year. On New Year Eve of 1915, Dr. Niles presented her case at the police headquarters, sitting tranquilly with great dignity for over six hours in the waiting room. A few hours before the beginning of the New Year, the arrears were paid totally in piles of $5.00 Canton bills.[73]

Since Dr. Niles specialized in gynecology and obstetrics and expected to devote her life to caring for women and children, she knew very little about education for the blind. As a result, she decided to translate Chinese characters into Braille, a writing system consisting of patterns of raised dots that were read by touch for vision-impaired or sightless people. She herself learned it with infinite care and patience in order to translate it into Chinese. Finally, a monumental achievement was made when the Braille system of writing was translated into the Cantonese language, for which Mary Niles's alma mater, the Elmira College, awarded her the degree of L. L. D. afterward.[74]

By 1928, the Mingxin School had six grades and offered courses in Chinese language, history, music, geography, society, nature, physical education, government, and so on. In addition, the School offered such skill-learning courses as handicraft, piano, family administration, massage, acupuncture, and so forth. The school employed new teaching methods, according to students' individual interests, to engage students in the learning process. The School issued diplomas to those students who had completed the requirements of the School. After their graduation, the sightless graduates, like sighted students, went to the middle school to continue their education, worked at the health centers as massagers, weaved straw mats, knitted sweaters, labored as housekeepers, or preached as priests. These blind people not only supported themselves but were useful in the society.[75]

At the beginning of the School, all money came from Dr. Niles' fundraising assisted by her friends in America. Later, local government officials, merchants, and businessmen were the major donors for the expansion of the school. To solve the financial problems, the School inaugurated a fund-raising drive in 1929 with a target of 4,000 yuan and had successfully collected an endowment of 10,000 yuan by 1930.[76]

Dr. Niles carried the responsibility of that school until her retirement in July 1928 after forty-six years of service in China, best known in China through her work for the blind. Similarly, she taught and took charge of the obstetric department at the Hackett Medical College and its hospital until the year 1923, after which she devoted herself entirely to the School for the Blind. In addition to these activities, Dr. Niles held several positions, such as trustee of the Refuge for the Insane and other positions in connection with missionary work in Canton. She breathed her last breath on January 18, 1933 in California, where she lived with her brother, Rev. John S. Niles. Her colleagues paid her this tribute: "Into dark places, full of pain and suffering she went, taking light and relief and beauty, and most of all, a loving heart."[77]

From 1908 to 1932, 113 girls and seventeen boys received training at the School and completed its courses. Of fifty-one graduates of the School in 1931, eight were massagers at hospitals; seven were weavers of mats or baskets; and twenty-one were teachers at schools. Eleven blind boys were also offered jobs as teachers and weavers. Some worked at churches, with well-to-do families, and so on. One of them had been engaged in education as the principal of a school for more than twelve years, her excellent work praised greatly by her students and teachers.[78] An incomplete survey of the graduates of the school for the thirty-year period of 1908-1938 suggests that the graduates of the Mingxin School earned their living by themselves and became useful persons in society.[79]

In brief, the Mingxin School for the Blind indicated American doctors' efforts to extend charitable service from the sick to the blind. This new modern philanthropic institution not only provided aid to the helpless blind children, but also helped them learn skills to make their own living. This School had an impact on the Cantonese. The significant achievements of this School gradually won first the financial support of the Cantonese elite and merchants, and then gained government endorsement when the Cantonese officials sent the blind children to the School with government subsidies. The Cantonese government began to regard it as a part of the welfare system in society and was willing to participate in the management of this philanthropic institution. The school that Dr. Mary Niles started was the first such institution in south China, although an English missionary William Murray established China's first school for the blind in Beijing in 1874. Thereafter, more blind schools were founded at the beginning of the twentieth century, In Jinan, the capital of Shandong Province, one school for blind was found in 1905 and one in Shanghai in 1907.[80] Today, the Mingxin School in Canton is the largest school for the blind in China.[81]

Kerr's Refuge for the Insane, 1899-1935

Many Chinese believed that the human body is a balance system, in which disease, including psychiatric disarray, was caused by a lack of balance, and in which self-control in emotional life was necessary. The Chinese took into account all of somebody's physical, mental, and social conditions in the treatment of illness, and their comprehension of the interrelationship of brain and body had a long history, too. Equilibrium and self-control resulted in health; overindulgence or dearth was the cause of ailment. Throughout Chinese history, coexisting with the great practice of Chinese medical and psychiatric thought was the public custom in communities, which emphasized the study of demons, ghost possession, the ceremony to drive out evil spirits, clearing the mind of oppressive feelings, and so forth. Most Chinese patients having mental syndromes were expected to be treated, if at all, in this public custom.[82]

The common therapy depended on the use of shackles and fetters. Herb medicines and acupuncture were the most normal solution to correct the body's irregularity, which was regarded as the reason for particular psychological problems. The common remedy included not only the use of allegedly magic words but also toxic liquid therapy, whippings, and even signs with burning irons. Many devastating ceremonies or spoken formulas were used with the intention of expelling evil spirits in their bodies or awakening the stricken patients. These ceremonies and methods of healing continued in China until the twentieth century.[83]

Officials considered madness as an urgent social problem, but the government did not put restrictions upon the mad people, provided that they were not caught in theft or they did nothing aggressive. If caught in the street doing anything out of the normal way, they were taken into custody and put into prison, basically the same as the lawbreakers. Even if the mentally ill were inoffensive and strayed in the streets, they were ridiculed and insulted, sometimes stones were thrown at them. Their families usually dealt with them as unfamiliar persons and locked them up in a dark room. If they ripped their garments or were dangerous, their families occasionally renounced them. Most mentally ill were shackled at home and were not permitted to leave their homes. As a result, few people, even their neighbors, knew about them. The mentally ill represented a very helpless class in imperial China.[84]

In the United States, in the second half of the nineteenth century American doctors began to regard the whip, the chain, the straitjacket (a garment with long sleeves that could be tied together, used to restrict arm movement), and the dark room as brutal, humiliating, and producing problems, instead of helping achieve a goal in treating the mentally ill. They advocated mental education, instead of corporal compulsion, to restore the confined mad person to mental health so as to return to society ultimately.

American medical missionaries, while practicing medicine in China, started to pay attention to the Chinese mentally ill and proposed the introduction of a mental hospital in China. As early as 1872, Dr. Enud Faber who was in charge of the dispensary at Humen in Guangdong Province reported a case of the mental illness. After reading this report, Dr. Kerr became interested in the study of this type of disease. He then appealed in a letter to the Medical Missionary Society for the creation of a mental hospital to provide rational treatment of this class of mental patient. He claimed in his report of 1872 that the government or missionaries had not addressed the need of the mentally ill, and that the asylum would be the first in all of China. According to the report of E. P. Thwing of the American Presbyterian Mission, Kerr's motivation for the refuge for the mentally ill was philanthropic, rather than religious to transmit Christianity.[85]

From 1876 to 1880, Kerr published several articles on the necessity and enormity of the formation of a hospitals for the mentally ill in China in the journal, *Wanguo gongbao* (Global News), such as "On Funding of the Mental Hospital," "The Ways the British Adopted Psychosis," and "The Earlier the Better: The Treatment of Madness."[86] Kerr wrote in 1878:

> In China there are thousands who perish annually in the streets of her great cities from disease, starvation and cold; and there is a reason to believe that the insane are often made away with when they are troublesome.... The multiplication of benevolent institutions is the glory of our religion, and herein is exhibited its superiority over all the pagan religions which have existed in any age or country.[87]

To Dr. Kerr, the creation of mental hospitals in China was to extend Christianity's benevolence to the unfortunate Chinese, who were suffering and dying. In 1886, Kerr repeated his suggestion of the significance of a mental hospital in China in celebration of the fifty-fifth anniversary of the Canton Hospital. Kerr's plan, however, won little support from either the Canton Medical Missionary Society or the Canton government, which had little interest in his proposal.[88]

Obstacles stood in front of Dr. Kerr, but these obstructions did not discourage Dr. Kerr from making an effort to realize his plan to establish an asylum for the mentally ill in China. At the 1890 conference of the China Medical Missionary Society, when the delegates were discussing the issue of mental illness, Kerr appealed on February 18 that so far China did not have any asylum for the mentally ill when many patients of mental illness, rich or poor, were dying every day from brutal treatments. He urged the benevolent missionaries to help the Chinese treat those unfortunate patients with modern medical technology and to launch a fund-raising campaign for the support of a permanent charitable asylum for the mentally ill in China. At the conference Professor E. P. Thwing of the American Presbyterian Mission also read a paper, "Western Methods with the Insane Chinese," and Dr. Kerr published a leaflet distributed to the delegates to promote the cause. The Conference seemed to have expressed its approval of this suggestion.[89]

The Society, for various reasons, was not ready for such a project, but Kerr refused to give up. After receiving contributions from his American and Chinese friends, he started an asylum on his own. He used his own money to purchase seventeen acres of land at Fangcun in southwestern Canton as a site for an asylum in 1892, where Wen Tianmou, a member of the Provisional Committee, soon started a dispensary on a piece of land of three acres in order to secure the goodwill of the neighbors. Kerr's hospital received offerings from many Chinese overseas, missionaries, and merchants. He received unpredicted assistance in 1894 when a medical missionary outside China handed over to Dr. Kerr an amount of money for medical charity from the Cantonese. The donors' endorsements were used for the erection of a building on the site, providing an accommodation of thirty beds in twenty-four rooms. More contributions later collected by the Provisional Committee and others were sufficient for the second building.[90]

Dr. Kerr also won strong support for his project from William Martin (William Martin was appointed later by Emperor Guangxu as the dean of the Imperial University, or later called Beijing University, which was founded on December 31, 1898). Since Kerr was probably the world's foremost surgeon in treating vesical calculi, in 1897, at the age of 70, Kerr was called to Beijing to perform a serious operation on the U.S. minister, Charles Denby, who had already gone to Europe for treatment, which had proved unsuccessful. After operating successfully on August 5 upon the minister, Dr. Kerr continued taking care of him in Beijing for several months. During that time, learning of Kerr's Refuge for the Insane, William donated $20 to the hospital and published an article, "A Record of a Refuge for the Insane in Guangdong," strongly praising Kerr's philanthropic efforts to create China's first mental hospital.[91]

Dr. Kerr's relation with the Canton Hospital was not very good in his later years because of the conflicting viewpoints between his younger colleagues and him. In 1898, he resigned from the Hospital and from the Medical Missionary Society in order to devote his whole energy to the work for the mentally ill. Kerr's Refuge for the Insane was formally opened in Fangcun in southwestern Canton after a lot of difficulties were overcome. For the first time in the history of China, a psychiatric hospital that attempted to provide modern psychiatric care was opened with thirty beds to attend to the mind-diseased patients. Dr. Kerr had the honor of founding the first refuge for the mentally ill in China, extending the charitable service to mental patients at the end of the nineteenth century. Most of the patients were taken to this special hospital in fetters. The first patient was chained to a stone for three years before going to Kerr's Refuge on February 20. The second patient was a woman found with a shackle around her neck. At the end of the year, Dr. Kerr and his wife moved over to the Refuge and started living there. Dr. Kerr took with him his class of male medical students, who were very helpful in carrying on the work at the Refuge, which had eleven patients at that time.[92]

Dr. Kerr believed that the asylum could do more than merely segregate lunatics from society and could restore the mental patients to health because madness came to be regarded as a condition that could be treated and cured by a course of therapy of moral persuasion in Western society. A change of emphasis from internment to therapy began at the Refuge. Dr. Kerr first declared the rules: the mentally ill patients were ill and should not be held responsible for their activities; they were in a hospital, not a prison; and the patients had to be treated as humans, not animals. He promised to offer a course of treatment based on persuasion rather than force, freedom rather than restraint, and an outdoor life in good physical shape with a maximum of recreation, warm baths, and compassion. He also had the goal to provide the patients with paid employment when workable. As a result, at the Refuge the patients were not chained, although most of them had been shackled and confined in secluded rooms before being taken to the Refuge. They were encouraged to participate in labor work, such as watering flowers, cooking food, growing vegetables, sewing clothing, and participating in entertainment and sport activities. Dr. Kerr also designed new devices to improve the living condition for the patients.[93] By September 1900, a home had been completed so that Dr. and Mrs. Kerr were able to move from their unsatisfactory quarters with the patients into a house. One-third of the expense was endowed by Chinese Christians.[94]

In 1900, Dr. Charles C. Selden joined the Refuge. Due to his poor health, Dr. Kerr was willing to hand over the administration of the Refuge to the competent man, Dr. Selden, who would be assisted by Dr. J. Allen Hofmann. By 1901, the Refuge for the Insane had treated seventy-nine patients; of this number twenty-one were cured and returned to their friends, and the buildings were able to accommodate fifty patients.[95]

Dr. Kerr lived to see fifty patients within the Refuge's walls, but at the age of seventy-seven, he died on August 10, 1901 after a memorable career of forty-seven years in Canton. He was buried at the Protestant cemetery outside of Canton on the way to White Cloud Mountain. Dr. Kerr was one of the foremost medical missionary pioneers of China. At his death his colleagues paid him a high tribute: "No man in all that empire, and perhaps no medical missionary in any mission field had accomplished so great a professional work as Dr. Kerr."[96]

Mrs. Martha Noyes Kerr started to take on what her husband had left, serving as an administrator and a fund-raiser for the asylum. In 1901, Dr. Selden was the superintendent of the Refuge, which had one nurse and seventeen nurse assistants. He played a significant role in constructing stronger buildings, structuring small cottages to create a community atmosphere, establishing a neat backyard, making available modern facilities, a chapel and more than enough space for doing exercises, and effectively overcoming the confusion of obstacles of different cultures to expand this Refuge. Selden's mental hospital emphasized social communication and liberty of movement. The patients at this hospital came from two sources. About one-half were sent by officials, while the others were brought by their families or friends.

The patients, including all classes of society, beggars, scholars, officials, and others, not only came from mainly Guangdong but from Shanghai, Tianjin, and other cities. The Refuge's office extended its service to the relatives and family of those afflicted, too.[97]

It had been Kerr's original plan to admit the patients who were brought by their relatives or friends. The Refuge remained a private institution until 1904 when a policeman brought a mentally ill man to the Refuge, together with a letter from the commissioner of the Police Department. The policeman asked whether the Refuge would admit this man for treatment and accept the payment of five dollars for the first month, and the Refuge accepted this man because any rejection of police referrals would be in opposition to its mission of unconditional benevolence. Thus began the relations between the government and the Refuge. The private-to-public transfer suggested more than only satisfying the mental requirement of a new recommendation, but also implied the change of the nature of the Refuge for Insane from private to semi-official function in the public security system.[98]

The police referral was significant in two ways. First, the Canton officials began to realize that the refuge for mental patients was an important part of the welfare system in the Cantonese society, and that the government would assume more responsibilities in this system. Second, the acceptance of official patients and public dollars ended the Refuge's identity as an entirely private Christian organization. The private-public union was unavoidable because American medical missionaries saw the police referrals as an opportunity to make possible the transfer of the insane asylum into Chinese control in the future while the government officials saw in realistic terms the philanthropic Refuge as a means to maintain stability and order in society.[99]

This connection was a sign of a second phase (1904-1926) in the development of the Refuge. After 1904, the policemen took the mental patients to the Refuge, together with fees; the patients were also admitted by directive of the local governments who, like the police, agreed to pay the expense for their cases. The relations with the Canton government were most harmonious from 1904 to 1926.[100]

In 1908, Dr. J. Allen Hofmann arrived in Canton, accompanied by his foster mother, Mrs. Olive A. Allen, who had for many years looked forward to coming to China as a missionary. As indicated by the report, Dr. Hofmann therefore "has proven himself to be a true yokefellow" while working at the Refuge. The day-to-day operational costs were covered by the patients' money, and the wealthy families paid the room rents and sometimes helped out those who could not pay by themselves. American superintendents' salaries were special gifts from the donors; mats for use were acquired via the endowments, too. Accommodations for housing the patients were sometimes not sufficient, and "a dozen to eighteen have been obliged to live in a mat shed," according to the missionary report.[101]

The Refuge for the Insane was making good progress. More and more patients caught in the streets were taken to the Refuge, and even the patients in Hong Kong were relocated there. In 1909, the Refuge received 194 patients, of whom ninety-nine were referred by the government or supported by the government. About two-thirds of the patients were men and one-third women. Some were reassigned from the Government Lunatic Asylum in Hong Kong, and some were captured by policemen in the streets in Canton. This asylum accommodated on the whole from 300 to 380 persons, men and women being separated. By that time, the Refuge had earned an international reputation that expanded its medical appointment base. Recommendations came from England, Germany, Singapore, and even as far as the United States, including a Columbia University student who suffered a mental collapse in New York City. These mentally ill Chinese living overseas were willing to visit the Refuge because they could receive better treatment in a society of Chinese culture.[102]

In 1918, the twentieth anniversary of the opening of the Refuge for the Insane was celebrated. Governor Wu Tingfang, military, naval, and civil officials, and prominent citizens occupied the seats on the platform of the pavilion erected for the event, and after the ceremony, all six hundred people paid a visit to the Refuge.[103]

The Refuge for the Insane helped treat many patients successfully. Painful stories were told in the hospital's reports. A girl of seventeen was brought in by a man who said she was his daughter. On a later visit, he confessed that she was not his daughter, but he had "bought her for business." In her situation, she was a valueless article of trade, and he threatened that "if she is not well by the end of the month, I will take her out and drown her." When the police were informed, her mean master lost his control of the girl. She restored fully to mental health, learned to read and write, turned into a smart young woman, and in the end became a Christian.[104] During the two-year period of 1920-21, 11,781 outpatient visits were recorded. Of those discharged, twenty-two percent were pronounced cured, twenty-one percent were improved to some extent, twenty-seven percent were not improved, and twenty-five percent died.[105]

The Refuge helped to promote the mental health movement in Canton, in addition to taking care of the mental patients. For example, in 1921 the Canton government organized a unique event in the mental health campaign. During the New Year celebrations, the public was invited to the Refuge for five days of lectures, drama, wrestling matches, and acrobatic shows. About 50,000 people attended the event and showed great interest in the patients and the methods of the treatment. The major goal of the campaign was to develop the public demand that their government assume the work of attending to the mental patients for the benefit of their welfare.[106] On each of the five days, concentration was given to one special category of the citizens, but the most popular was the mental patients. Every day a doctor of Western medicine delivered a lecture on mental hygiene. The event was very successful, as one organizer said, "We wished to show the people what could be done for the insane and to teach them something in the line of preventive measures."[107]

The Refuge was a philanthropic institution. At the start, to maintain its operations, the Refuge depended on donations from the churches, including land and resources, and relied mostly on foreigners' offerings. Later, more and more Chinese bestowed funds to the Refuge. The operating cost of the institution, exclusive of the physicians' salaries, was completely paid by the patients. The city officials paid certain amount for their patients' food and clothing as well as other general expenses.[108]

The Refuge in normal times accommodated from seven to eight hundred patients, though the doctors in charge made every effort to reduce the numbers in view of the difficulties. From 1898 to 1927, 6,599 patients (4,428 males and 2,171 females) stayed once at the Refuge; 5,913 (4,100 males and 1,813 females) were cured. The Refuge had 686 patients in 1927, 200 of whom were self-supported.[109] In 1927, the staff of the Refuge was: Charles C. Selden, superintendent; Robert M. Ross, treasurer; R. J. McCandliss; and G. R. H. Dittmann, business manager, as well as two Chinese doctors and one Chinese business manager.[110]

Due to the increasing number of mental patients, American doctors urged the Chinese government to set up more mental hospitals in China. They also encouraged the Canton government to assign more land to enlarge the Refuge and offer more financial support for it. Dr. Robert Ross suggested making Kerr's Refuge as a model for more psychiatric hospitals in China, "at least 1,000 in proportion to China's population."[111]

Partially urged by Americans, the Canton municipal government erected a new refuge for the mentally ill in 1926 because the Refuge for the Insane was no longer able to accept more mentally ill sent by the Department of Health. The First Municipal Insane Asylum founded by the municipality had a capacity for 400 psychological patients, of whom 113 insane were transferred from the Refuge for the Insane and 270 were sent by government agents or their families. Most of the patients were Cantonese residents, and some came from other districts or other cities within the Guangdong province.[112] The employees' strike in 1926 paralyzed the Refuge for the Insane. American doctors at the Refuge called for official arbitration in the strike and intervention in this charitable institution.

Due to the hospital's internal crisis, the Canton government decided to take over the Refuge for the Insane in 1927 at the request of the Board of Trustees of the Refuge. The Refuge's administration thus was transferred from American medical missionaries to the Department of Health of Canton and was renamed the Second Municipal Insane Asylum, but the ownership of the hospital was still in the hands of the trustees of American missionaries.

Official takeover of the administration of the Refuge for the Insane was a sign of a third phase (1927-1935) in the development of the Refuge. By that time, the Refuge had four doctors, two nurses, seventeen nursing-assistants, and seventy workers. By 1927, the Refuge had admitted 6,599 cases (4,428 men and 2,171 women) and discharged 5,913 cases (4,100 men and 1,813 women).[113] The Refuge for the Insane was the only well-equipped and efficiently run private institution for the mentally ill of any size in China.

The Canton government took over the entire care of the Refuge and changed its name, but its mission remained the same as before. Dr. Robert M. Ross, then the superintendent of the Second Municipal Insane Asylum, in a letter of March 27, 1929 to Chen Mingshu, the civil governor of Guangdong Province, listed several objectives of the Asylum:

- It was founded as a private Christian institution in order to demonstrate the scientific methods of treating the mentally ill;
- To interest individuals in the need for establishing many such hospitals;
- To provide courses of training for medical students and nurses in the subject of psychiatry, especially for those who intend to run such hospitals;
- To translate psychiatric literature and facilitate the spread of knowledge of the importance of this form of medical work through hospitals, schools, and public welfare organizations; and
- To publish psychiatric and mental health literature.[114]

Both asylums had been working well since the commencement. Most of the male patients between the ages of twenty and thirty and the women patients between thirty and fifty were at the First Insane Asylum, but younger women were found in the Second Insane Asylum. About thirty percent of the inmates were originally smart, arriving at their condition as a result of overstretching their mental abilities or too much concern about financial issues. Indeed, among the patients were college students, former military officers, government officials, merchants who failed in trade, and numerous women neglected by their lovers. The aggressive patients who were generally sent to the First Insane Asylum had to be given properly sedating medical therapy; their hands and feet were shackled to put a stop to serious fights.[115]

Dr. Selden, seventy-one years old, retired on February 10, 1932. He served the Refuge as the superintendent between 1901 and 1929; working at Kerr's Refuge for thirty years, he guided the hospital through hard and exciting times. He contributed significantly to the development and expansion of China's first mental hospital.[116]

Since the Second Insane Asylum became eminent all over China, in March

1935 the Canadian government asked the Asylum to accept sixty-five Chinese Canadian patients who were between fifty and eight years old, most of whom were unemployed thanks to the Great Depression. After careful treatment, some mentally ill patients returned to Canada, but some remained at the Hospital. In June, the Canton municipal government decided to purchase the property of the Second Insane Asylum from the Board of Trustees of the Second Insane Asylum after negotiation for several years. An agreement was signed by both parties with the American consul as witness. The ownership of the property of the Second Insane Asylum was transferred in August to the Canton government. The Chinese combined it with the First Insane Asylum and renamed it as the Municipal Mental Hospital. This Hospital had a capacity of serving 800 patients and employed four doctors, thirty-four nurses, and forty-four other workers, the largest modern mental hospital run by a local government in China at that time.[117] Nowadays this mental hospital remains a leading mental hospital in China.[118]

The establishment of Kerr's Refuge for the Insane had an effect on Chinese society, more mental hospitals, private or official, appearing in China. Sponsored by the Southern Presbyterian Mission, Dr. James R. Wilkinson opened a second psychiatric clinic in China in 1911 at the Elizabeth Blake Hospital in the city of Suzhou, one hundred miles west of Shanghai. This institution, however, had very poor achievements because of its lack of scientific psychiatric care.[119]

Official hospitals for the mentally ill began when the Refuge for the Insane was established in Beijing in 1906. The Refuge was then attached to the Municipal Hospital and was in the charge of both a foreign-trained Chinese doctor who received his education in Japan and an old-style practitioner. This alleged Refuge was nothing more than a prison because its patients, highly antisocial and aggressive, were impounded and at times were chained without sympathy. In 1912, the Refuge had only seventy-five patients. It was transferred in 1933 to the Health Department, named Beijing Refuge for the Insane. By special arrangements, this 200-bed Refuge was used as a teaching hospital of the medical college for training their students in this line of medicine, combining the staff of the Beijing University Medical College with the Beijing City Psychiatric Hospital. In other cities, the Shanghai Municipal Psychiatric Hospital, a 200-bed facility, was founded with the assistance of the Nationalist government in 1934. The Hangzhou International Hospital had only one ward for the psychological patients, but sadly it did not have sufficient equipment for appropriate mental attention.[120]

In summary, Kerr's Refuge for the Insane indicated American doctors' effort to extend charitable service from the sick to the mentally ill. This mental hospital was so successful that the Canton government began to send the mental patients to the hospital with financial support and later erected another mental hospital partly urged by Americans. The Canton municipal government finally took over the Refuge for the Insane after realizing the significance of this philanthropic institution in maintaining order in society. By that time the Cantonese believed that the government needed to assume responsibility for the establishment of charitable enterprises and a welfare system in Canton. Kerr's Refuge for the Insane had an effect on the Chinese. For the first time China had a psychiatric hospital to take care of mental patients, who were treated scientifically with Western medical methods. Thereafter, more Chinese realized the importance of the scientific treatment of mental patients, and several mental hospitals were established in China.

Americans' Medical and Health Work of Charity in Canton, 1900-1935

At the beginning of the twentieth century, the charitable work made good progress in Canton; more and more Cantonese contributed endowments to the philanthropic institutions, societies, and organizations. In the field of medicine and health, medical institutions increasingly provided more free medical and health care to the poor and the needy, and American doctors continued playing a part in the philanthropic movement in Canton.

The Hackett Medical College for Women

Dr. Fulton was the first Presbyterian woman medical missionary sent to China. Once in Canton, she was engaged in various medical services at no cost to those patients who could not pay, taking account of different kinds of medical illness as well as the common surgical operations: kidney stones, tumors, and cataracts. She took care of many of the sick, especially the obstetric patients, in their homes. When Chinese tradition refused her endeavors to turn down payment, she used the gifts of food or livestock, such as a goat, a big buffalo, and a young cow, to support the patients' families. If the cash payments were given in large amount, she contributed them to the hospital. From different patients, Dr. Mary Fulton once received the sum of $2,500, and in the end she used that amount of money to purchase a piece of land for the Hackett Medical College for Women. Like her brother, Dr. Fulton was a very good fund-raiser. Her furloughs in America, from the late 1890s to the early 1900s, were a time of fund-raising. By means of the endeavors of both Albert Fulton and Mary Fulton and the charity of Cantonese citizens and officials, who greatly appreciated both of them, the Fultons were able to erect a complex of spiritual and remedial institutions: a roomy brick and rock-solid building designed the hot weather.[121]

The David Gregg Hospital was an actively generous institution. Each year almost 20,000 patients, more of whom were women and children, came to the Gregg Hospital to seek medical advice from physicians, gynecologists, and pediatricians, who required no payment or little. On March 9, 1924, Dr. Margaret Taylor Ross of the Gregg Hospital opened the Child Welfare

Clinic because many babies were in poor health due to poor hygiene and a lack of health care. The Hospital had to "do something to safeguard and build up the chances of health for children," in the words of Dr. Ross.[122] The clinic had been made known to patients in the Obstetric Department in the hospital for three months but only five or six babies were brought each clinic day, all of them actually coming from the Obstetric Department. Later, the number of children brought to the clinic increased so rapidly that from March 1924 to June 1926, the total enrollment was 525 babies. The nurses of the hospital made impressive services available to their parents in weighing, measuring, taking temperatures, and giving information on baby hygiene. Not only the nurses, but also the fourth-year students of the Hackett College, took an impressive part in the work, which was supervised mainly by the assistants of Dr. Taylor Ross and Dr. Liang Yiwen. The charge for participation in the clinic was almost a token: fifty cents for three months, paid on registration, with a small charge for any medicines prescribed, making it possible for the poor and wealthy to be attended on the same basis. To help the poor patients, Hackett students also willingly made small beautiful hats during the weekends and sold them so they could buy mosquito nets for those in the wards, who did not have any.[123]

Hackett not only provided free medical services to the poor but also participated in the charitable campaign in Canton. In June 1906, an immense and terrible flood caused by long rainstorms engulfed several districts and many places along the route of the east and north rivers in Guangdong Province. More than 20,000 people became dispossessed and had to run away to the hilly areas for lodging, where they were exposed to sun and rain without garments and provisions, and were assaulted by bandits, who raided and carried off the women and children. The suffering that they had endured was too awful for words. To make the situation worse, a big tropical storm lasting several hours destroyed a large number of houses and boats and killed several thousand people on July 25, thus increasing their suffering. Accordingly, professionals, merchants, and other classes of people emulated the Western countries to inaugurate a flea market for the sale of items, the first time in Canton. The David Gregg Hospital transferred its patients into the college building; the recently remodeled buildings were used for the marketplace, showing its profound kindness for the people in this terrible time of need. The Hackett College students sold over 10,000 dollars' worth, including over fifty gold medals, at their booth. The Hackett's students and professors made an embellished picture showing the distress caused by the flood and sold it for 1,800 silver dollars. The accomplishment of the flea market held at the David Gregg Hospital grounds and adjacent lots primarily resulted from the tireless hard work of the Cantonese women. The Cantonese were grateful to Dr. Fulton because she relocated her patients and unlocked her gates, charitably and unreservedly giving her compound for the use of fund-raising. A grateful statement was sent later, writing, "China has had many illustrious women, but none greater than Dr. Mary Fulton...so may our coming generations follow Dr. Mary Fulton's example."[124] In 1919, the Hackett students raised funds to open a primary school for poor children in western Canton, the First Charitable School of Hackett College.[125]

Owing to Hackett's charitable service and contribution to the society partially, the alumnae demonstrated their lifelong devotion to their old school when raising or pledging $100,000 toward the construction of a new building for Hackett. In 1935, Hackett gained more strength when a new, modern hospital building was constructed.[126]

The Henan Hospital

The Henan Hospital in Canton was active in the medical and health charitable work in south Canton, too. Throughout the Nanjing era of 1927-1937, Dr. William W. Cadbury, Lingnan University physician, remained active in the Lingnan community church and continued to make medical philanthropic expeditions into the countryside. Li Fulin, a former bandit but enrolled in the Nationalist army during the 1911 Revolution, became a general after the revolution in charge of all the troops in Henan Island, Canton. A supporter of Chiang Kai-shek, Li offered important services to the Lingnan College, not only rescuing those who had been taken into custody by bandits, but also building on the campus a small hospital where the patients from the nearby villages could be cared for. Thereafter, Dr. Cadbury received a total of $13,000 for construction of a new hospital, $10,000 from General Li. The completed Hospital, intended for the treatment of the villagers in the rural area adjacent the Lingnan University, was formally opened in the presence of General Li on April 21, 1925. Drs. Cadbury and H. P. Nottage, as well as two Chinese physicians, worked at the Henan Hospital, assisted by four Chinese nurses.[127]

Dr. Cadbury continued his philanthropy by establishing clinics in the nearby villages, in addition to taking care of the college community of over 2,000 persons. His hands-on relief activity at the clinics helped him understand the distress beyond the enclosed space of the well-supported Lingnan University. At one deserted house, for example, Dr. Cadbury found a young woman chained to a chair because she was mentally ill, and her family did not have enough money to pay for treatments at Kerr's Refuge for the Insane. Dr. Cadbury later found the necessary funds by some means and sent her to the Refuge, and the woman was restored to health in a month.[128]

The Hospital and its clinics treated different diseases, including leprosy, beriberi, malaria, bacilla dysentery, bubonic plague, cholera, and smallpox, providing medical and hygienic works of charity to the poor peasants on the Henan Island. The woman physician of the Hospital was competent to be engaged in, within a brief time, the obstetric work among the villagers.

A Chinese visiting nurse of the Hospital made calls on five hundred patients in nine villages in only one year, and the serious cases were taken to the Hospital. A woman with advanced leprosy, after months of indecision, in the end showed willingness to come for therapy; the disease was stopped and several lepers started to seek medication at the Hospital. During the first year, there were ninety childbirths in the Hospital.[129]

The Cantonese's Medical and Health Work of Charity, 1912-1935

After the Republic of China was established in 1912, the charitable work made good progress in Canton; more and more Cantonese contributed funds to the philanthropic institutions, societies, and organizations. In the field of medicine and health, under American influences to some degree, medical institutions increasingly provided more free medical and health care to the poor and the needy in the 1920s and 1930s. The charitable institutions in Canton had more than thirty hospitals, but more of them adopted Chinese medicine, only several of which adopted Western medicine.[130]

Fangbian Hospital was the first medical, charitable institution in Guangdong province. Originally, it had only sixteen wards for the patients and was set up to collect the dead and plague victims in the streets, but later it not only provided free medical treatment, free distribution of medications, free delivery of babies but also gave relief to the poor, delivered free coffins, and buried the dead. More and more poor people were going to this humanitarian institution for help, and its operation was enlarging daily at the beginning of the twentieth century.[131]

The Hospital, following the Canton Hospital, established a council composed of several directors elected by different guilds, and adopted modern management skills of charitable work. The general director was in charge of the business of the Hospital. Fangbian did not adopt Western medicine until 1926, and after that the patients had two choices for their treatment: Western or Chinese medicine. By 1935, the Hospital had been enlarged significantly and had 1,054 beds, most of which were free, eighteen doctors of Chinese medicine, four doctors of Western medicine, about forty staff members, sixty midwifes, and 110 janitors. Different departments of special treatment were established, too. In the 1910s, only about 1,000 patients visited the hospital daily and the death rate was seventy percent, including those dead bodies picked up in the streets; in the 1930s, more than 15,000 patients went to the hospital daily and the death rate was only thirty percent.[132]

Fangbian Hospital, relying on contributions to maintain its daily function, regarded fund-raising as one major task for its leaders. The superintendents of the Hospital often appealed to the Cantonese merchants, professional people, businessmen, government officials, even the overseas Chinese for donations.[133] On June 2, 1913, the Hospital dispatched more than ten persons divided into several teams to the streets door by door, asking for contributions to the Hospital. In December 1925, Fangbian organized a lottery and a sports competition to raise funds.[134] Many Cantonese were willing to donate their houses to Fangbian after their deaths because of Fangbian's significant contributions to Cantonese society.[135] Mr. Frank Samson, for example, a Chinese gentleman of Sydney, who died in 1915, left his entire estate to the Canton Hospital.[136] The fund-raising drives were so successful that social donations covered half of the total income of Fangbian in 1935, which received more than 450,000 yuan in 1936, in comparison to only 6,000 yuan in 1899.[137]

Fangbian Hospital was considered the most outstanding philanthropic institution that had been most vigorous in charity work in the Guangdong province, especially in the city of Canton. The Hospital became the largest charitable institution in south China in the 1930s, spending most of the funds on philanthropic works. In 1935, about 170,000 patients received free treatment or medicine from the Hospital.[138] Practicing humanitarianism, the Hospital played a significant role not only in relieving the sick or injured persons, healing the wounded, and rescuing the dying, but also in providing relief to the people in a disaster area by bringing patients out of danger, treating and curing them. Numbers of medical workers hurried to the disaster area to give treatment to the sick and wounded and to deliver relief food and funds in the city of Canton and other towns in Guangdong Province. The Hospital even sent ambulance corps to Cambodia, Laos, and Vietnam when the plague erupted there. In 1936, for example, the Hospital spent 200,000 yuan on sending out medical teams and giving aid to the people in urgent need.[139]

Guanghua Medical College was enthusiastic in charitable medical and health work, offering free medical care and service and medicine to the poor and to the lower classes with the charge of a small amount of fees or no fees.[140] In January 1918, Guanghua Hospital provided free services to 377 inpatients and 1,667 outpatients between September and December.[141] In 1933, to facilitate charitable enterprise, two free dispensaries were opened in Henan district for the poor.[142]

Lianguang Baptist Hospital was a charitable Christian institution, providing free medical care, surgery, and medicine to poor patients. The Hospital not only provided free medical treatment to the poor, helpless, old patients, but also dispatched doctors and nurses to countryside to offer medical assistance. In 1924, only 6,210 patients received free medical treatment from the Hospital, and in 1935, 27,076 patients did.[143]

In addition to the medical charity work of the private institutions, several government hospitals had been established by 1933 to offer free medical services. All these medical clinics were under the administration of the Department of Social Welfare of Canton, which was established in 1929. The statistics showed that an average of 40,000 cases was treated without any charges yearly by the first and the second clinics.[144] By the 1930s, medical charitable work in Canton was conducted by both the government and private organizations, and a comprehensive modern philanthropic system of medicine and health was established in Canton.

Conclusion

Modern missionary hospitals created in the nineteenth century served as the medical centers as well as philanthropic and religious institutions in Europe and the United States. When American medical missionaries arrived in China, they founded the Canton Hospital and other dispensaries. The Canton Hospital, providing free medical care and healing to many poor Cantonese patients, became the first modern medical charitable institution in China. Under American influence to some degree, charitable giving was becoming a new trend in Canton, and the Chinese donations became one of the very important financial sources of the Canton Hospital. American medical missionaries contributed to the modern medical and health work of charity in Canton.

American missionary doctors, advocating Christian benevolence, encouraged the Chinese to found modern charitable institutions along Christian lines. Partially influenced by American doctors' Christian charitable philosophy and impressed by the Canton Hospital to some measure, the enlightened Cantonese elites began to develop modern charitable thought and launch a modern philanthropic movement in Canton. Beginning in 1871, the modern charitable institution, Shantang, a Chinese-style association, appeared in Canton, which was a combination of both a Chinese traditional charitable institution and a Western benevolent institute. Shantang was a modern benevolent society, not kin-clan oriented and administered by both professionals and merchants with modern management skills, which provided free services to the poor and the needy on a year-round basis. Shangtang carried out moral teachings of Confucius and professional education, provided social relief and medical services to the poor, and played an important role in preventing epidemic spread and alleviating people in stricken areas in time of natural disaster. American medical missionaries were one of the forces that inspired the Cantonese to found such new form of philanthropic institutions, although many forces motivated the Cantonese elite to launch a modern charitable movement in Canton.

American medical missionaries played a role in the modern philanthropic movement in Canton. The establishment of the Mingxin School for the Blind by Dr. Mary Niles in 1889 and Kerr's Refuge for the Insane in 1899 indicated American doctors' efforts to extend charitable services from the sick to the blind and the mentally ill. The Mingxin School, the first school for the blind in south China, not only provided aid to helpless blind children, but also helped them learn skills to make their own living. The graduates of the school became useful persons in the society. Kerr's Refuge for the Insane, the first mental hospital in China, adopted scientific treatment based on persuasion, freedom, and a healthy outdoor life, rather than force and restraint. For the first time in Chinese history, a psychiatric hospital took care of the Chinese mental patients who were treated scientifically with Western medical methods.

American doctors' new charitable institutions and Americans' medical and health charitable work in Canton in some way contributed to a new philanthropic movement in Canton at the beginning of the twentieth century. More and more Cantonese contributed funds to the philanthropic institutions, societies and organizations. In the field of medicine and health, more Chinese hospitals and dispensaries increasingly provided free medical and health care to the poor and the needy. A new form of medical philanthropic institution—Fangbian Hospital—appeared, and became the largest philanthropic institute in south China. Fangbian developed from a traditional charitable medical house and adopted modern management skills and modern fund-raising methods, providing treatments of both Western and Chinese medicines to the poor and having the characteristics of both Chinese and Western charitable institutions.

American medical missionaries influenced not only the Cantonese elite, but also the Canton government in the modern charitable movement. The Mingxin School for the Blind was so successful that the Cantonese government began to send blind children to the School with government financial support, regarding it as a part of the welfare system in the society and participating in the management of this philanthropic institution. Kerr's mental hospital was so successful that the Canton municipal government began to send the mental patients to the hospital with government financial support and finally took it over. In addition, the Canton government founded another mental hospital because the Cantonese officials regarded this institution as important in maintaining social order in society, and believed that the government needed to be involved in the charitable enterprise and to build up a welfare system in Canton. Therefore, in the 1930s, charitable medical and health work in Canton was conducted by both government and private organizations, and a modern system of medicine and health was established in Canton. American doctors played a part in the modern charitable movement in Canton, which had an effect on Chinese at the beginning of the twentieth centuries when more mental hospitals and schools for the blind were founded in China.

American missionaries transplanted into China modern hospitals, a new form of modern philanthropic institution. They aimed to change the Chinese attitude toward the Westerners through their hospitals so that they would be able to teach the Chinese Christianity. The medical missionaries encouraged the Chinese to found modern charitable institutions in China with an intention of promoting God's benevolence among the Chinese. Thereafter, the Cantonese elite combined the traditional Chinese benevolent institution on the basis of brotherly love advocated by Confucius with the Western counterpart, rather than only copying totally the Western charitable institutions. The Cantonese reformers adopted and modified the features and functions of Western charitable institutions and created a new form of modern Chinese charitable institution of their own style. In this regard, American medical missionaries worked as the transmitters of modern technology in cultural globalization in China.

Notes

1. For an overview of Chinese charitable and welfare activities in Chinese history in the nineteenth century, see Arthur Henderson Smith, *Chinese Characteristics* (Shanghai: North China Herald and S.C. & C Gazette, 1890), especially Chapter XV, Benevolence, 68-73.
2. T. J. Preston, "The Chinese Benevolent Institutions in Theory and Practice," *Chinese Recorder and Missionary Journal* 28 (1907): 245-53.
3. Medical Missionary Society, *The Medical Missionary Society in China: Address, With Minutes of Proceedings* (Canton, 1838), 25.
4. *The Hundred Years History of the Canton Hospital* (Organization Committee of the Sun Yat-sen Medical College, Lingnan University, Canton. 1935), 11-12.
5. John Glasgow Kerr, "Self-Support in Mission Hospitals," *China Medical Missionary Journal* 9, 3 (1895): 136.
6. Canton Hospital, *Annual Report for the 106th year of Canton Hospital, 1940-1941* (Canton: Canton Hospital, 1941), 73-5.
7. E. C. Bridgman to R. Anderson, Canton, May 2, 1836 and P. Parker to R. Anderson, Canton, March 27, 1836, Papers of the American Board of Commissioners for Foreign Missions (ABCFM), Missions to China (ABC 16.3), Houghton Library, Harvard University, microfilm, reel 256, ABCFM.
8. George H. Danton, *The Culture Contacts of the United States and China, 1784-1844* (New York, 1931), 103.
9. *Papers Relative to Hospitals in China* (Boston: J. R. Butts, 1841), 5-6.
10. Peter Parker, *Statements Respecting Hospitals in China*, 192.
11. R. H. Graves, *Forty Years in China in Transition* (Baltimore: Woodward, 1895. Reprint, Scholarly Resource at Wilmington, Delaware, 1972), 240.
12. *The Hundred Years History of the Canton Hospital*, 11-12.
13. Jia Yuehan (John Kerr), *Qizheng lueshu* (On special treatment) (Canton: Canton Hospital, 1886).
14. Ibid.
15. "Canton Hospital: Celebration of the Eightieth Anniversary," *The Hong Kong Daily Press*, December 21, 1916.
16. Canton Hospital, *Annual Report for the 106th year of Canton Hospital, 1940-1941*, 79.
17. "Canton Hospital: Financial State for 1923," Folder 8, Box 27, Record Group 82, Presbyterian Church in the U.S.A. Board of Foreign Missions. Secretaries Files: China Missions, 1891-1955, Presbyterian Historical Society, Philadelphia, Pennsylvania.
18. J. G. Kerr, "The Native Benevolent Institutions of Canton," *China Review* 2 (Sept./Oct. 1873), 88-95.

19. Ibid.
20. John Glasgow Kerr, "Medical Missions," *Records of the General Conference of the Protestant Missionaries of China Held at Shanghai, May 10-24, 1877* (Shanghai: the Presbyterian Mission Press, 1878), 114-17.
21. J. G. Kerr, *Medical Missions: At Home and Abroad* (San Francisco: A. L. Bancroft, 1878), 89.
22. R. H. Graves, *Forty Years in China or China in Transition*, 244.
23. Zheng Guanying, *Zheng Guanying ji* (Works of Zheng Guanying), vol. 1, ed. Xia Dongyuan (Shanghai: Shanghai renmin chubanshe, 1982): 27-28.
24. Ibid., 525-7.
25. Ibid., 527-34.
26. Xia Dongyun, *Zheng Guanying zhuan* (Biography of Zheng Guanying) (Shanghai: Huadongshifan daxue chubanshe, 1981).
27. Kang Youwei, *Datong shu* (Great Harmony) (1902, reprint, Beijing: Beijing guji chubanshe, 1959).
28. Kang Youwei, *Datong shu* (Great Harmony) (Shanghai: Shanghai zhonghua shuju, 1935).
29. Tang Zhijun, *Kang Youwei zhenlun. shangji* (Kang Youwei's political essays, vol. 1) (Beijing: Zhonghua shuju, 1981): 129-30.
30. Ibid., 187.
31. Kang Youwei, *Datong shu* (Great Hamony) (Zhengzhou: Zhongzhou guji chubanshe, 1998).
32. Tang Zhijun, *Kang Youwei zhenlun. shangji*, 187.
33. Chen Xiqi, ed. *Sun Zhongshan nianpu changbian* (A chronicle record of Sun Yat-sen's life) (Beijing: Zhonghua shuju, 1991), 66.
34. Sun Zhongshan, *Sun Zhongshan quanji* (Comprehensive works of Sun Yat-sen), vol. 1(Beijing: Zhonghua shuju, 1981): 297; ibid., vol. 2 (Beijing: Zhonghua shuju, 1982): 22; ibid., vol. 6 (Beijing: Zhonghua shuju, 1986): 523; ibid., vol. 9 (Beijing: Zhonghua Shuju, 1986): 124. See also Sun Zhongshan, *Sun Zhongshan xuan ji* (Selected works of Sun Yat-sen), vol. 1 (Beijing: Beijing renmin chubanshe, 1956): 89; ibid., vol. 2: 570.
35. Liang Qichiao, "Yixue shanhui xu," in *Wuxu bianfa* (1898 reform), *Zhongguo jindai shi ziliaocongkan*, vol. 4 (Shanghai: Shanghai renmin chubanshe, 1961): 449-53.
36. Liang Qichao,"Lun guohui" (On parliament), in Liang Qichao, *Yinbingshi wenji* (Works of Liang Qichao), vol. 3 (Beijing; Zhonghua shuju, 1989): 73.
37. Deng Yusheng, *Quanyue she hui shi lu* (A record of the Guangdong society) (Canton: Guangdong xuewu gongsuo, 1910): 2-3.
38. See http://baike.baidu.com/view/1529102.html.
39. *The Hundred Years History of the Canton Hospital*, 19-20.
40. John G. Kerr, "Benevolent Institutions of Canton," *China Review* 3 (1874-1875): 108-114.
41. J. G. Kerr, "A Chinese Benevolent Association," *The China Medical Missionary Journal* 3, no. 4 (1889): 152-55.
42. Medical Missionary society, *Report of the Medical Missionary Society in China for the Year 1871* (Canton, China: The Medical Missionary Society, 1872): 7-10.
43. John G. Kerr, "Benevolent Institutions of Canton," *China Review* 3 (1874-

1875): 108-114.

44. John Glasgow Kerr, "Is It an Advance?" *China Medical Missionary Journal* 3, 2 (1889): 66-67.

45. *Guangdong minzhen gongbao* (Guangdong civil government bulletin) (Guangzhou: The Department of Civil Administration of Guangdong, 1929): 211.

46. *Nanhai xianzhi* (A gazetteer of Nanhai county), vol. 6:10a.

47. Ibid., 10-13.

48. Deng Yusheng, *Quanyue she hui shi lu* (A record of Guangdong society) (Canton: Guangdong xuewu gongsuo, 1910), 2-3.

49. John G. Kerr, "Benevolent Institutions of Canton," *China Review* 3 (1874-1875): 108-114.

50. J. G. Kerr, "The Native Benevolent Institutions of Canton," *China Review* 2 (Sept./Oct. 1873): 88-95.

51. Deng Yusheng, *Quanyue she hui shi lu* (A record of Guangdong society) (Canton: Guangdong xuewu gongsuo, 1910), 3-5.

52. J. G. Kerr, "A Chinese Benevolent Association," *The China Medical Missionary Journal* 3, no. 4 (1889): 152-55.

53. John G. Kerr, "Benevolent Institutions of Canton," *China Review* 3 (1874-1875): 108-114.

54. Ibid.

55. For an account of the medical school, see *Minsheng ribao* (People's living daily), March 3, 1913; ibid., March 11, 1913; ibid., March 12, 1913; ibid., March 17, 1913; and ibid., April 4, 1913.

56. In 1872, Aiyu shantang provided free 836 coffins in 1872 and distributed 547 in 1873 to the dead, most of whom were found in the streets, unidentified and unclaimed. Aiyu gave one hundred free jackets to the unfortunate in winter in 1872 and 526 in 1873, spending a lot of resources on remedy, teachers' incomes, school equipments, tomb diggers, gravestones, and rituals to pay tribute to the deceased. See John G. Kerr, "Benevolent Institutions of Canton," *China Review* 3 (1874-1875): 108-114.

57. A significant difference between dispensaries and hospitals was that hospitals received patients round the clock, through the year while dispensaries operated on a limited daily or weekly schedule and usually were staffed only during those months when the people in charge predicted that the need would be greatest.

58. Aiyu shantang hired four physicians and provided free prescriptions of $1,797.36 in 1872 and hired three physicians and provided free prescription of $1,225.29 in 1873. 37,750 patients were treated at the dispensary in 1872. The dispensary attended 103 patients every day; each of the attending physicians saw twenty-four patients. See John G. Kerr, "Benevolent Institutions of Canton," *China Review* 3 (1874-1875): 108-114.

59. Just only from March to September 1908, for example, Chen took care of eight-two cases of delivering children, 144 cases of brain disease, 267 cases of feet disease, 467 cases of stomach disease, 264 cases of heart disease, 244 cases of five internal organs (lungs, hearts, livers spleen, and kidneys), 130 cases of high temperature, eight-four cases of amenorrhea, sixty-four cases of abnormal behavior, twenty-four cases of milking baby problems, three cases of uterus tumor, 245 cases of scabies, and 480 cases

of child scabies. See Deng Yusheng, *Quanyue she hui shi lu* (A record of Guangdong society) (Canton: Guangdong xuewu gongsuo, 1910), 2-3.

60. *Guangdong sheng zhi. minzhenzhi* (Annals of Guangdong Province. Annals of the civil administration) (Guangzhou, Guangdong renmin chubanshe, 1993), Chapter 5: Natural Disaster Relief, 113-15.

61. *North China Herald*, June 15, 1894, 946.

62. Mary Niles, "Plague in Canton," *China Medical Missionary Journal* 8 (June 1894): 116-19.

63. Canton Hospital, *Annual Report for the 106th year of the Canton Hospital, 1940-1941* (Canton: Canton Hospital, 1941), 79.

64. John Henry Gray, *Walks in the City of Canton* (Hong Kong: De Souza, 1875), 523-25.

65. Heng You," "Alice Carpenter and the Chinese Ming Sum School for the Blind," *Journal of Presbyterian History* 58 (Winter 1990): 259.

66. *History of the South China Mission of the American Presbyterian Church, 1845-1920* (Shanghai: The Presbyterian Mission Press, 1927), 67-68.

67. *Ming Sum School for the Blind, the 50th Anniversary Report, 1889-1939* (Hong Kong: Standard Press, 1939), 13.

68. Ibid., 11.

69. "Ming Sum School for the Blind, 1919," File 430, Catalogue 1, Record Group 92, Guangdong Provincial Archives, Guangzhou, China.

70. *History of the South China Mission of the American Presbyterian Church, 1845-1920* (Shanghai: The Presbyterian Mission Press, 1927), 116-17.

71. Ibid., 118-19.

72. Ibid., 143-44.

73. *Ming Sum School for the Blind, 50th Anniversary Report, 1889-1939*, 14.

74. "The Graduate Roster and History of Ming Sum School for the Blind, 1908-1928," File 430, Catalogue 1, Record Group 92, Guangdong Provincial Archives, Guangzhou, China.

75. Ibid.

76. "Ming Sum School for the Blind, 1929-1930" File 430, Catalogue 1, Record Group 92, Guangdong Provincial Archives, Guangzhou, China.

77. "Mary W. Niles," *Chinese Recorder* 64, 3 (March 1933), 176.

78. "Ming Sum School for the Blind, 1933-1934," File 430, Catalogue 1, Record Group 92, Guangdong Provincial Archives, Guangzhou, China.

79. Evangelistic work in schools, hospitals, churches: 27; Teachers in schools for the blind: 21; Teachers in schools for the seeing: 9; Massagers in hospitals: 4; Industrial work (knitting, etc): 30; Married, housework: 22. See "Records of the Board of Trustee of the Ming Sum School for Blind, 1918-1945," File 1, Catalogue 71, Record Group 17, Guangzhou Municipal Archives, Guangzhou, China.

80. "Establishment of Schools for the Blind and Deaf," *Shen bao*, February 25, 1905; "Regulations of the Schools for the Blind and Deaf," *Shen bao*, October, 16, 1907. See also Wei Waiyang, *Xuanjiao shiye yu jindai zhongguo* (The missionary enterprises and modern China) (Taibei: Yuzhou guang chubanshe, 1992).

81. After 1949, the Mingxin School was combined with other schools for blind in Canton and was renamed the Guangzhou Municipal School for Blind in the 1980s. It has more than 320 students and offers courses to students

of kindergarten, elementary school, middle school, and professional school in the present day. See http://www.hudong.com/wiki/%E5%B9 %BF%E5%B7%9E%E5%B8%82%E7%9B%B2%E4%BA%BA%E5%AD%A6 %E6%A0%A1.

82. V.W. Ng, *Madness in Late Imperial China: From Illness to Deviance* (Norman, Oklahoma: University of Oklahoma Press, 1994), 67.

83. John J. Kao, *Three Millennia of Chinese Psychiatry* (New York: The Institute for Advanced Research in Asian General topic of insanity in traditional Chinese medicine, 1979), 7-17.

84. J. Lincoln McCartney, "Neuropsychiatry in China; A Preliminary Observation," *China Medical Journal* XL, 7 (July 1926): 617-26.

85. E. P. Thwing, *China Medical Missionary Journal* 7 (March 1893): 140.

86. *Wanguo gongbao* (Global news) 383 (April 15, 1876), 577 (May 15, 1880), and 611 (October 23, 1880).

87. J. G. Kerr, *Medical Missions: At Home and Abroad* (San Francisco: A. L. Bancroft & Company, 1878), 8.

88. Chas C. Selden, "The Story of the John Kerr Hospital for the Insane," *The Chinese Medical Journal* 52 (1937): 705-14.

89. John Kerr, *The First Report of the Refuge Insane for the Insane in Canton*, vol. 38, 1-2, Presbyterian Church Board of Foreign Missions, *China Letters, 1837-1900*, microfilm, Presbyterian Historical Society, Philadelphia, Pennsylvania.

90. C. C. Selden, "The Story of the John G. Kerr Hospital for the Insane," *The Chinese Medical Journal* 52, 1 (November 1937): 707-14.

91. After the Refuge was formally open to the public, William wrote another article, appealing to the Chinese and foreigners for endowments to the hospital. See *Xinxue yuebao* (Monthly journal of new learning), vol. 3 (July 1897) and vol. 10 (February 1898).

92. K.C. Wong, "A Short History of Psychiatry and Mental Hygiene in China," *Chinese Medical Journal* 68, 1 (Jan.-Feb. 1950): 44-49.

93. Patients often made a lot of troubles when tearing their clothing. Dr. Kerr introduced a little lock-button device to prevent the unbuttoning and removal of clothing. When pressed, it snapped easily, but it could only open by means of a very simple key. Dr. Kerr introduced another device as well—wire netting—very efficient and humane at the same time. In the daytime, it was seldom used, as patients sometimes felt uncomfortable with it. But for the night it proved to be most satisfactory from the standpoint of both the attendant and the patient. Under this wire netting, the patient was comfy on his bed and could turn back and forth freely, but he could not get up. It was used during the wintertime for those who continued removing their clothing at night, or those who were very active, moving around the whole night. This device assured break for them as well as for the others and reduced the number of the attendants. See C. C. Selden, "III. Treatment of the Insane," *China Medical Journal* 23, 6 (November 1909), 374.

94. C. C. Selden, "II. Treatment of the Insane," *China Medical Journal* 23, 4 (July 1909): 221-22.

95. Born in 1861 in Erie, Pennsylvania, Selden finished his undergraduate studies at Harvard and decided to pursue a career in medicine. He com-

pleted his two-year medical residency in New York City at the Brooklyn Hospital from 1895 to 1897. After the State of New York granted Selden his medical/surgical license, the Selden newlyweds sailed for China in 1897, sponsored by the Presbyterian Mission Board. The sponsorship, however, was only symbolic because Selden refused to accept a salary from the Board in order to exercise his skills as he saw fit and requested that his salary be sent to missionaries who needed. Both planned to practice medicine together, hopefully in an orphan asylum. Once in Canton, they planned to pay a courtesy visit to Kerr's asylum. Excited when learning they were coming, Dr. Kerr wrote reiterating his offer. Impressed significantly by Dr. Kerr, Dr. Selden agreed to fulfill Kerr's vision of developing psychiatric care in China. They finally joined the Refuge and moved to Fangcun in 1901. See C. C. Selden, "Work among the Chinese Insane and Some of its Results," *China Medical Missionary Journal* 19, 1 (1905): 2-3.

96. *Annual Report of the Presbyterian Board of Foreign Missions* (New York: The Board of Foreign Missions, Presbyterian Church in the U.S.A., 1902), 40.

97. *History of the South China Mission of the American Presbyterian Church, 1845-1920* (Shanghai: The Presbyterian Mission Press, 1927), 97.

98. Chas C. Selden, "The Need of More Hospital for Insane in China," *China Medical Journal* 24 (1910): 326.

99. C. C. Selden, "The Story of the John G. Kerr Hospital for the Insane," *Chinese Medical Journal* 52, 1 (November 1937): 707-14.

100. K. C. Wong, "A Short History of Psychiatry and Mental Hygiene in China," *Chinese Medical Journal* 68, 1 (Jan.-Feb. 1950): 44-49.

101. *John G. Kerr Hospital for the Insane, Report for the Years 1907-1908* (Canton: China Baptist Publication Society, 1909): 2-5.

102. C. C. Selden, "A Work for the Insane in China," *Chinese Recorder* XL (May 1909): 262-69.

103. *History of the South China Mission of the American Presbyterian Church, 1845-1920*, 145-46.

104. *John G. Kerr Hospital for the Insane, Reports for the Years 1918-1921* (Canton: Wai Hing Printing Co., 1921), 3.

105. In 1921, a total of 439 inpatients were received and 380 were discharged. Ibid., 7, 9, 15.

106. *History of the South China Mission of the American Presbyterian Church, 1845-1920*, 145-46.

107 . *John G. Kerr Hospital for the Insane, Reports for the Years 1918-1921* (Canton: Wai Hing Printing Co., 1921), 4-5.

108. The Refuge provided three levels of charges. The charges for patients with normal room and board were low, $5 for one month including clothing. The wealthy patients paid all charges for their private rooms or for places in private wards. C. C. Selden, "The John G. Kerr Refuge for the Insane: The Opening of the Insane," *China Medical Journal* 23 (March 1909): 82-91.

109. "The John G. Kerr Hospital for the Insane, Canton," *China Medical Journal* 41(1927): 164-68.

110. "Materials Relating to Weiai Hospital, 1926-1927," Group Number 65, File 33, Guangdong Provincial Archives, Guangzhou, China.

111. Robert M. Ross, "Mental Hygiene," *China Medical Journal* 1 (January 1926): 8-13.

112. "Material Relating to the Hospital for the Instance," Group Number 65, File 73, Guangdong Provincial Archives, Guangzhou, China.
113. C. C. Selden, "The Story of the John G. Kerr Hospital for the Insane," *Chinese Medical Journal* 52, 1 (November 1937): 707-14.
114. "Material Relating to the Hospital for the Instance," Group Number 65, File 73, Guangdong Provincial Archives, Guangzhou, China.
115. Deng Chanxian, "General Report of the Second Municipal Hospital for Insane," *Guangzhuo weisheng* (Guangzhou health) 1 (October 1935): 107-10. See also Edward Bing-Shuey Lee, *Modern China* (Shanghai: The Mercury Press, 1936): 104-5.
116. Selden left Canton in early 1938 and retired in America. He died of heart attack on June 16, 1938 in Oberlin, Ohio while traveling to visit his children on the East Coast. See *Guangzhou shi jingshen binyuan shi, 1899-1998* (The History of the Guangzhou Municipal Mental Hospital, 1899-1998) (Guangzhoushi jingshenbing yiyuan yuanshi weiyuan hui, 1998): 4-21.
117. *Guangzhou weisheng* 1(October 1935): 83-92.
118. Today this hospital called the Guangzhou Municipal Mental Hospital has a capacity for 2,000 psychological patients and 900 employees of doctors, nurses, and staff, a major mental hospital in China. See http://gzsnkyy. h.51daifu.com/introduce.shtml.
119. K. C. Wong, "A Short History of Psychiatry and Mental Hygiene in China," *Chinese Medical Journal* 68, 1 (Jan.-Feb. 1950): 44-49.
120. Gregorio Bermann, "Mental Health in China," in A. Kiev, ed. *Psychiatry in the Communist World* (New York: Science House, 1968): 233-34.
121. *Xiage yike da xue sanshi zhounian jinian lu* (The Thirtieth Anniversary of the Hackett Medical College for Women (Guangzhou: xiage yike daxue, 1929): 11-16.
122. Margaret Taylor Ross, "A Child Welfare Clinic," *The China Medical Journal* 41 (1927): 250-54.
123. Ibid.
124. Mary H. Fulton, *"Inasmuch": Extracts from Letters, Journals, Papers, Etc*, 101-102.
125. Guan Kaixi, "Wo duiyu muxiao zhi jinxi guan" (My perspectives on my alma in the past and the present), in *Xiage yike da xue sanshi zhounian jinian lu* (The Thirtieth anniversary of the Hackett Medical College for Women) (Guangzhou: Xiage yike daxue, 1929).
126. Mrs. J. F. Karcher "Dear Friends" letter, Canton, November 18-December 22, 1936, Folder 17, Box 53, RG 82, Presbyterian Historical Society, Philadelphia, Pennsylvania.
127. Not a Christian, but General Li wanted his son to be raised in a Christian society. Consequently, he asked Dr. Cadbury and Mrs. Cadbury to provide parental care for his infant son, and both agreed to do so, though they had three daughters of their own. Thus, his son became a member of Dr. Cadbury's family and took a trip with them to America. As a token action of thanks for their personal care, General Li decided to build a larger hospital with from two to three hundred beds near the campus in New Phoenix Village on Henan Island because medical treatment for the people living near Lingnan was not available. Dr. Cadbury would be in charge of this hospital because the reputation of Dr. Cadbury's medical mission appealed

greatly to the villagers. See W. W. Cadbury, *Lingnam Hospital for the Care of College Workmen and Neighboring Villages* (Canton: Knipp Memorial Press, 1925), 2-4.

128. "Ling Nam Hospital, Canton," *Chinese Medical Journal* XL, 4 (April 1926), 402.

129. Ibid.

130. Zhongping, "Lun shantung yiyuan yi she xiyi," (On adoption of Western medicine by charitable hospitals), *Zanyu yuekan* 22 (1922): 4.

131. *Guangzhou shi diyirenmin yiyuan shi* (The history of the first Guangzhou municipal hospital, 1899-1999). (Guangzhou shi diyirenmin yiyuan yuanshi weiyuan hui 1999), 3-9.

132. "Report on Income and Expenses in 1935," *Fangbian yuekan* (Fangbian monthly journal) 1 (1936).

133. "History of Fangbian Hospital, 1934," Group Number 18, File 8, Volume 136, 32, Guangzhou Municipal Archives, Guangzhou.

134. "Fangbian Hospital's Entertainment Park," *Guangzhou minguo ribao* (Guangzhou republic daily), December 9, 1925, 2

135. "On Fangbian Fund Raising," *Guangzhou minguo ribao* (Guangzhou republic daily) February 3, 1926, 2; "Charity Donations," Ibid., May 13, 1928, 2.

136. "Canton Hospital: Its work in 1919," *South China Morning Post*, July 31, 1920, 8.

137. Interview with Dr. Quangxin Xu at Guangzhou on May 31, 2006.

138. "Fangbian Hospital in West Canton," *Fangbian yuekan* (Fangbian monthly journal) 2 (1936).

139. "Guangzhou's Fanbian Hospital," *Guangzhou wenshi ziliao*, vol. 8.

140. *Guanghua yishi weisheng zazhi* (Guagnhua medical and health journal) 3 (October 1910), 1.

141. *Guanghua weisheng bao* (Guanghua health journal) 1 (July 1918), 79-81; *Guanghua weisheng bao* (Guanghua health journal) 4 (January 1919), 64-66.

142 . *Sili Guangdong Guanghua yixue yuan gai kuang* (The outline of the private Guangdong Guanghua Medical College history) (Canton, Guanghua Medical College, 1936), 1-10.

143. *Liangguang jinhui yiyuan sanshi zoulien tekan* (Special issue of the thirtieth anniversary of two guang Baptist hospital (Canton: Liangguang jinxinhui yiyuan, 1947), 3-4.

144. The first one was erected on November 10, 1931, the second one in June 1, 1932, and the third on November 15, 1933. See *Guangzhuo zhinan* (The guide to Canton) (Guangzhou: Guangzhou municipal government, 1934).

5

American Doctors and the Modern Health and Hygiene Movement in Canton, 1835-1935

Poor hygiene was a serious problem in late Qing and early Republic China. Some books and articles have been written on this subject, but they do not focus on Canton. The modern health and hygiene movement in Canton is not well researched.[1] This chapter focuses on how American medical missionaries encouraged the Cantonese to change their unhygienic habits and to improve the unsanitary environment of Canton, conducted vaccination work, fought the plague, treated opium addicts and lepers, and promoted rural hygiene and health work. This chapter also studies how the Cantonese elites, encouraged by Americans and impressed by Western preventive medicines and measures to some degree, advocated sanitary modernization, and how the Cantonese medical professionals and the Canton government worked together to launch a public health and hygiene movement in Canton in the 1920s and 1930s.

The Sanitary Problems in Late Qing China

Modern hygiene was to improve public health through official and public efforts, including such elements as environment sanitation, food hygiene, clean drinking water, promotion of knowledge of personal hygiene, encouragement of modern medicine, and control of contagious diseases. In nineteenth-century China, the Chinese generally lacked concepts of public sanitation and regulations on environment cleanliness, and few people cared about the environment. Consequently, refuse, trash, filth, rubbish, dung, droppings, and compost were on the narrow streets everywhere and dirty water ran all over the place in the cities due to the lack of a sewage system. The lack of environment sanitation without a public health system resulted in widespread plagues and diseases, which contributed to the high mortality rate in China.[2] Many Chinese were weak and not healthy, and they were called shamefully "Sick Men of East Asia" by Westerners.[3]

Westerners began to pay attention to the public hygiene issue and develop the concept of state medicine and sanitation; its central tenets were that the state had primary responsibility for protecting the public's health and therefore had the right, even the duty, to impose hygiene regulations on private citizens for the public good. As a result, in Western countries underground sewage systems and water plants were built, and flush toilets and water closets were adopted.[4]

In the mid-nineteenth century, using the microscope to identify several viruses and developing the bacteriology and parasitology, Western scientists and physicians believed that germs played a role in the transmission of diseases and that preventive medicine was important in stopping the spread of disease. They also contended that strict asepsis and sanitation were necessary to protect public health, making great efforts to encourage their governments to adopt measures to prevent the spread of contagious disease. Thus, sanitation was becoming an important part of Western medicine. The local and municipal governments started to pass laws on the subject of food safety and the control of smallpox. Modern public health systems were inaugurated, and public health works got underway. To implement public health policy on a national basis, England was at the forefront of the national medical movements, the first nation to enact centralized public health legislation. Sanitary conditions and public health were significantly improved, and the mortality rate was reduced to less than fifteen percent in Western countries in the nineteenth century.[5]

When arriving in China, Westerners felt intensely uncomfortable with sanitary matters in the cities and the countryside, due to dirty surroundings, unclean drinking water, bad hygienic habits, and outbreaks of transmittable diseases. The Chinese were ignorant as to public sanitation, as indicated by Westerners' observations. Dr. R. H. Graves of the Southern Baptist Convention of America, who had practiced medicine in south China for over twenty years, wrote in his book published in 1895:

> Their cities and towns are unspeakably filthy, many of their busy thoroughfares being but elongated cesspools. Every householder is at liberty to throw any kind of abominable refuse into the public street before his own door, and sanitary laws, if they exist, are neither understood nor enforced. The dwellings of the poor are minus everything that makes for comport or conduces to health, and in times of sickness the condition of the sufferers, especially if they have the misfortune to be women, is extremely deplorable.[6]

Canton also had unsanitary conditions. Located on the border of the Torrid Zone, the city of Canton of more than a million inhabitants dwelling in a space of four and one-half square miles was absolutely bereft of all the requirements for public sanitation in modern cities. The city did not have any public provisions for cleaning either streets or ditches. The owners of stores only cleaned the parts before their doors if they did any cleaning at all. When sections of the ditches were cleaned, nobody paid attention to opening an outlet to the river or canal. On the sides of many narrow lanes, uncovered ditches were stuffed with refuse and dirty water, on the top of which was scum, demonstrating the chemical development in process underneath.

American Doctors' Influence in the Hygiene Campaigns in Canton

American Doctors' Criticisms

American doctors in Canton criticized the unsanitary environment and unclean personal hygiene. After living in Canton for more than thirty years, Dr. Kerr wrote in his article, "The Sanitary Condition of Canton," published in 1888, that Canton had "no water supply and no drains, no inspector of nuisances, and no municipal government to look after the health of the people."[7] Dr. Kerr stated, "Doubtless a lesson is to be learned from the condition of this [Canton] and hundreds of other cities and towns in China where generation after generation has passed without benefit of sanitary measures which are considered so essential in Western cities."[8] To Kerr, many Chinese cities, like Canton, had contaminated conditions, which were threatening the Chinese's health. In terms of personal hygiene, "the poorer classes wear the same garments for weeks without change" in the cold weather, as indicated by another article by Kerr published in 1894.[9] Dr. Mary Fulton, in a letter to Dr. H. W. Boone on May 8, 1894, wrote about the horrible, unclean environment of Canton with such observations:

> The accumulated filth seems to increase daily. As I see the decaying debris piled high on almost every corner and see the utter lack of any sanitary regulations, and think of the ignorance of the people regarding laws of hygiene, I am not so astonished to hear of the death of hundreds, as I am to find the multitudes living on, in spite of neglecting such important factors pertaining to health. According to all hygiene teaching, the whole race ought to have become extinct![10]

It seems that cultural superiority and Westerners' awareness of the germ theory of disease led Westerners to describe the Chinese as unclean in contrast to Western cleanliness.

The Model of Modern Hospitals

The founding of modern hospitals in Canton helped the Cantonese witness the Western hygienic culture. The Cantonese learned of modern preventive measures from the hospitals as well as others. Separation, for example, was one important measure to prevent spread of contagious disease, and the Canton Hospitals had separation rooms or wards for the patient, who carried communicable diseases. Disinfection was another modern method to kill bacteria and viruses. The Canton Hospital sterilized with alcohol, bleaching powder, high temperature, or other disinfectants. Patients' clothes, utensils, blankets, and other items were sterilized, especially in the operating theaters.

The Cantonese also learned personal and public hygiene in part from modern hospitals. The Canton Hospital was clean, well organized, and orderly, a modern sanitary model for the Chinese. To contain contagious disease and to provide efficient therapy and treatment, American doctors needed the cooperation of their patients. American doctors encouraged their patients to wash their hands before eating, drink clean water, eat fresh fruits, stop spitting in the street, and take showers regularly. Patients first learned those hygienic customs from the hospital and then applied them in their communities after returning home. Therefore, the Cantonese began to change their personal hygienic customs, an essential prerequisite for public sanitation.

Kerr's Call for Modern Hygiene

To encourage the Chinese to develop a modern system of hygiene, the medical missionaries were determined to take the lead in the campaign, believing that their hospitals could become a model of cleanliness and order in an unclean society. Their physicians could train Chinese medical professionals, and their medical organizations could help transmit modern knowledge of hygiene to the Chinese as well as encourage them to change their unhygienic habits and launch a modern hygiene movement. They also believed that promotion of modern hygiene and adoption of preventative medicine and measures would not only benefit the Chinese, but also would reduce the medical missionaries' workloads as a result of an improvement in people's health. Dr. John Kerr was the first medical missionary to call for modern hygiene in China.

Dr. John Kerr was very concern about sanitary matters at the Canton Hospital. As he complained, "Certainly it is difficult to keep patients from expectorating on the floor and from storing food, articles of clothing, and tobacco and pipes in the bed."[11] In 1875, Kerr published a book, *Weisheng yaozhi* (Essentials to Hygiene) in Chinese. The purpose of this book, in the words of Kerr, was to lay emphasis on prevention of illness and to awaken the Chinese to pay attention to modern hygiene issues. John Kerr wrote that many Chinese were poor and unhealthy because they ate unhealthy food and lived too crowded together in badly ventilated houses. Consequently, when it was hot and humid, diseases proliferated and caused the healthy and strong people to get ill, while the old and weak were so sick that they frequently died.[12]

To improve Chinese health, Kerr suggested that garbage be prevented from being thrown to the streets and rubbish be moved out of houses so as to avoid starting disease and spreading it; sick pigs and cows be slaughtered and buried in order to avoid contagious viruses proliferating; human excrement be removed from houses at regular times in an effort to keep houses clean. This book also contended that the people had to turn their attention to personal hygiene, frequently taking a bath, often changing clothes, regularly taking a rest, and drinking clean water. Kerr continued that the best water to drink was spring water, the second was river water, and that since water in the cities was mostly polluted and very harmful to public health, the running water project needed to be implemented so as to safeguard the residents' health. Kerr also stressed eating healthy food, such as vegetables, grains, rice, wheat, cereal, milk, fresh pork, beef, fish, and others.[13]

One of very important points of *Weisheng yaozhi* (Essentials to Hygiene) was that the hygiene issue was not only a personal matter or individual problem, but also a government matter and social duty. Dr. Kerr recommended that sanitary officers be appointed with the purpose of taking care of hygiene matters, and local officials and village leaders be responsible for keeping the communities clean and taking preventative measures to contain spread of disease in the cities and towns. This book advocated that state government should employ inspection officials to examine foreign ships once they were at the Chinese ports so that contagious viruses would not be transmitted from other countries to China, and that the Chinese government establish offices of vaccination to enforce compulsory vaccination. This book also asserted that preventive work on a vast scale implied laws, and enforcement of laws was essentially the function of the government, underscoring that the government had to pass laws to prohibit the sale of sick domestic poultry in the market by punishing those illegal merchants. Without local government's support and cooperation, large-scale campaigns and projects could not be carried out in China because the Medical Missionary Society had neither sufficient resources nor adequate manpower to do those, as Kerr claimed.[14]

Weisheng yaozhi (Essentials to Hygiene) encouraged the Chinese to learn modern hygiene from the Westerners. First, Kerr praised the medical examination system of Western countries and encouraged the Chinese government to establish licensing examinations for physicians so as to prevent quacks from practicing medicine. This book claimed that if such medical examinations were organized by the state, more and more people would receive good medical care by good doctors, and the Chinese people's lifespan would be extended. Second, Kerr underscored that Western nations had been improving public health through official and public efforts. This monograph stressed that Westerners, no matter rich or poor, paid attention to environmental sanitation, dietetic hygiene, street cleanliness, epidemic prevention, clean drinking water, and personal hygiene, and that Western governments played a significant role in modern hygienic work. Finally, this book, mentioning mental hygiene in the West, claimed that since the Western women received more education than the Chinese women, they had healthy minds and knew how to adjust themselves to hard situations, rather than the Chinese women who often committed suicide in critical situations.[15] Kerr's book was the first book in Chinese on modern hygiene, not only introducing modern hygiene knowledge but also stressing government and social responsibility in public sanitary and health work.

Huaxue weisheng lun (On Chemical Hygiene) was another imperative book on hygiene in China at that time. This book was published in 1853 by James Johnston and translated by the English missionary John Fryer into Chinese in 1881 and republished in several issues of *Gezhi huibian* (Chinese Scientific Magazine) of 1881-1886.[16] This book had a great impact on the Chinese reformers and revolutionaries, such as Sun Yat-sen, Liang Qichao, and others. Unlike Kerr's book, this book did not mention the principal element of modern hygiene—the relationship between hygiene on one side and government, laws, police, and the public on the other.[17]

Huaxue weisheng lun had a greater impact on the Chinese than *Weisheng yaozhi*, but John Kerr, with the help of his Chinese student, had translated in 1870 a book on chemistry into Chinese, *Huaxue chujie* (Elementary chemistry), which was ten years earlier than *Huaxue weisheng lun*. According to Kerr, one of the objectives of this book was to help the Chinese understand the importance of chemistry because Western medications were manufactured according to chemical principles. In this book, Dr. Kerr mentioned a lot of elements in the nature, which were important to health and hygiene, such as oxygen, hydrogen, albumen, boron, iodine, nitrogen, acid, and others. This is the first book in Chinese on relations between chemistry and hygiene.[18]

In addition to books, Kerr published several articles on modern hygiene after 1875. Kerr believed that medical missionaries not only healed patients of diseases, but also helped them learn how to prevent disease by removal of its causes, and that missionary hospitals should be an example of sanitation. According to Kerr, medical doctors needed clean environments in the hospital, not only to practice medicine, but also to help Chinese patients learn modern hygiene to become healthy citizens. In an article, "Cleanliness," Kerr wrote,

> Anyone who lived in China for any length of time must be convinced that much of the disease and suffering here is due to dirt. Should we not set a good example by excluding dirt as far as possible from our wards? To be successful surgeons, we must use clean instruments and clean dressings. In our medical work, if we are going to attain the highest success possible, both spiritual and physical, we must place our patients amidst clean surroundings. We preach to our patients a gospel of purity and love. We strive to live lives of purity before

them; then let us emphasize such teaching by clean wards and by cleanliness and order in all the hospital surroundings.[19]

The American doctor also encouraged the Chinese to learn Western hygienic measures, as Kerr wrote in an article published in 1890, claiming that in the West the sanitary measures adopted by states and municipalities for the protection of inhabitants and travelers had helped keep a tight rein on the spread of epidemics. Kerr admitted that if the Chinese people had cultivated their hygiene habits and understood the negative consequence of illness, the sanitary environment would have been improved in China.[20] Dr. Kerr suggested in another article to the medical missionaries that much attention should be given to make food and beverages satisfying to the appetite in order to have good health.[21] Kerr was one of the first Westerners to encourage the Chinese to pay attention to the hygiene issue and played a role in promoting modern hygiene awareness among the Cantonese.

The Cantonese Reformers' Modern Hygiene Thinking

Impressed by modern hospitals and American doctors' cry for modern hygiene, to a certain extent, the Cantonese elite began to promote modern hygiene to keep the Chinese healthy, encouraging the Chinese to adopt Western preventive medicine and measures as well as modern hygienic habits and cultures, although many forces inspired them to launch a hygiene modernization in Canton.

Zheng Guanying

Cantonese reformer Zheng Guanying began to develop modern hygienic thought in the 1880s. First, he criticized Chinese's unhygienic habits and unsanitary living conditions and underscored the government's responsibilities in environmental hygiene. He claimed that the Chinese had known the significance of drinking and eating for health, but had paid little attention to the importance of fresh air and sunlight to people's health. He stated that many Chinese always closed the windows of their houses so tightly that they received little light and little fresh air, and that, because the Chinese did not pay attention to the sanitary environment outside their houses, rubbish and trash were in the streets everywhere in the cities and towns, where there was no running water and no sewage system.[22] He also testified that the Chinese peasants lived together with domestic animals in small and crowed houses in the countryside where garbage, filth and dirt were everywhere, and that waste products, garbage, filth, rotten food, and dead domestic animals in their living areas had contributed to the sickness of many residents living there. Under such conditions, according to Zheng, plague erupted and swept over places, and hundreds of thousands of people died of such epidemics, more than those dying of wars and hunger, which had become one of the major causes of the high mortality rate in China.[23] The Cantonese progressive reformer further encouraged the local government to intervene in sanitary matters. In 1884, when suggesting to the county magistrates in Canton to improve sanitary conditions, Zheng wrote:

> Every year during the time between summer and autumn, plague occurred in Canton and spread quickly to other places. The change of climate is one reason for the occurrence and spread of plague, but uncleanness is another major reason…. Dirtiness brought disaster to the people, and local governments are responsible for such calamities. Local government officials should advocate hygienic habits among inhabitants, and both Nanhai and Panyu county magistrates had to order local militias, nobles, merchants, and others to move and clear rubbish in the streets out of the city of Canton.[24]

Zheng Guanying was the first Chinese who linked health with cleanness of streets and urged the government official to take charge of the hygiene issue. His new word, *Weisheng* (hygiene), in his book had new meaning, and the concept of modern hygiene began to appear among the Chinese elite.

Second, Zheng encouraged the Chinese to study Western hygienic science. Admiring the cleanness of streets in Western countries in his article titled "Construction of Road" in his famous book, *Shengshi weiyan*, Zheng wrote that the municipal governments in Western countries had established special offices in charge of environmental matters, and that in many cities the drainage systems were built, carts were used to collect garbage, sprinkle-cars were utilized to spray water on streets, and running water was provided. In his book, *Zhongwai weisheng yaozhi* (Sino-Foreign Essentials to Hygiene), published in 1890, the fourth volume, "*Taixi weisheng yaozhi*" (Western Essentials to Hygiene), introduced five elements of hygiene (air, drinking water, food, heat, and light) and praised Western learning for its ability to analyze and to discern the actual nature of food substance and the process of digesting food. He wrote,

> They [The Westerners] utilize microscopes to examine the structure of everything to identify how much oil, sugar, starch, and protein they hold. They could not only find out whether foodstuff was helpful to physical condition, but also clarify how much helpfulness foodstuff hold. Western knowledge is capable of confirming how much foodstuff enters the body and how much it excretes out from the body in the type of sweat, urine, and feces.[25]

It seems that Zheng had accepted as true that Western hygienic measures were scientific and excellent.

Finally, Zheng advocated compulsory vaccination with government regulations, the first Chinese stressing the government's role in contagious disease control. Since the Qing government still had not passed any regulations on vaccination by the late nineteenth century, Zheng, in his book, *Zhongwai weisheng yaozhi*, wrote that everyone had to be vaccinated; the person who had not been vaccinated could contract smallpox and spread it to other people, which was dangerous not only to the person himself, but also to others. He maintained that government officials had to check whether poor families' children had been vaccinated, and that those who refused to be vaccinated would be prosecuted by the government as committing crimes.[26]

Liang Qichao

The Cantonese reformer Liang Qichao advocated endorsement of Western hygienic measures. In his survey of translated hygiene texts, Liang praised John Kerr's *Weisheng yaozi* (Essentials to Hygiene), James Johnston's *Huaxie weisheng lun* (On Chemical Hygiene) and others for their account of the scientific ways of maintaining a good physical condition. In his article "Du xixueshu fa" published in 1896, Liang wrote, "Unlike the Chinese, Westerners greatly paid attention to public health and cleanliness, such as unpolluted environment, food hygiene, and so on. Those who sought health in excellent bodily shape had to adopt hygienic measures specified in recently translated books, such as *Weisheng yaozi, Huaxie weisheng lun, Juzhu weisheng lun* (On Hygiene of Residents), *Youtong weisheng lun* (On Children's Hygiene), and so on."[27] Liang urged the Chinese who cared about their lives to keep an eye on the methods of modern hygiene and to adopt healthy personal habits so that they would improve their health significantly.

Liang also clarified the role the government played in the field of public health. He regarded government's support of medical science and public health as a key factor contributing to prosperity of the powerful Western nations.[28] Liang began to realize that the government should play an important role in safeguarding people's health by introducing modern medicine, including preventive medicine, to the Chinese. He wrote in 1897 that if the Qing government had regulations to preserve people's health, more than 30,000 to 40,000 peoples' lives would have been saved in China annually, and that the Japanese government already had established the Department of Health to protect peoples' health.[29]

In his consideration of both personal hygiene and the nation, Liang further claimed the hygiene problem was a national issue, although the solution was personal. According to the Cantonese reformer, personal hygiene was not the government's responsibility but citizens' responsibility as they ate, drank, and ordered their daily lives, but individual hygiene became a national issue when it was directly combined with national survival, put in the situation of national crisis. Comparing the serious decrease in the Chinese population with the fast increase in the European population, which posed a menace to racial survival, Liang affirmed that to safeguard the Chinese nation from being destroyed by other peoples, the Chinese had to improve their physical stature in addition to their intellectual stature.[30] At this point, Liang tried to create a picture of deficient Chinese bodies that were in need of Western hygiene to avoid the extinction of a nation. Under the influence of Darwinism, this critical philosopher, paying more interest to the conceptual issue of the nation than Chinese personal lives, promoted personal hygiene in order to meet the requirement of national endurance.[31]

Sun Yat-sen

As a doctor of Western medicine, Sun had been advocating modern hygiene. Sun regarded prevalence of infectious disease, in addition to hunger, flooding, and insecurity of lives and property, as one of the four major sufferings the Chinese had in the nineteenth century. In 1897, Dr. Sun pointed out in his article, "China at Present and in the Future," that the origins of the prevalent plagues and contagious diseases in the Qing Empire resulted from the Chinese people themselves, due to a lack of hygiene organizations and official hygienic offices to battle transmittable disease in the overcrowded cities and towns where a lot of dirt and garbage existed.

Sun also blamed the corrupt officials for poor sanitary conditions in cities when taking the city of Canton as an example. He wrote that since there was no running water in the cities and towns throughout the Qing Empire, city residents only drank water directly from rivers or wells. He claimed that in the 1890s, a company was trying to open a water plant in Canton in an attempt to supply residents with clean water, but this plan had not materialized and had to be abandoned because a high-ranking official in Canton demanded a huge amount of bribery from the company concerned. Sun suggested all big cities in China had to adopt water plans to provide clean water to their residents.[32]

Sun was forced to resign from the presidency of the Republic of China in February 1912, but he was still concerned with the possibility of the outbreak of plague when signs of epidemic occurred in some areas in China. On March 26, he submitted to the Provisional Parliament a bill, "Preventive Measures against Contagious Disease," in an effort to encourage the government to pass sanitary laws and to let the people take preventive measures to battle diseases.[33]

Sun also encouraged the Chinese to eat more vegetables, instead of meat and oily food, and to abandon such unhygienic habits as having long nails, spitting, sneezing, farting in public places, dumping garbage anywhere, and taking no showers for a long time. He believed that when the Chinese realized the meaning of modern sanitation and made good progress in the movement of hygiene, the Chinese would be a stronger race in the world.[34]

Kang Youwei

Enlightened reformer Kang Youwei disapproved of the living environment in China. In his annotated bibliography of Japanese books, *Riben shumu zhi*, published in 1897, Kang alleged that since the Tang dynasty, Chinese cities had declined, roads had deteriorated, uncleanness had existed everywhere, diseases had prevailed, people's health had got worse, and their life spans had become shorter.[35] He poured scorn on unsanitary conditions in the capital of Beijing in the late nineteenth century, writing, "Since Beijing does not have any public toilets, anyone can discharge urine anywhere in the streets, which creates an unhygienic environment in the city." Kang also criticized Chinese's unhygienic habits, as he wrote, "The pigtails of the Chinese head hairs are unclean because the Chinese rarely wash them, which contributes to many diseases and sickness."[36]

Alumni of the Canton Hospital

Liang Shenyu, a graduate from the Canton Hospital's medical school, started to publish a monthly journal in 1908 on public health, *Yixue weisheng bao* (Medical Hygiene Journal). Liang wrote in an article in the first issue of the journal that many Chinese did not mind personal hygiene: worked hard without breaks, ate too much or too little on an irregular basis, drank unclean water, rarely cleaned their clothes, and lived in houses without fresh air. Liang also claimed that in terms of environmental sanitation, due to there being no hygiene laws in China, filth, rubbish, waste, and trash were piled up everywhere in the streets, underground sewage systems were not working, human waste was in the streets, which resulted in disease proliferation. He wrote that in Western countries, people paid attention to public sanitation and personal hygiene because Westerners were better educated, and that the Western governments had established offices in charge of environmental sanitation. He also claimed that many Chinese were determined to revive China, but they were so weak and unhealthy that they could only sacrifice themselves for their country instead of rescuing it. Finally, this Canton Hospital's medical school alumnus asserted that modern hygiene included not only diet and care of body but also public hygiene, advocating that public sanitary works could produce healthy and intelligent people, who could create a powerful state.[37]

Liang Peiji, Dr. Kerr's student, stressed the importance of modern hygiene education. He wrote in an article of 1909 that the independent associations should give more public speeches on sanitation and the government needed to promote public lectures on hygiene, and that, if necessary, compulsory education laws should be enforced to help the public understand the cleanness policy. He asserted that it was necessary to use enforced means to keep public places clean because the Chinese people had not realized the importance of public cleanness. He maintained that public lectures were vital because they would help the people understand the official cleanness regulations. Liang claimed that modern hygiene helped make people healthy, keep away disease from their bodies, and revitalize the Chinese race, and that the introduction of modern sanitary, like the promotion of industrialization, was to make China equal to other countries in the world.[38]

In 1918, Liang, when discussing the impact of medicine and hygiene on the state, wrote that healthy people were essential to build a strong state, modern sanitation would nurture healthy people, and medical science was a source of modern hygiene. Liang asserted that since there were close relations between medicine and the state, good medicine would produce a strong state while bad medicine would produce a weak one. On the word of Liang, the Chinese had to learn modern medical and sanitary knowledge, cultivate personal hygiene habits, and promote public sanitary works; otherwise, a strong Chinese state would not be established. Liang claimed that the rise of modern Japan was a good example when medical science took the lead in the reform movement in nineteenth-century Japan.[39] Both Dr. Ye Fangpu and Dr. Ye Peichu, alumni of the Canton Hospital's medical school, echoed Liang's points of view in their articles, "On the Relationship between Hygiene and State" and "Warning against Spitting," published in *Yixue weisheng bao* in 1918.[40]

The Cantonese elite also published one of the earliest journals on modern hygiene in order to publicize knowledge of modern hygiene. Both Canton's *Yixue weisheng bao* (Medical Hygiene Journal) and Shanghai's *Weisheng baihua bao* (Public Hygiene Journal) were the two earliest public journals on hygiene propaganda in China, which played a significant role in introduction of modern hygienic knowledge to the Chinese masses at the beginning of the twentieth century. The objectives of this journal were to seek the therapeutic and recuperating ways, introduce Western countries' laws regarding medical practices and public health so as to promote administration of public health, and publish new experiments of medical science in an effort to help the masses understand the principles of public and personal hygiene. To persuade the public to discard the social customs in opposition to a hygienic way of life and to promote good health practices, *Yixue weisheng bao* published many articles in plain language so as to appeal to the public, rather than the medical professionals.[41] In the following years, more and more journals on public health appeared in China; by the 1930s, there were sixty journals. Canton, like Shanghai, took the lead in promoting mass education on public and personal hygiene.

The progressive Cantonese reformers, alumni of Canton Hospital's medical school, and foreign-trained doctors were promoting modern hygiene, healthy habits, sanitary environment, and Western-style public health reforms. The Canton officials eventually moved to institute Western-style public health measures, and Canton had become one of the cradles of the modern hygiene movement in the Republic of China in the first three decades of the twentieth century.

American Doctors' Vaccination Work

Contagious disease control is an important part of modern hygienic work. American doctors not only advocated modern hygiene, but also actively participated in campaigns against contagious disease in Canton, introducing Western preventive medicine and adopting preventive measures. American doctors' contribution to the vaccination campaign in Canton was one of the examples.

Early forms of inoculation were developed in ancient China as early as 200 B.C. The earliest documented examples of vaccination are from China in the seventeenth century, where vaccination with powdered scabs from people infected with smallpox was used to protect against the disease. The smallpox vaccine, the first successful treatment ever to be developed against smallpox disease, was first perfected in 1796 by Edward Jenner who acted upon the observation that milkmaids who caught the cowpox virus did not catch smallpox. Western vaccination methods were first introduced to China by a Portuguese, who carried the vaccine from Manila to Macao in the spring of 1805. In that year, Dr. Alexander Pierson, the senior surgeon of the British East India Company, introduced vaccination into China, training several Chinese assistants, who continued to vaccinate the Chinese after Pierson left the country.[42]

Canton was the first city in China to use Jenner's method of inoculation when a dispensary was opened in 1815 by the Cantonese merchants to vaccinate the poor. When American doctors practiced medicine in Canton, they continued the vaccination work. Dr. Kerr opened a vaccine department at the Canton Hospital in 1859 to not only offer weekly free vaccination to the poor, but specially to supply fresh genuine virus, which could be distributed readily to all parts of south China. In 1860, the Vaccine Department vaccinated approximately 700 children and sent lymph to the open ports of China as well as Japan and Siam. Despite those achievements, Dr. Kerr complained that, due to a lack of official and public support, the masses failed to pay attention to vaccination, and that those who practiced it were unable to preserve the virus, relying on fresh supplies transported from England.[43]

The Canton Hospital and the outstations of the Medical Missionary Society carried out vaccination work. Early in 1861, vaccine operations were started at the Zhaoqing Dispensary, sixty miles west of Canton. In the spring 1863, a vaccine station was opened at the Yanbu Dispensary, five miles from west of Canton. In 1864, a pupil of the Canton Hospital opened an institute to carry out vaccine operations in an eastern suburb of Canton under the patronage of a wealthy Cantonese. A former pupil of Dr. Kerr was engaged in similar work at Daliang, Shunde County, thirty miles south of Canton, supported by an association of rich men. In 1868, 671 children were vaccinated; in subsequent years free vaccinations were continued at both the Canton Hospital and the outstations of the Medical Missionary Society.[44] Dr. Huang Kuan gave the following interesting and satisfactory survey in 1878:

> When a doctor is called to a family to perform vaccination he [Kerr] takes a child with him to furnish the vaccine, for which he generally gets 50 cents or $1 as fee, and the child 25 cents for the lymph. Poor people may be vaccinated for 10 or 25 cents.[45]

The Canton Hospital was the only institution in China where a supply of lymph was kept on hand for the purpose of supplying vaccine to native practitioners and institutes at that time.[46]

Kerr endorsed vaccination education for the Chinese. To help the Chinese understand the significance and performance of vaccination, Kerr published a brochure, *Zhongdou yaojue* (Essentials to Vaccination) in 1859.[47] To promote a vaccination campaign, Kerr voluntarily organized several classes to teach the Chinese physicians how to perform vaccination and maintain good vaccine in tubes. He discouraged the Chinese from taking vaccines directly from the human body while providing fresh vaccine to the Cantonese practitioners in order to raise the survival rate of vaccines. Those Cantonese practitioners, after leaning Kerr's method, persuaded their sons to learn and to provide vaccination to other children. Kerr also taught his students how to perform vaccination at the Canton Hospital's medical school, and after learning such skills, they were able to perform vaccination for hundreds of thousands of Cantonese children. The 1866 Medical Missionary Society Report stated:

> Many Chinese have also been taught to preserve the lymph in capillary glass tubes, in which it can be transmitted to distant parts, thus enabling them to dispense with the uncertain and troublesome method in common use of taking a child that has been vaccinated to the place where the children are to undergo the operation.[48]

The 1867 report testified that instruction was given and lymph was supplied to two Chinese vaccinators who endeavored to replace the old style method with Jenner's art in the southwest districts of Guangdong Province. In 1888, an epidemic of smallpox occurred. Because of the prevalence of smallpox, Dr. Kerr persuaded a native hospital, Aiyu charitable institution, to include vaccination in its activities and trained a group of vaccinators by giving them a three-month course of instruction so as to popularize this form of preventive medicine, which was becoming common among the people.[49]

Dr. Kerr not only promoted the vaccination campaign but also urged local governments to play a significant part in this work. Kerr wrote in his book, *Weisheng yaozhi* (Essentials to Hygiene), that the government should establish offices to sponsor vaccination and open vaccination clinics to offer free vaccination to all children at regular time in order to control smallpox disease, a very contagious disease killing many babies. He also asserted that babies in Western countries had to be vaccinated and, sometimes, to be vaccinated again two years later; consequently, numerous babies' lives were saved, a policy that China should implement.[50] The Guangdong government, partially encouraged American doctors, took an active interest in vaccination as a means of stamping out smallpox. Zhang Shusheng, the viceroy of Guangdong and Guangxi provinces, established a new vaccination station in 1881 and sent forty men to seventy-two districts in Guangdong Province to teach vaccination. Due to the government's support, in 1887 only one case of smallpox was brought into Canton Hospital when one of the dressers caught it. The patient was immediately isolated and was nursed by the captain after a boat was therefore secured, attended by Kerr when necessary.[51]

After the 1911 Revolution, vaccination became more popular, and most Cantonese people regarded it as an absolute necessity. It was said that about 100,000 children received vaccination in Guangdong Province every year. An institute for cowpox manufacture was founded in Canton in 1912, and the work was started under the guidance of the local government and continued as a municipal enterprise.[52] In 1926, Canton had 50 vaccination stations. A rough estimate of the total number of vaccinations performed would be between 50,000 and 60,000 annually.[53] Distribution of vaccine to children through the schools and the public health stations also helped reduce mortality rates from cerebrospinal fever in Canton. In 1928, deaths resulting from cerebral spinal fever amounted to 210 and reduced to 78 in 1931, a similar number in 1932, and only 20 in 1933.[54]

The vaccination campaign was successful in Guangdong. Canton was the first city in China to not only practice Jenner's method, but also host the first genuinely Chinese institute for cowpox manufacture. The Canton Hospital played an important role in the vaccination campaign in Guangdong overall and in Canton in particular. The successful campaign against smallpox attack had an effect on China when the Cantonese practitioners introduced Kerr's method of vaccination to other provinces to promote vaccination work.

American doctors played an important role in promoting vaccination in Canton, but the Cantonese played a more significant part in this campaign because the Chinese had developed the forms of inoculation many centuries before the invention of vaccination. As a result, the Cantonese, who already had a lot of experiences in inoculating, had little difficulties accepting this new form of inoculation. More importantly, many Cantonese physicians of Chinese tradition reinterpreted and modified this new technology, which made it easier to be accepted by the Cantonese.

American Doctors in the 1894 Bubonic Plague

Widespread diseases often occurred in Canton due to its humid climate. Bubonic plague approached nearer and nearer to Canton in the nineteenth century and finally invaded this city early in 1894. American doctors played a role in the campaign against plague in Canton.[55]

The plague epidemic began in Canton as early as February, but there was no public announcement of the outbreak until a Chinese-language newspaper mentioned it on March 14. The plague, if truth be told, started in the old inner city in the Mohammedan quarter, one hundred dying on one street. In this district, the filth was the densest and the houses were the most crowed. Many people died of the plague because the disease spread very fast. The disease soon spread to the outer portions and then reached the countryside when many Cantonese residents left their homes and fled from the city to other cities or countryside, although they did not know which way to flee.[56]

During the anti-plague campaign, some Cantonese used superstitious ways to fight the plague at the beginning. As many Cantonese residents died, the superstitious people attributed the disease to a lack of harmony between the elements. As a result, some worshipped the idols in an exaggerated and frantic manner. The dragon was carried from door to door, accompanied by the beating of gongs and bursting of firecrackers to scare and chase off the wicked spirits and ward off their harmful influences. Some believed that if they could smell a malodor from a small xiangbao (a small bag filled with perfume), they would be completely out of harm's way from any contamination. The superstitious officials even went to the temple of the tutelary God to pray for the people and donate money to many different idol parades.[57] In 1895 Dr. Graves of the Canton Hospital described those people's activities in details with such observations:

> During the epidemic of the "black plague" in Canton, in 1894, processions with their idols and music paraded the streets day and night. The Chinese frequently let off fire-crackers to drive away the evil demons, which they suppose cause the illness, and whenever a patient becomes delirious, fancy that an evil spirit is possessing him, and call in the magicians to drive away the demon by the noise of their charms and brandishing of swords.[58]

While some people used the superstitious efforts, the Cantonese philanthropists tried to direct relief efforts and mobilize residents against the plague. They took necessary measures, setting up special hospices for the treatment of the plague victims where only classical Chinese therapies were used. But little progress was made. The plague continued spreading and the epidemic at Canton reached its height in May because the plague patients were not isolated from their families. The failure of the Chinese traditional ways to battle the plague contributed to the rational effects on the Chinese mind and urged the civil leaders to adopt modern quarantine measures. As a result, a provisional plague hospital was erected in western Canton, which was thoroughly ventilated and kept very clean. It was a large mat-hut built on a mound of bamboo over the water, an ideal hospital for plague, but the loose structure made a lot of sound when somebody walked on it.[59] The epidemic eventually began to disappear at the end of July, though sporadic cases were still reported. The mortality rate was high, and it was estimated that as many as 100,000 or 150,000 died in a population of about 1.5 million, although there were no precise figures of the mortality.[60]

American Doctors' Role

American doctors played a significant role in the anti-plague campaign in Canton. First, Dr. Mary Niles first identified the outbreak of the plague and speculated about its causes. On January 16, Dr. Niles was called to a government officer's home to help cure his daughter's illness after the patient had been treated unsuccessfully by a Chinese physician. Dr. Niles identified the patient with symptoms of plague, the first case reported in Canton in 1894. After identifying the causes of the illness as the bubonic plague, she lost no time reporting the seven cases to the local government so as to take preventive measures against the spread of plague.[61] Dr. Niles also suggested rats as one of the major transportation means for the spread of disease and rat migration as a missing link in the chain of plague transmission, although at that time it was not known whether rats had anything to do with the distribution of this disease. Dr. Niles, complaining that there were too many rats in Canton, recorded that in a house where she went to see a plague patient, eight dead rats had been taken out the day before, and that she still unintentionally stepped on a rat which screamed but did not run away and died soon after.[62]

Second, American doctors identified the sanitary issue as one of the major causes of the epidemic. Dr. John Kerr lamented that in "the great city of Canton...there was no sanitary board, the government adopted no sanitary or preventive measures, there was no isolation of cases, no removal of filth or rubbish, no water supply, no system of drainage, and...Chinese medicine and Chinese superstitions had full and unrestricted sway."[63] The American consul in Canton, Paul Seymour, also considered that the disease was probably not directly contagious but could be contracted from the personal effects of Cantonese residents. Articulating the belief that plague was transmitted via the living space of the Chinese, he wrote in June 1894:

> I am persuaded that with the observance of proper precautions, especially in assuring the supply of pure water for cooking and washing, and for flushing drains in times of drought; there should

be no such thing as this "plague," except where natives in congested localities cause pollution of the air by overcrowding and filth, and violation of sanitary conditions for safety.[64]

Americans also criticized the Chinese's superstitious ways in the plague while addressing the sanitary issue. Dr. Fulton wrote, "If we could have hundreds of dispensaries scattered broadcast, we could impress the people with the fundamental necessity of cleaning their homes and streets at such a terrible time as this, instead of spending additional thousands of dollars in begging idols to cause an abatement of the epidemic."[65]

Third, American doctors encouraged local government to play a part in the anti-plague campaign. From an American perspective, Canton lacked the kind of efficient governmental involvement deemed essential to the effective prevention and control of an epidemic, and the Chinese response to plague was inadequate precisely because the campaign was organized and directed largely by civic leaders, rather than officials. American doctors believed that modern medicine, government's role, and sanitary regulations on the Chinese community would play an essential role in the anti-epidemic campaign, civil activism alone being insufficient. Dr. Niles proposed that official engagement, in addition to social support, was critical to solve the sanitary problem in the anti-plague battle. Encouraged partially by American doctors, the local officials began to take anti-epidemic measures. On April 11, officials issued a proclamation that the streets in the city be cleaned and all rubbish be prohibited from being thrown into the river. The population was reminded of a regulation that all night soil be taken away before 10 a.m. every day and be carried in covered buckets, and that slaughtering pigs and fishing in the river be prohibited. The authorities also mandated that the clothing of plague victims be burned.[66]

Convinced by Dr. Niles' speculation in part, the Cantonese assumed that these rodents had brought the diseases as the envoys of the devil, and that their death implied the forthcoming evil. The local officials thereafter launched a campaign to annihilate rats. As part of their common endeavors to clean up the city during the plague, several officials offered rewards for the collection of dead rats. Twenty workers then were hired to clean up the city, picking up and burying the dead rats outside the city. The campaign was successful. As indicated by Dr. Niles, one of the officials offered from his personal money a payment for every dead rat brought to him—he accumulated 35,252 in just one month and 2,000 were brought in one day.[67]

Finally, American doctors used preventive medicine to provide scientific treatments of the patients during the critical situation. Dr. Kerr and Dr. Niles worked day and night during the epidemic without catching the infection and used a boat anchored in the river as a hospital. Twenty-four cases were attended at this informal hospital, and only ten recovered. Since various measures to prevent contagion were not very effective during that time, some Cantonese refused to let any foreign doctors attend to the sick. But after comparing the thirteen patients who restored to health after being treated by American physicians with only one patient who was getting well after being treated by the physicians of Chinese medicine, the Cantonese gradually concluded that Western preventive measures were more effective than the Chinese measures, and that it would be better to bleach their plague-ridden walls and disinfect their foul drains. They, subsequently, changed their minds and allowed American physicians to help and advise them.[68]

Official Protection

American doctors' scientific treatments of patients helped them win official protection. As the epidemic was still flourishing in May, some Chinese started the rumor that no foreigners died of the plague because they had poisoned the water used only by the Chinese. Some placards appeared in Canton, stating that the foreigners were distributing poison in the form of amulets. Then the rumor claimed that the scent-bags distributed by foreign missionaries to Chinese Christian women were then given to Cantonese around the city. Those people, after smelling the bags, passed away. Convinced by gossip that Westerners' poisons put in the wells and in these small bags contributed to the plague, some Cantonese threatened to burn down foreign businesses, and many foreigners were in a rush to migrate out of town.[69]

Anti-foreigner sentiments rose when the plague was mushrooming. On June 11, two American women physicians who attempted to treat plague victims were stoned and attacked by a mob in Canton.[70] As a result, the consuls of Britain, the United States, France, and Germany all protested to Viceroy Li Hanzhang, who thereafter ordered military officers to tear down all posters and sent about forty agents to arrest those who spread the rumors.[71] The viceroy also issued a proclamation ordering immediate suppression of such stories and asked the foreign consuls to tell the medical missionaries not to offer services to the Chinese community so as to avoid attacks. He further ordered the temporary closure of all missionary hospitals and dispensaries, including Dr. Kerr's hospital, where for forty years he had attended to the pain of the residents in this city.[72]

Sanitary Authority

In June, the Cantonese native doctors began to identify some Chinese medications, which were helpful in treating the patients.[73] As an article of *North China Herald* reported, "The Chinese doctors seemed better able to manage the disease, so that many lives" were saved by them.[74] The plague finally diminished in July 1894.

Afterward, the Cantonese officials, realizing the importance of disease prevention, began to pay attention to the anti-epidemic measures and to carry out new prevention policies to enforce environmental sanitation. Canton thus became the cleanest city in late Qing dynasty in terms of street cleanness, as John Stoddard, a well-known English traveler, wrote in 1897 with such remarks:

> Canton is said to be superior to many Chinese cities.... One writer has declared that, after walking through the Chinese quarter of Shanghai, he wanted to be hung on a clothes–line for a week in a gale of wind. Tientsin is said to be still worse for dirt and noxious odors. Even Peking, from all accounts, has horrible paved and filthy thoroughfares, and its sanitary conditions are almost beyond belief.[75]

In June 1901, the magistrate in Canton ordered the residents to clear all garbage, trash, refuse, and rubbish in the streets, dispatched agents to check cleanness of the streets, and collected cleanness fees from inhabitants.[76] The Bureau of Police in Canton began to enforce sanitary regulations. Those rulings prohibited the residents from throwing garbage, urinating, and burning anything in the streets and encouraged the stores to put all their rubbish in their buckets instead of throwing it onto the streets. The Bureau of Police dispatched the police to the streets to check the residents and business communities, and punished those who violated the sanitary regulations.[77] Canton thus became the first local government to adopt sanitary regulations and to use police to enforce sanitary authority in China at the beginning of the twentieth century.

American doctors played a significant part in fighting the 1894 bubonic plague in Canton. They identified the major causes of the plague scientifically, encouraged the Cantonese to improve sanitary conditions, used preventive medicine to treat plague victims, took scientific measures (quarantine, sterilization, and others) to prevent the spread of the disease, and promoted local government intervention in the control of the plague. Encouraged by American doctors to some degree, and impressed in part by Western preventive meditations and scientific measures to prevent contagious diseases, the physicians of Chinese medicine adopted some modern preventive medications to treat their patients while using traditional Chinese medications. Their efforts to adopt both Western and Chinese preventive medications helped control the spread of bubonic plague.

American Doctors in Canton and the Anti-Opium Campaign

Opium, like disease, posed a threat to public health, and the treatment of opium addicts was an important part of public health work in China from 1840s to 1930s. Following China's defeat in the Second Opium War in 1858, the Chinese government was forced to legalize opium, massive domestic production began in China, and the import of opium peaked in the late

1860s. Opium use continued to increase in China, and a quarter of the male Cantonese were addicted at the end of the nineteenth century.

American doctors took part in the anti-opium campaign in Canton. They made efforts and worked hard to cure opium-addicts at the Canton Hospital. After several years of experiment and study, Kerr was sure that the only effective measures, with the exception of Christian ethics, for treating those hooked on the wicked habit of opium smoking was the founding of asylums, similar to those for intoxicated persons in America. Therefore, Kerr opened a ward for the treatment of fifty opium smokers who tried to break the habit at the Canton Hospital. Those addicts varied in age from twenty to fifty-nine years old and had been addicted to the drug from one to twenty years. Each of them had to make a deposit of $1 as security for an adequately long continuation of the therapy. The patients usually wanted to get rid of the habit that had driven them to the threshold of destruction and seriously hoped that ten to twelve days were sufficient to divest themselves of the drug. In 1868, at least 117 smokers were treated, only three of whom forfeited the money. Kerr believed undoubtedly that many were relieved for good.[78]

In 1873, Dr. Kerr looked rather less positive that some patients certainly were cured for good, but at the start some patients were given pills including a small amount of opium besides camphor and ipecacuanha. The 1874 report claimed that two of the 212 addicts admitted were women. Dr. J. F. Carrow recorded in his 1878 report that a special ward was given to treat opium smokers in 1877 and over 250 had been received, and that the Hospital knew little about the patients after they were discharged from the Hospital, although one-third of them confessed that they had been effectively healed. The number of the patients decreased in 1881, of whom twelve departed in several days, giving up their deposit money and going back to smoking.[79]

Dr. Swan was treating opium addicts with new medications at the Canton Hospital. In his article published in 1889 on opium treatment, he claimed that in his two cases of opium poisoning, he had attributed success to the use of atropine, a poisonous alkaloid obtained from the belladonna plant. These two successful cases were significant because the doctors met often with cases of opium poisoning in China at that time and differed on the real value of belladonna or its alkaloid in cases of opium poisoning.[80]

In addition to offering scientific treatment of the opium addicts, American doctors strongly condemned the evils of opium from the perspective of health. Dr. Kerr, in his 1862 report on opium smoking, believed that opium-smoking cases were worse than death, seeing that it brought damage and shame to the family. In his article, "The Opium Habits," published in 1889, Dr. Kerr detailed some of the direct and indirect evils of opium smoking that "a poison like opium, when daily received into the system, permeates the blood, the nervous system and all the organs, exerting a mortifying power in proportion to the amount imbibed and the susceptibility of the individual and that the opium habit causes torpidity of the bowels, including, of course, torpidity of the stomach and liver." He concluded,

> Opium smoking is attended with shallowness of countenance and loss of flesh, the results of injury to digestion, which vitiates the action of the nervous system in its relations to the physical, intellectual and moral nature of man, marks the symptoms of disease in its early states, aggravates disease in its advanced states and counteracts the effects of medicine, and shortens life.[81]

American medical missionaries in Canton, together with other medical missionaries in China, were enthusiastic in the anti-opium campaign. In May 1890, Dr. Kerr, together with Drs. Thomson and Fulton, attended the National Missionary Conference in Shanghai, which afforded an opportunity for many medical missionaries to meet together for the first time. The conference in Shanghai was a forum for opposition to the opium trade. The missionaries discussed the opium problems because many Chinese still connected Christianity with opium to a certain extent on account of the awkward situation that many early Protestant missionaries arrived in China on opium clippers. At a meeting chaired by Dr. H. W. Boone on May 19, Dr. Kerr read his paper, dealing at some length with the social evil and opium smoking. He stated, "In regard to the use of opium, there is no difference of opinion. Its evil effects are so obvious that all can see them."[82] To Kerr, opium resulted not only in physical disease but also in the distortion of man's moral character.

After much debate and negotiation, the conference passed a resolution, the wording of which was "studiously temperate," continuing their opposition to the opium traffic and urging Christians in China to arouse public opinion against it. They thereafter established the Permanent Committee for the Promotion of Anti-Opium Societies, of which John Kerr was a member.[83]

Regional missionary conferences were forums for opposing the opium trade, too. At the Canton conference in June 1891, Dr. Kerr, the chair of the Committee on the Opium Traffic, reported that it was thankful for the increasing knowledge of Christians in Britain and that the issue had been discussed lately in the British Parliament. Dr. Kerr remarked that "the Christian Church in China is practically an anti-opium society" and that missionaries needed to rescue opium addicts and to prevent others from becoming addicts. He urged the Chinese government to understand "the desirability of suppressing the production of the native opium, and of effectually stopping the import of the drug from India."[84] The Conference was determined to work for the destruction of both the opium traffic and the farming of the poppy in China.

During the early years of the Republic of China, Canton witnessed a relatively successful campaign against opium smoking. In 1907, the recently established Anti-Opium Association was successful in appealing for an end to many opium smoking rooms in Canton.[85] The Canton Hospital was vigorous in the anti-Opium Campaign. In 1921, the chief officials of Canton were greatly interested in and, in fact, were promoting the newly formed Anti-Opium Society. The Society had several meetings at the Canton Hospital to discuss how to put forward the anti-opium campaign, according to Dr. J. Oscar Thomson's report.[86]

In the 1920s and 1930s, the Canton Hospital continued to provide treatments for opium addicts. According to the regulations of the ward for opium treatment, opium addicts had to deposit money at the Hospital and pay the treatment fees after signing the agreement. If the patient completed the treatment, the Hospital would refund all his deposit money; if not completed, the Canton Hospital would not return his deposit.[87]

In brief, for the sake of the Chinese health, American doctors in Canton not only strongly condemned opium smoking and helped cure those opium addicts with Western medicine and scientific measures, but also made an effort to prevent the development of the addiction by eradicating the temptation. They played a role in such a social reform movement to eliminate the evils in Cantonese society. Their efforts had an impression on the anti-opium campaign in China in general and in Canton in particular.

American Doctors and the Cantonese Reformers in the Anti-Footbinding Crusade

Women in traditional China were, without doubt, placed in a subordinate status, and the low standing of Chinese women was commonly recognized. The horrible footbinding custom plus the other cruel treatment of the Chinese women persisted for more than one thousand years until the missionaries called for women's rights in the late nineteenth century to abolish such evil customs that hurt severely women's bodies and health. The crusade against footbinding, like anti-opium-smoking, was an enlightenment movement and part of the early modern women's movement in China to assert women's rights to be in good physical shape.[88]

American Doctors in the Campaign against Footbinding

American medical missionaries played a role in the anti-footbinding crusade in Canton. Dr. John Kerr established his authority over this issue when making a list of several pieces of evidence about footbinding in his article, "Small Feet," published in 1870, including the cruelty, the crippling impact, the pain, and the malformation. He denounced footbinding from a health viewpoint, pointing out to the pain belonging to the binding procedure itself and medical problems of all sorts. He claimed that foot contagions were the most usual problem, and that blood poisoning and paralysis could be also brought about by unsuitable dressing and inappropriate attention. He also alleged that internal maladies and low-back problems were common because the woman's weight went on the heel when walking and tended to upset the spine, and that tissue decay was one of the most horrible symptoms and amputation was required in some cases.[89]

The Canton Hospital was treating women patients whose bound feet had developed problems at that time. In 1874, Dr. Kerr was treating a female patient whose feet had disintegrated from wintry weather and were blown off as a result of dry tissue decay. She handed them over to Dr. Kerr, and implored him to stitch them back on her legs again. After convincing her that the feet could not be reconnected, Kerr surgically removed the stumps carefully. When the woman's feet were quite healed, she was so astonished that she could walk rather well. The patient later offered her feet to Dr. Kerr, who sent one to a physician in England, and the other to the College of Physicians of Philadelphia in the United States in an attempt to illustrate the atrocious result of the footbinding practice. Missionary M. Johnstone told the story in the report of 1891, "Dr. John Kerr told us of a case he had in his hospital at Canton: a woman came to him with her feet in her hands, asking him to put them on again. One foot is now in a museum in America, the other in England."[90] Mrs. Archibald Little, wife of the English commissioner of customs of Shanghai, wrote about this case once more in her book, *In the Land of Blue Gown.*[91] Afterwards, Dr. Kerr made use of this case to advise women who bound their feet that it was very pointless for them to waste so much time and suffer so greatly in constricting and squeezing their feet, and that, if they actually did not need them, they might come to the Canton Hospital where he could sever them with no trouble.[92]

American doctors were enthusiastically involved in the crusade against footbinding in Canton, too. Mrs. Little came to Canton in 1900 to promote the anti-footbinding movement. When she was giving a lecture on anti-footbinding during a meeting chaired by the British consul, both Mary Fulton and John Kerr were dynamically distributing many anti-footbinding brochures to encourage the audience to take part in the Canton's Tianzu hui (Heavenly or Natural Feet Society), and many listeners did join the society during the meeting. In July 1900, Dr. Mary Fulton, Mrs. Little, and others went to see Li Hanzhang, the viceroy of Guangdong and Guangxi provinces, so as to get his support for their work of unbinding women's feet. Li was in support of not only the anti-footbinding movement, but also the Hackett Medical College for Women. "The Viceroy with his own hand wrote his name, saying he would send a hundred dollars to our women's Hospital," according to Dr. Fulton's record.[93]

Cantonese Reformers in the Anti-Footbinding Crusade

American doctors' anti-foot binding stance had an impact, to some extent, on the Cantonese reformers. Like the reform movement, the pioneers in the anti-footbinding crusade were the most enlightened Chinese reformers

Kang Yuwei and Liang Qichao, both the most leading activists in social transformation in the late nineteenth century. Kang Youwei began to develop his anti-footbinding thought and take action in 1880s, the most radical in Chinese society and the first man in Canton to condemn footbinding activities. Becoming aware of the injury the practice affected, Kang condemned footbinding as an evil of the Chinese society. Thus, both his daughters did not bind their feet, a remarkably brave action in view of the contempt they endured for it from a number of their family members.[94] In 1883, Kang and local members of the gentry established China's first anti-footbinding society, Buguozu hui (Anti-Footbinding Society), near Guangzhou.[95]

Zheng Guanying, another Cantonese reformer, strongly condemned footbinding. Zheng published in 1892 his influential book, *Shengshi weiyan* (Admonitions for a Prosperous Time). In his book, Zheng launched a conventional attack on footbinding, regarding it as very hurtful to women's health, as he wrote: "It is even more unfortunate to be born as Chinese women, for their limbs are mutilated, their bones are restricted and crushed, and flesh is shattered and bloody, as they are afflicted with the most serious illness."[96]

Cantonese reformer Liang Qichao also committed himself in this movement. Like Kang, he refused to bind the feet of his daughters. In 1896, Liang published an essay attacking footbinding in *Shiwubao* (World News) on behalf of the Jiechanzu hui (Society for Outlawing Bound Feet) to which he belonged. This essay, in which Liang showed his strong opposition to footbinding from the viewpoints of human health, the Chinese nation, the compassion and affection of the family, and others, exemplified not only Liang's strong criticism of the footbinding practice but also his adoption of missionaries' point of view of opposing punishment of the body.[97] Liang's article was evidently exceedingly important in changing public opinions, as Lin Yutang portrayed that one father was so stimulated by Liang's article that he was determined not to bind his daughter's feet.[98]

The anti-footbinding societies began to sweep across China when Western women missionaries started a movement for the natural foot just about the same time. Kang Youwei and his brother Guangren organized a new anti-footbinding society in Guangdong in 1895. In 1897, Kang Guangren helped establish an anti-footbinding society in Macao, and Liang and Kang Guangren founded a Canton-based Buchanzu hui (Anti-Footbinding Society) in Shanghai. This organization claimed 300,000 members with many branches in many cities in China in just one year.[99]

Canton became the most active in the anti-footbinding movement in China.[100] The Hundred Days' Reform brought an extra element to the campaign against footbinding. Remaining as a straightforward opponent of footbinding, Kang Youwei submitted to Emperor Guangxu his "Memorial Requesting a Ban on the Binding of Women's Feet" on August 13, 1898.[101] This memorial clearly showed the direct effects of missionary ideas in general and medical missionary inspiration in particular, on his reform ideology. By that time Kang had accepted the ideas of persistent advancement and the modern concept of health, entirely fundamental to the idealistic perfective cores of Presbyterian missionaries and completely unknown to Chinese traditions.[102]

The reform movement of Kang Youwei and Liang Qichao disintegrated with the downfall of the Hundred Days Reform. The anti-footbinding society was brought to an end, and the crusade for a time had to break up. The Cantonese reform leaders, though officially disgraced and expelled from the country, began again to condemn footbinding in their writings.[103]

American doctors in Canton not only treated the women patients whose bound feet had problems, but also participated enthusiastically in the anti-footbinding crusade. They published articles condemned footbinding, encouraged the Chinese to abandon such an evil habit, and sought to persuade the officials to support their crusade. Inspired by modern concepts of health to some extent, and aroused by American medical missionaries to some degree, the Cantonese reformers played an important role in the anti-footbinding movement in China, although many forces motivated the Cantonese. Canton became the cradle of the crusade against footbinding in China in the late nineteenth century.[104]

American Doctors and Chinese Lepers in Canton

Leprosy scourged China for thousands of years. The Chinese understood the need to isolate lepers from healthy people because most people were afraid of contagion and felt very uncomfortable with lepers' horrible physical appearance. Since public opinion held that leprosy was a result of some transgression, lepers, a special class of the sick, were not only physically abhorrent but also morally detestable. The wide prevalence of leprosy in south China was due to its semi-tropical climate: the intense heat and prevailing humidity, but the intermingling of lepers with unaffected people, in conjunction with a lack of sufficient medical remedy, undoubtedly was a key reason for the distribution of the disease.[105] Since science did not find any means of prevention for the dreaded disease—leprosy, at that time the only method of putting a stop to infection was still separation. Leper asylums provided refuge and monetary support for the afflicted and secluded lepers from society.[106]

The English medical missionaries were the first to be aware of the issue of lepers in China. While practicing medicine in Canton, Dr. Benjamin Hobson was doing research on leprosy in the 1860s. He believed that leprosy was a hereditary disease, particularly prevalent in the humid areas.[107]

The beginning of the leper asylum in Canton was mentioned when John Henry Gray, the British consular chaplain in Canton, noted down in detail the various buildings and institutions of that city and published his comments in 1875 in his book, *Walk in the City of Canton*. He noted that the asylum was supported by the government, but the daily business was administered by two resident lepers.[108] Dr. James Cantlie arrived at a leper asylum in Canton with his student Sun Yat-sen and made the same observation in 1897, claiming that, in 1873, "there were two leper asylums near Canton."[109] Dr. Kerr also offered a concise account of the asylum in Canton in the 1870s, disclosing the minor corruption that was to be found even in the institutions that operated apparently for sufferers of leprosy and for the good of society. He alleged that the government had not taken any effective measures to either thwart the transmission of the disease or heal the sufferers of the bacteria or alleviate their pain, and that the asylums, generally speaking, were short of medical care facilities or any therapy programs, and only the wealthy lepers could receive doctors' attention or medicines.[110]

The First Leper Village in Canton

American medical missionaries began to watch lepers closely in the late nineteenth century. In June 1886, after Miss Martha Noyes was married to Dr. Kerr, her work was transferred from the True Light Seminary to the Canton Hospital's school, which she opened under her care. Later, Mrs. Kerr established a leper village outside the East Gate of Canton, with the help of one of her students from the Canton Hospital's school. The work for the leper village developed rapidly and was later transferred to both Rev. Andrew Beattie, who took care of the work for the male lepers, and Dr. Mary Niles, who cared for the females. In 1894 only one village for lepers existed near Canton, as Dr. Cantlie wrote in 1897 "There was a leper village a mile or two outside the East Gate of Canton."[111]

In 1902, Dr. Beattie reported that a new chapel at the leper village, largely the gift of the Leper Mission of Edinburgh, was opened for services in July 1902 and about one hundred lepers attended the opening ceremony.[112] Missionary R. D. Thomas, witnessing the existence of such leper village, recorded that a leper village located below the city of Canton was positioned on the bank of the Pearl River and received revenue for the village by levying a "leper's toll" on boats heading toward or leaving the city.[113]

On May 6, 1905, a home for uncontaminated children of lepers was opened. This building was filled with Chinese and foreigners and was formally opened by American Consul General Julius Lay, who gave a very interesting address during the opening ceremony. Ten children were in the home supported by the Leper Mission of Edinburgh. In 1910, the Presbyterian Mission opened another home for unaffected children nearby the leper colony outside of Canton, and William Noyes, Dr. H. W. Boyd, and Dr. Mary Niles were in charge of the work.[114]

By 1907, this leper village was had been named Fafong yuan (Refuge for the Insane). The Refuge contained "382 leper inhabitants, and close by is a newly-built Leper Asylum, containing 76 rooms (wards with accommodation for about 200 patients)." The new building, the property of the Chinese government, was placed at Dr. Adolph Razlag's disposal for one year.[115] Thus American doctors established the first leper village in Canton.

Modern Treatments for Leprosy

Special treatments for leprosy were carried out at the Canton Hospital. According to James Cantlie's report, Dr. Kerr denied that leprosy had spread with vaccination because the Canton Hospital provided free vaccinations to many Chinese at that time.[116] Several cases of this disease were quarantined in an isolated portion of the hospital building. In May 1902, Dr. Adolph Razlag, a graduate of the University of Vienna, attended to a young patient with fully developed tubercular appearance on his face for four months. The treatment was highly successful. When this patient had occasion to visit the Hospital on business, he was completely liberated from the disease in good health. Dr. Razlag claimed that many lepers, if not all, were open to medical treatment. He warranted great recognition for his unselfish work, which had been done on a scientific basis and for the most part at his own cost. Razlag gave an account of the treatment, as he wrote:

> The treatment—symptomatic, systematic, and prophylactic—is a combined and complicated one. In the main, it consists of external and internal medicines (disinfectants, tonics etc.), including electro and sero-therapy, bathing, the employment of leeches, etc.[117]

The Canton Hospital gave several lepers systematic injections of a chaulmoogra oil mixture in 1915 and inaugurated a regular outpatient clinic for lepers every Thursday morning in 1916. In 1918, Dr. Cadbury began a year's experience in the treatment of lepers, who attended as outpatients. He injected deeply into the muscles of the buttock a mixture of chaulmoogra oil, resorcin, and camphorated oil, which was first used in the Philippines and later in Honolulu. Reporting the results in his article, "New Methods in the Treatment of Leprosy," published in *The China Medical Journal* in 1920, Dr. Cadbury wrote:

> We must state that the various remedies, as outlined above, while in most cases of leprosy they have definite therapeutic value, yet unless the patients are cared for in a sanatorium, given proper food, together with baths and attention to personal hygiene, a complete cure can hardly be looked for. Where these conditions are unobtainable the weekly injections offer the only hope for improvement we can give to the patient.[118]

The Canton Hospital treated approximately one hundred lepers annually. This was the first organized leprosy clinic in China, although previously much work had been done for these poor ill-fated people in leper colonies all over the country.

Other than the medical treatment of lepers in Canton, American doctors attended to lepers in other cities in Guangdong. Dr. W. H. Dobson, for example, with the aid of the Mission to Lepers, started to attend to the unfortunate victims of leprosy in 1915 at the Fumin Hospital. The patients were housed in the "Emperor Mother's Village," named after the mother of a former emperor, who herself had been a victim, in miserable huts. With the resources from America, wooden sleeping boxes with screened windows were constructed to isolate a number of patients, and therapy was provided to the extent that was possible.[119]

Official Control of the Leprosarium

Besides the American medical missionaries' leprosarium, other Western missionaries opened leprosarium in Guangdong, too. French Catholic missionary P. Comrardy opened the Shilong Leprosarium in 1907, ninety miles east of Canton, which was able to house seventy patients, China's largest leper asylum. With local government financial support, the Shilong Leprosarium was enlarged to accommodate more than 600 patients in 1915. German missionary John E. Kuhne founded another one in Xiaotan in 1907, one hundred miles east of Canton.[120] Since Guangdong Province had more lepers than other provinces had, in the 1920s there were thirteen leprosy hospitals in Guangdong Province, nine in Fujian Province, and six in Jiansu Province, about two-thirds of China's cases of leprosy in these three provinces.[121]

Realizing the significance of the leprosarium in the modern health movement, the new Canton government began to undertake and support the work of caring for lepers. Following the inauguration of a modern form of municipal government in Canton in 1920, the administration of the leprosarium in the eastern suburb outside East Gate of Canton was transferred from the Department of Police to the Department of Health of Canton. In 1931, the leprosarium was expanded and named the Municipal Leprosarium of East Suburb.[122] Other leprosarium was taken over by the Canton Municipality in the 1920s, too.[123]

To suppress the spread of leprosy, the Canton government launched an anti-leper campaign in August 1933, and fifty-seven lepers were arrested and then sent to Shilong Leprosarium.[124] In 1935, the Second National Conference on Lepers held in Canton passed the resolutions to encourage more government funding for leper treatment and research, sending Chinese doctors to Western countries to study the treatment of leprosy.[125]

American medical missionaries played a role in establishing the first leper asylum in Canton area and providing the scientific treatment of the lepers. Inspired by Americans as well as others and motivated by the public pressure to establish a new image of Chinese health, the new Canton municipal government, having realized the importance of the leprosarium in both public hygiene and the welfare system, was determined to take charge of the care of lepers, an imperative step in Canton's hygienic modernization.

The Canton Hospital and Public Health Work, 1921-1935

The Canton Hospital was vigorously engaged in public health education, an important part of public health work, at the beginning of the twentieth century. Dr. Frank Oldt of the United Brethren Mission, while working mostly at the hospital of the United Brethren Mission in the small town of Xiaolan, twenty miles south of Canton, started to give lectures on public health to the students of the South China Medical School, the first course of such a kind in China. In the 1920s, Dr. Oldt began to offer courses of preventive medicine and public health to students at the Gongyi Medical School, and the Hackett Medical College for Women.

In October 1921, the Canton Hospital opened the Department of Public Health and appointed Dr. Oldt as the chair of the new department. The appearance of Dr. Frank Oldt on the staff of the Canton Hospital for public health work added new momentum to the work of educating people against the dangers of trachoma and emphasizing the importance and efficiency of surgical treatment. Dr. Oldt also promoted public health education. He, for example, took a prominent part in organizing a clean-up campaign against prostitutes (sexual evils) in the autumn of 1921, supported by the Canton Christian Council.[126]

Public Health Research

From 1921 to 1927, public health research at the Canton Hospital was carried out, and particular attention was paid to the prevention and cure of hookworm disease. The hookworm was a parasitic nematode worm that lived in the small intestine of its host, which might be a mammal such as a dog, cat, or human. Hookworm was a leading cause of maternal and child morbidity in Guangdong Province, especially in the countryside. In susceptible children, hookworms caused intellectual, cognitive, and growth retardation, intrauterine growth retardation, prematurity, and low birth weight among newborns born to infected mothers.

In 1909, the Rockefeller Sanitary Commission for the Eradication of Hookworm Disease was organized as a result of a gift of one million dollars from John D. Rockefeller and began a five-year program. This program, a remarkable success and a great contribution to American public health, nearly eradicated hookworm. Afterwards, with new funding the Rockefeller Foundation's International Health Division was founded. Sent by the International Health Board of the Rockefeller Foundation, Dr. W. W. Cort arrived in China in 1924 and made his headquarters at the Lingnan Hospital of Lingnan University for six weeks' research on hookworm infestation in Guangdong Province.[127]

Dr. Oldt devoted all his time for several months to this investigation and rendered valuable assistance, not only in conducting the survey but also in compiling the monograph in 1924, entitled, "Researches in Hookworm in China." Later published in *American Journal of Hygiene* in 1926, this report asserted that the growers of mulberry trees were the most seriously infected people in the province while vegetable farmers came next, and the least infected were rice growers.[128]

Dr. Oldt also conducted research on the effects of mixing ammonium sulphate with night soil for use as a fertilizer, a mixture that would destroy the vitality of hookworms' eggs in the night soil without impairing its fertilizing usefulness. To help the farmers learn more about the impact of this disease, Dr. Oldt gave an illustrated lecture in 1925 on hookworms and hookworm disease and showed a film on the common housefly and its danger to public health.[129] Dr. Oldt went on furlough in June 1927 and with the re-opening of the Canton Hospital in 1929 resumed his activities in the public health movement, especially hookworm research. The Canton Hospital and Dr. Oldt contributed to the public health work in Canton.

Rural Public Health Work

American medical missionaries were the pioneers of the rural public health program in south China when engaged in the dispensary movement to provide medical services to the Chinese in the nineteenth century. American doctors in Canton continued carrying out the rural public health projects in the twentieth century.

At the beginning of the twentieth century, more than 80 percent of roughly 450 million Chinese lived in the countryside. The virtual absence of modern health care in rural areas encouraged the National government in Nanjing to develop a modern health-care system in China—a program including the development of three phases of health care services (village stations, sub-district health stations, and district health centers), the education of village health workers, and the collection of essential statistics. The National Health Administration was interested in cooperation with mission hospitals to develop such a system, including a project with the Canton Hospital so as to expand rural health all over Guangdong province.

After the Lingnan University took over the Canton Hospital and renamed it the Sun Yat-sen Memorial Hospital, the Lingnan Hospital and its outpatient clinic for the villagers were transferred to the Sun Yat-sen Memorial Hospital in September 1932, and its work was under the care of the Lingnan University physician, Dr. W.W. Cadbury. New dispensaries were also started at a small house possessed by the Lingnan University in New Phoenix village. The Lingnan Hospital became the center for the rural work in southern Canton, which had a rural population of 70,000 in fifty-two villages. The Lingnan Hospital initiated the early development of a rural health program and organized a model of three-level service thereafter. The first level was village dispensaries where the general practitioners visited three days a week, and the nurses tracked the patients at their homes. The second one was the Lingnan Hospital where more grave patients were transferred for additional thorough therapy. The final was the Sun Yat-sen Memorial Hospital where those patients were referred, who were expecting major surgical procedures, special diagnostic examinations, X-rays, and so on. Thus, a model for a complete rural health program was established in southern Canton. The Lingnan Hospital, accommodating about twenty patients, became a model of what might be constructed and upheld in any large rural community in China.[130]

The Association of Family Health Promotion of Guangdong established in 1931 also played an important role in promoting public and family sanitary work in the villages around the city of Canton. Dr. Oldt was one of the seven members of its executive committee, who was employed as the professor of public health of the Medical College of Lingnan University in that year. He, together with three male Chinese health workers and two Chinese women physicians, was responsible for public sanitation education. This Association launched a campaign for public health in outlying villages, laying especial emphasis on eradicating trachoma among schoolchildren, a program carried on in cooperation with Dr. Hayes of the Eye Department of the Sun Yat-sen Memorial Hospital. To promote rural public health work, the Sun Yat-sen Hospital, together with the Association of Family Health Promotion, established an office in 1934 on the campus of Lingnan University. The office, employing an assistant physician and two nurses of public health, did a lot of public health work on the Henan Island.[131]

In 1933, Guangdong Health Center Association was founded, of which the David Gregg Hospital was a cooperating unit, providing maternal and child welfare in nearby villages and carrying on a large maternity service for village women. The Bureau of Agriculture and Forestation of the Construction Department of Guangdong Province also participated in the rural public health work by opening dispensaries in two villages near Lingnan University. The Sun Yat-sen Hospital sent doctors to take care of the maternity and pediatric clinic of the new dispensaries and took charge of the physical welfare of the students in three rural schools.[132]

In 1935, the Sun Yat-sen Memorial Hospital developed a rural health system. The Hospital sent doctors to conduct regular check-ups for about 1,300 students at eight middle and elementary schools in Henan while opening dispensaries at schools to provide free medical treatment for students. The Hospital also sent nurses and doctors to visit peasants' homes in eight villages near Lingnan University to help women gain more information on public hygiene, prevention of diseases, child health, and family hygiene. During the visits, many villagers came to seek advice from the doctors and nurses. Besides, the Hospital provided to the students of Lingnan University and the villagers free smallpox vaccination as well as cholera, diphtheria, hydrophobia vaccines in order to prevent the spread of contagious diseases, 3,000 villagers receiving free vaccination. It also sent out doctors and nurses to hold public hygiene exhibits at the villages and the schools when local governments or organizations started public hygiene campaigns, calling the attention of the villagers to the need to safeguard their health.[133]

The Hygiene Administrations in Canton, 1903-1935

Before the end of the nineteenth century, the Qing government did not have any medical administration but had provisions of laws with regard to medicine, such as prohibition on quacks' practice, use of poisons to kill people, production of poisonous wine and drugs, sale of unclean drinking water, and others. The Qing dynasty did not have any sanitary laws and hygiene administration until the beginning of the twentieth century. In September 1905, the Qing government opened a Hygiene Office under the Ministry of Police to administer public health. For the first time in the Chinese history, the term of *Weishen* (Hygiene) was adopted by the central government as an office name. In 1909, the Beijing government published detailed regulations on street cleanness and on food hygiene. After the Manchu government was overthrown and the Republic of China was founded in 1912, the Beijing government formed the Department of Health in charge of the national public health, under the Ministry of Internal Affairs. On October 10, 1915 the Beijing government published regulations on the administration of medical salesmen, the first regulations on medicine administration in the Republic of China.[134]

In provinces, the public health work was slow at the beginning of the twentieth century. Due to a lack of special health departments, provincial police departments usually carried out the basic sanitary functions. Since Canton was the first city in China to introduce Western medicine, and by that time had twenty Western hospitals, the enlightened Cantonese, inspired by modern public health concepts, created the Office of Health under the Department of Police of Guangdong in 1906, the earliest provincial public health administration in China. The establishment of the Office of Health signaled the beginning of the modern hygiene movement in Guangdong.[135]

The success of the 1911 Revolution causing the downfall of the Manchu dynasty gave momentum to the public heath movement under Chinese leadership. The enterprising Cantonese, who took the lead in the Revolution, inaugurated in 1912 the Department of Health, which was independent from the Department of Police, the first health administration on a provincial level in China. Appointed as the health commissioner of Guangdong Province, Dr. Li Shufen, a graduate of Edinburgh University, was assisted by five foreign-trained Chinese physicians.[136] After publishing regulations on medicine and public sanitation, the Department of Health launched a campaign to enforce cleanness in the major cities in Guangdong Province in 1913. The Guangdong government took measures in the following years to prevent the spread of contagious diseases.[137]

Department of Health of Canton Municipality

In Republic of China, no municipal health departments existed before 1920, and health administration was generally under the authority of city police departments. The progressive Cantonese were among the first to become imbued with the new spirit and soon put their ideas into practice. Public health work at Canton was placed upon a firm basis when a municipality was established in Canton through the promulgation of a charter in 1920, the first modern form of the municipal government in China. The Canton municipal government thereafter created the departments of public security, social work, engineering, health, and others.

Dr. Hu Xuanming, a Western-trained physician, was appointed as the first Commissioner of the Department of Health. Dr. Hu, who studied medicine in the United States in 1910 and received his Ph.D. degree in public health, was a public health expert. After visiting public sanitary facilities in Western countries, he advocated the formation of official public health offices in China, alleging that since the Chinese lacked knowledge of public sanitation and did not understand the importance of public health, China was far behind Western countries in terms of public health work, and that the Chinese government had to develop public health projects.[138]

The Department of Health was subdivided into two divisions (sanitation and prevention) and two offices (public health education and statistics). The activities of the Health Department were governed by the municipal regulations promulgated in 1921, which dealt extensively with the matter. The total expenditure of the Health Department in 1921 was about one-ninth of the total expenditure of the Canton municipality.[139]

Six public health stations were opened in 1921 in various parts of the city of Canton so as to cover all the city's areas within easy access. Those stations had the functions of dissemination of general information on sanitation, injection of vaccine, collection of statistics, investigation of sanitary conditions, registration of births and deaths, and other duties.[140]

Canton was the first city to start the public health work in China. To put into effect the public sanitary regulations, the Department of Health of Canton organized a public health police squad in 1925 to patrol on the streets, annihilating diseases and safeguarding inhabitants' healthiness and fitness, a police-directed model of public health.[141] By 1925, the total Canton government annual expenditure on health was 325,000 yuan; the Shanghai government's was 270,000 yuan and the Beiping (Beijing) government's was 160,000 yuan.[142]

To promote health and prevent disease, it was necessary to combat ignorance. One of the basic tools was education; this emphasis led to recognition of health education as a major task in the community health program. The Department of Health, the private hospitals, and the associations made great endeavors to pass on health information and guidance and to launch a hygiene education program to teach the people how to get rid of their unhygienic habits and to develop public health knowledge. The Canton Hospital, the Hackett Medical College for Women, the Gongyi Medical School, the Guanghua Medical College, and the Two Guang Baptist Hospital often sent out doctors to give lectures on public and personal hygiene to students and government employees and distributed leaflets on infant care and diphtheria.[143]

American doctors helped the Canton health administration improve public health work. For example, Dr. W. C. Cadbury had kindly given "valuable information" on public health in Canton, according to Dr. Li Ting'an. Dr. Cadbury suggested "that acute gastroenteritis and dysentery should be placed among the most important causes of death, and that tetanus neonatorum is very common cause of death in the first month of life." The Canton Health Department afterward adopted his suggestions to battle the disease.[144]

Canton became the first city in China to have an official hygiene administration, an important office of the modern municipal government. Influenced by Western medicine, the Cantonese foreign-trained medical elite founded a municipal health administration to carry out hygiene modernization in Canton. Dr. Li Ting'an wrote with such observations:

> The Canton government has tried to encourage public health more than can be found anywhere in China. A special building has been built for the health work of the city. Modern ideas beneficial to health are willingly accepted.
>
> ... Canton has stood in China as the leader in this new and important enterprise.... It is the only city in China that has even had a well organized municipality, that put health on an equal plane with other lines of municipal work, and that has built a separate building for health work.[145]

The establishment of the Canton municipal health administration had an effect on China. A Department of Health was established in Tianjin in 1906, but it was a regional health office, not a municipal health office, because it enforced sanitary regulations not only in Tianjin, but also in the surrounding cities. Shanghai did not create a Department of Health until 1928, Nanjing did so in 1932, Beiping in 1934. Thereafter, more municipal public health administrations were founded in China in the 1930s.

The Modern Hygiene Campaigns in Canton, 1921-1935

Hygiene modernization is an important part of modernization. Canton's health administration played a significant part in enforcing regulations on public sanitation, adopting modern hygiene measures and technologies, popularizing health education, and administering medical work. It took the lead in hygiene administration on a municipal level in China.

Environmental Sanitation

The Cantonese began to build streets in 1886, and streets were cleaned occasionally only by residents themselves without government support. In 1903, the Bureau of Police of Guangdong established the Department of Health and hired street cleaners to clean streets in the cities. After the city wall was demolished in 1921, more streets were built and old streets were widened. The system of drainage works was completed; dirty water was running through canals or drainage pipes to the Pearl River.[146]

Since environmental sanitation was a major aspect of the public health program in the cities in China in the twentieth century, it became a significant part of the work of modern municipal administration. Dr. Hu Xuanming, the director of the Department of Health, put more resources into public sanitary work, setting up a special office in charge of environmental matters. Since its commencement, street cleaning was a regular function of the Department of Health. Since sanitary regulations were important in environment cleanliness, by 1924, a set of regulations on environmental hygiene had been published. They covered matters such as cleaning public lavatories, constructing more public lavatories, forbidding shop workers from throwing garbage into the streets, and maintaining the cleanliness of laundry shops, hairdressers, theaters, and minor streets. In December 1925, the Canton municipality published the laws banning spitting in public places, such as schools, restaurants, hospitals, hotels, tea houses, and so on, providing that anyone violating these laws would be fined five yuan. This was the first law banning spitting in China. The 1926 report of the Health Department on street cleanliness work was encouraging.[147]

The street cleanliness campaign at the beginning of the 1920s was very successful. Huang Yanpei, the leading educator and the director of the Bureau of Education of Jiangsu Province, in his book, *Yisui zhi Guangzhoushi* (One-Year Old of the City of Guangzhou) made informative comments in 1922 on public sanitation of Canton. He remarked:

> After reading Canton municipal communiqués, one could find that most of the regulations were on public health and sanitation issues. At that time, most cities in China did not have any administrators of public health, but the Canton municipality had already established the office of health and hired specialists on sanitation to enforce scientific sanitation regulations in order to prevent diseases and to promote health of the inhabitants of Canton.... As far as I know, the streets of Canton are much cleaner than those of any other cities all over China. Since the Canton municipality was determined to

adopt scientific measures to improve sanitation, it had contributed an excellent chapter of the public health administration to the Chinese history.[148]

Li Zonghuang (1887-1987), a prominent official of the Yunnan Province in 1919, highly praised Canton's sanitary work, too.[149] Li commented in 1922:

> There were two major reasons for great hygiene progress in Canton. First, the Department of Health had promoted public health education by using posters, exhibits, books, popular songs, pictures, and others. Second, the Department of Health won the support of medical doctors of hospitals, public and private, to promote public health education and to prevent the spread of contagious disease.[150]

Inspired by Western concepts of hygiene and preventive medicine, Cantonese medical professionals trained in Western countries established a modern administrative system of environmental sanitation. This not only helped establish a better and cleaner environment in Canton, but also helped control and reduce the spread of contagious disease. In 1935, the Canton municipality had to spend about half of its whole year's health budget on such activities as street cleaning and refuse removal. Canton became a role model of environmental cleanliness for other cities in China.

The Ministry of Health of the Nanjing government promulgated regulations for street cleaning and refuse removal in 1928, but such activities remained largely an urban phenomenon. Only in such large cities as Nanjing, Shanghai (particularly in the International Settlement), Beijing, Tianjin, Qingdao, and Canton, was the work carried out systematically with the support of special funds.[151] In 1928, the Health Ministry published "The Outline of Public Health Administration" to support the formation of public health departments in every province and public health bureaus in every city, and had detailed plans for sanitation and infectious disease control, but the enforcement of the regulations was not encouraging.[152]

Epidemic Prevention

Protection of the community against communicable diseases was a major aspect of the public health program. The Canton municipality adopted strict measures in epidemic prevention after 1920. When cases of typhus, yellow fever, diphtheria, or scarlet fever were reported to the Health Department, immediate steps were taken to send the patients to the infectious disease hospitals run by the municipality. If deaths occurred, the health authorities would see to it that the former living quarters of the victims were properly fumigated and their clothing was burnt. By 1924, the Canton Municipality had published epidemic prevention regulations on quarantine service. To prevent disastrous bubonic plague, the Department of Health, since its formation in 1920, had been conducting vigorous campaigns to eradicate rats.[153]

In May 1924, the hospitals in Canton reported thirty cases of bubonic plague. The Canton health authorities immediately sent doctors, nurses, and public health propaganda teams to put up posters in well-frequented places to encourage people to pay attention to the need to protect their health. They also delivered a lot of flyers, encouraging every resident to take responsibility for suppressing the disease and to adopt such measures as raising more cats to eliminate rats.[154] The epidemic was thus placed under effective control after the government had enforced tight regulations to contain the disease at the end of May. The government played an important role in control of the spread of bubonic plague with the scientific measures. Following the year 1925, systematic smallpox prevention campaigns were conducted by the health authorities twice yearly in all public health centers, public gathering places, schools, factories, and hospitals.[155]

Cholera was an acute and often fatal intestinal disease that produced severe gastrointestinal symptoms and was usually caused by the bacterium vibrio cholera. Preventive measures against typhoid fever and dysentery were taken by the Department of Health in the 1920s because these two diseases were related to cholera. Cholera cases were rather rare in Canton, which had a population of one million, but the Cantonese were threatened when a cholera epidemic swept over twenty-three provinces and 312 cities in China in May 1932, and 100,000 cholera patients were reported, 3,400 of whom died in June.[156]

Some superstitious Cantonese used traditional ways to battle the epidemic. They organized religious ceremonies to get rid of the epidemic, inviting Daoist monks to take the lead in the parades, and hoping gods would come out to help them suppress cholera. During the parades, the monks distributed magic figures or incantations and sprayed water on the heads of the people watching the parade so as to help them avoid any diseases. Some did go to the temples of city gods to pray for the suppression of cholera.[157]

The Canton government took preventive measures in several steps, while trying to identify any scientific and efficient treatment of cholera disease.[158] The Department of Health sent letters both to the physicians of Western and Chinese medicines, inviting them to the meetings to identify the causes and the treatment of cholera. Some Cantonese physicians proposed different prescriptions and published them in the newspapers. Even Chen Jitang, the governor of Guangdong Province, claimed to have identified a prescription to cure the disease. The Health Department appeared more confident in Western scientific treatments when writing a letter to the medical association of Western medicine stating, "since the great progress of Western medicine in recent years, you should have found a new treatment for cholera." The Cantonese used both the Western and Chinese prescriptions to fight the epidemic. The epidemic was finally brought under effective control in July 1932.[159] The anti-cholera campaigns were henceforth held every summer. It is clear that the scientific preventive measures taken by the Canton municipality were one of the major causes of stopping spread of the cholera disease in Canton in 1932.

Food Hygiene

The Beijing government published regulations for food hygiene and established a public health police, but those laws were only on paper without being carried out in the first two decades of the twentieth century. Canton was the first city in China to separate food hygiene from environmental sanitation. By 1924, the Canton municipality had published fourteen food hygiene regulations on catering service, cleaning services, and food service. The hygiene policemen enforced these food hygiene regulations after they were issued.[160]

The cleanliness of markets was another issue the Canton municipality had to address. The first modern market—Yushan—a spacious building housing all stores under one roof, was built in Canton in 1920 on the site of a former temple and administered by the Canton municipality. Unlike the side-street markets, this modern market had a supervisor in the person of a representative of the Health Department to keep an eye on food hygiene. The result of the Yushan market experiment was successful. By the 1930s, many markets, both municipal and private, were erected in all corners of the city.

Meat inspection was one of the important parts of food hygiene. China had not developed a meat inspection system by the 1920s, which posed a threat to public health and limited meat sales overseas because Western countries refused to import China's uninspected meat products. Beginning in 1928, a veterinarian official and three veterinarian assistants were in charge of inspections of domestic animals and meats at three slaughterhouses in east, west, and south Canton.[161] During the food hygiene campaigns, the Canton municipality published comprehensive food hygiene regulations and efficiently, if not completely, enforced them in the 1920s and 1930s—a major step toward hygiene modernization.

Modern Waterworks

The Chinese custom of drinking only boiled water in the form of tea existed for many centuries, but many Chinese died of drinking and using dirty water every year, which posed a threat to public health. After the sanitarians developed the water and sewage technologies, modern waterworks were started in Europe in the nineteenth century, and running water became available, one of the most widely diffused technological achievements in human history. The availability of clean tap water brought major public health benefits. Waterworks were introduced to China when Shanghai established

China's first water plant in 1875, but no other cities had such facilities until the beginning of the twentieth century.

In late nineteenth-century Canton, like other Chinese cities, the residents were drinking and using dirty river or well water. A gentleman in the English consular service claimed that he had seen two Canton women in adjoining boats, one washing in the river the bedclothes of her husband, who had died of cholera, the other dipping up water in which to cook the family dinner. John Stoddard reported his experience in Canton in 1897, "I have a vivid recollection, too, of walking over slimy planks, of breathing pestilential odors, and of looking down on patches of repulsive water, so thick with refuse that they resembled in the lamp-light tanks of cabbage-soup."[162]

Realizing the urgent need of waterworks for the city of Canton, the enterprising viceroy of both Guangdong and Guangxi provinces, Cen Chunxuan, organized a company in 1905. The system was actually put into operation, and the residents were provided with Zilaishui (running water or tap water) in 1908. Canton became one of the earliest cities in China to have a modern water supply.[163] The establishment of modern waterworks significantly improved health of the Cantonese by providing clean water, an imperative infrastructure for public heath in a modern city. By 1935, at least eighteen cities, including Shanghai, Canton, Nanchang, Xiamen, Nanjing, Chongqing, Tianjin, and Beijing, had been served by their own water-supply companies.[164]

Conclusion

Medical missionaries, while providing treatment to patients, promoted modern hygiene campaigns in Canton. On the subject of public health, American medical missionaries condemned the wicked habits of the Cantonese and unsanitary environment of Canton, which contributed to poor health and distribution of diseases. American medical missionaries promoted hygiene campaigns with their medical knowledge and experience. American doctors actively participated in campaigns against transmittable disease in Canton, introducing Western preventive medicine and adopting preventive measures to help the Cantonese. They made achievements in such areas as smallpox prevention, treatment of opium addicts, women's bound-feet problems, epidemic control, public health education, and rural hygiene work.

The modern vaccination campaign fighting smallpox was very successful in Guangdong generally and in Canton particularly, in which Dr. John Kerr and other American doctors played a role. Canton had the honor not only of having been the first city in China where Jenner's vaccination method was widely practiced, but also of having harbored the first genuinely Chinese institute for cowpox manufacture in China.

American doctors played a part in fighting the 1894 bubonic plague in Canton. They encouraged the Cantonese to improve sanitary conditions, identified the major causes of the plague scientifically, used preventive medicine to treat plague victims, took scientific measures (quarantine, sterilization, and others) to prevent the spread of the disease, and promoted local government intervention in control of the plague.

Opium also posed a grave threat to the Chinese health. American doctors in Canton were not content to deal with the opium question merely by attempting to cure those addicts with Western medicine and scientific measures, but also made an effort to prevent the formation of the habit by removing the temptation. Their efforts had an impact on the anti-opium campaign in China in general and in Canton in particular.

Chinese women's bound feet created a severe menace to their health. American doctors took part in the anti-footbinding movement. They first condemned footbinding from a hygiene viewpoint and then persuaded the Cantonese to eliminate this social evil so as to help improve women's physical condition. Inspired in part by American doctors and modern hygiene concepts, the Cantonese progressive reformers launched the anti-footbinding movement in Canton first. Later, it evolved into a campaign for women's freedom and a social reform movement against the traditional wickedness in Chinese society. Canton thereafter became the cradle and the center of the anti-footbinding crusade in China in the late nineteenth century.

American medical missionaries established the first leper asylum in Canton and provided the scientific treatment of the lepers. Since many lepers could not find any institutions to take care of them in Canton, in part due to a lack of well-equipped facilities to fight contagious diseases, Americans founded China's first organized leprosy clinic at the Canton Hospital, and devoted themselves loyally to the care of these unfortunate victims.

American doctors continued playing a role in promoting rural public health in the Canton area in the twentieth century. They popularized hygiene education in the countryside and provided medical care to the people in the rural area.

The establishment of modern hospitals helped the Cantonese witness the Western approach to hygiene, and the Cantonese learned of modern preventive measures to some extent from Americans and other Westerners. The patients first learned those hygienic customs from the hospitals and then applied them in their communities after returning home. Since Canton's prevailing humid climate with the intense heat, semitropical in nature, resulted in wide prevalence of epidemic diseases, the Cantonese were more enthusiastic than other Chinese people to adopt modern hygienic measures against different kinds of diseases. Therefore, many Cantonese began to change their personal hygienic customs, an essential prerequisite for public sanitation.

Inspired by Western medicine and preventive measures, the enlightened Cantonese reformers, members of the elite, alumni of the Canton Hospital's medical school, and foreign-trained physicians began to pay attention to the sanitary issue. They advocated modern hygiene to improve the health of the Chinese and urged the Chinese to adopt hygienic habits, create clean environments, and adopt a Western-style system of hygiene.

The Canton officials eventually moved to institute Western-style hygiene measures. The Canton authority adopted Americans' scientific measures to prevent contagious diseases during the 1894 plague. After the plague, when the Bureau of Police in Canton began to enforce sanitary regulations in 1901, Canton became the first local government to enforce sanitary authority in China and became the cleanest city in the late Qing dynasty in terms of street cleanliness.

China's first municipal health department was formed in 1920 when China's first modern municipality was established in Canton. Canton's health office started environmental sanitary work in the 1920s, a time of impressive investment by the Canton municipality in environmental quality in terms of water supply, waste disposal, well-paved clean streets, ventilated and roomier dwellings, and other areas. These efforts not only helped establish a better and cleaner environment in Canton, but also helped control and reduce the spread of contagious diseases. Canton was also the first city in China to separate food hygiene from environmental sanitation. In addition, the Canton government took charge of the care of lepers in the 1920s and took scientific preventive measures efficiently to stop the spread of cholera in 1932, an important step and a major accomplishment in hygiene modernization.

Canton, one of the cleanest major cities in China in the 1920s, became a role model for other Chinese cities and continued subsequently to be the most enthusiastic place in the modern hygiene movement in the Republic of China. Western medicine and American doctors helped transform Canton into a modern hygienic city, but the Cantonese played a crucial role in this transformation.

This transformation was a process of combining both Western preventive medicine and Chinese preventive medicine. The Cantonese physicians of Chinese tradition reinterpreted and modified vaccination, which contributed to the successful campaign again smallpox in Guangdong. The enlightened Cantonese elite and the physicians of Chinese medicine took Western preventive measures and medications to battle contagious diseases while continuing to use Chinese traditional ways and methods, a combination of the Sino-Western preventive measures and medications, which was efficient and practical to some degree in the epidemics. In this regard, this transformation was part of modern medical globalization in China.

Notes

1.   See Carol Benedict, *Bubonic Plague in Nineteenth-Century China* (Stanford: Stanford University Press, 1996); Ka-che Yip, *Health and National Reconstruction in Nationalist China: The Development of Modern Health Services, 1928-1937*, Monograph and Occasional Paper Series (Ann

Arbor: Association for Asian Studies, 1995); Yangwen Zheng, *The Social Life of Opium in China: A History of Consumption from the Fifteenth to the Twentieth Century* (Cambridge University Press, 2005), Yu Xinzhong, *Qing dai Jiang nan de wen yi yu she hui: yi xiang yi liao she hui shi de yan jiu* (Plague and society in south China during the Qing Dynasty) (Beijing: Zhongguo ren min daxue chubanshe, 2003), Zhang Daqing, *Zhongguo jin dai ji bing she hui shi: 1912-1937* (A social history of diseases in modern China) (Jinan: Shandong jiao yu chu ban she, 2006), and Yu Xinzhong, ed., *Qing yi lai de ji bing, yi liao he wei sheng: yi she hui wen hua shi wei shi jiao de tan suo* (Disease, medicine, and hygiene since the Qing Dynasty: A study from a social and cultural perspective) (Beijing: Shenghuo, dushu, xinzhi sanlian shudian, 2009).

2. Huang Zifang, "Zhongguo weisheng zhouyi" (On sanitation of China), *Zhonghua yixue zazhi* 13, no. 5 (1927): 339.

3. Xiong Yuezhi,, *Xi xue dong jian yu wan Qing she hui* (The dissemination of Western learning and late Qing society) (Shanghai: Shanghai renmin chubanshe, 1994), 490-493.

4. Jeanne Brand, *Doctors and the State* (Baltimore, Md.: John Hopkins University Press, 1965), 5.

5. Elizabeth Fee and Dorothy Porter, "Public Health, Preventive Medicine and Professionalization: England and America in the Nineteenth Century," in Andrew Wear, ed. *Medicine in Society: Historical Essays* (Cambridge, Eng.: Cambridge University Press, 1992), 249-75 and John Duffy, "History of Public Health and Sanitation in the West since 1700," in Kenneth Kiple, ed. *The Cambridge World History of Human Disease* (Cambridge, England: Cambridge University Press, 1993), 200-206.

6. R. H. Graves, *Forty Years in China or China in Transition* (Baltimore: Woodward, 1895. Reprint,Scholarly Resource at Wilmington, Delaware, 1972), 226-27.

7. John Kerr, "The Sanitary Condition of Canton," *The China Medical Missionary Journal* 2, 3 (September 1888): 134-35.

8. Ibid.

9. J. G. Kerr, "Visical Calculus in Canton Province, China, Including the Report of a Personal Experience in 1894 Operations," *China Medical Missionary Journal* 8 (1894): 104-16.

10. Mary H. Fulton to Doctor Boone, May 8, 1894, *China Medical Missionary Journal* 8 (1894): 142-43.

11. J. G. Kerr, "The Native Benevolent Institutions of Canton," *China Review* 2 (Sept./Oct., 1873), 88-95.

12. This book was divided into seven chapters: Chapter 1, On Long Life Span; Chapter 2, On the Causes of All Diseases; Chapter 3, On How to Identify Sickness; Chapter 4, On Good Doctors to Heal the Sick; Chapter 5, On How to Keep Good Health; Chapter 6, On How to Promote Modern Hygienic Work in the Communities; and Chapter 7, On Government's Role in Public Hygiene. See Jia Yuehan (John Kerr), *Weisheng yaozhi* (Essential to hygiene) (Yangcheng boji yiju, 1875). It was republished in 1884.

13. Ibid.

14. Ibid.

15. Jia Yuehan (John Kerr), *Weisheng yaozhi* (Essential to hygiene) (Yangcheng boji yiju, 1884) 2b, 34b-35a, and 37a-38b.

16. This book introduced several aspects of modern hygiene in Western countries, discussed relations between chemical science and human's ordinary lives, pointed to environment pollution caused by industrialization, and concentrated on chemical elements in food, water, wine, ciguatera, opium, soil, and grain, all very important to people's health. As James wrote in this book, "The common life of man is full of wonders, Chemical and Physiological. Most of us as through this life without seeing or being sensible of them, although everyday our existence and our comforts ought to recall them to our minds." See James F. Johnston, *Chemistry of Common Life* (New York: D. Appleton and Company, 1853), 1.

17. For a study of the impact of this book on Liang Qichao and Zheng Guanying, see Ruth Rogaski, *Modernity: Meanings of Health and Disease in Treaty-port China* (Berkeley; California: University of California Press, 2004), 15-20,104-64.

18. Jia Yuehan (John Kerr), *Huaxue chujie* (Elementary chemistry), 4 volumes, (Yangcheng boji yiju, 1870).

19. John Kerr, "Cleanliness," *China Medical Missionary Journal* 11, 3 (September 1888): 156-57.

20. J. G. Kerr, "Introductory—Medical Missionaries in relation to the Medical Profession," *China Medical Missionary Journal* 6, 3 (1890): 87-99.

21. John Kerr, "Preservation of Health: A Duty," *China Medical Missionary Journal* 5, 1 (March, 1891): 1-2.

22. Zheng Guanying, *Zheng Guanying ji* (Works of Zhang Guanying), vol. 1 (Shanghai: Shanghai renmin chubanshe, 1982), 660.

23. Zheng Guanying, *Zheng Guanying ji* (Works of Zheng Guanying), vol. 2 (Shanghai: Shanghai renmin chubanshe, 1988), 49-55.

24. Ibid., 350.

25. Zheng Guanying, *Zhongwai weisheng yaozhi* (Chinese and foreign essentials to hygiene) (1890, 1895).

26. Ibid.

27. Xiong Yuezhi,, *Xi xue dong jian yu wan Qing she hui* (The dissemination of Western learning and late Qing society) (Shanghai: Shanghai renmin chubanshe, 1994), 492.

28. Ralph Croizier, *Traditional Medicine in Modern China: Science, Nationalism, and the Tensions of Cultural Changes* (Cambridge: Harvard University Press, 1968), 59-63

29. Liang Qichao, "Diqiu renshi ji"(The record of human beings and the events), *Qingyi bao* (China discussion), vol. 41.

30. Liang Qichao, *Yinbingshi heji* (Works of the ice cream house), vol. 2 (Beijing: Zhonghua shuju, 1989), 120-26.

31. Liang Qichao, "Yixue shanhui xu" (The Discussion of the medical philanthropy society), *Shiwu bao* 38 (August 11, 1897).

32. Sun Zhongshan, *Sun Zhongshan quanji*, vol. 1: 89, 93-106.

33. Sun Zhongshan, *Sun Zhongshan quanji*, vol. 2: 281.

34. Sun Zhongshan, *Sun Zhongshan quanji*, vol. 6: 162, 64-45; ibid., vol. 9: 248-49.

35. Kang Youwei, *Kang Youwei quanji* (Works of Kang Youwei), ed. Jiang Yihu, vol. 3 (Shanghai: Guji chubanshe, 1992), 599-601.

36. Kang Youwei, "On Parliament Government's Hands off Public Customs," *Jindai zhongguoshiliao congkan* (Historical materials of modern China), ed. Shen Yulong, vol. 38 (Taiwan: The Wenhai Press, 1988), 8.

37. *Yixue weisheng bao* (Medical and hygienic daily) 1 (1908), 5-14.

38. Liang Peiji, "To organize Public Lectures on Medicine to Enforce Cleanness Policy," *Yixue weisheng bao* (Medical and hygienic journal) 7 (1909): 55.

39. *Guanghua weisheng bao* (Guanghua health journal) 1 (July 1918): 1-3.

40. Ibid., 12-23, 44-47.

41. *Yixue weisheng bao* (Medical and hygienic journal) 1 (1908), 1-3.

42. A. Pearson, "Report submitted to the Board of the National Vaccine Establishment, respecting the introduction of the practice of vaccine inoculation into China, AD 1805," *Chinese Repository* 2 (May 1833): 35-41.

43. John Kerr, "Report of the Medical Society's Hospital at Canton for the Year 1860," in Medical Missionary Society, *Report of the Medical Missionary Society in China for the Year 1860* (Canton, Friend of China Press, 1861), 5-6.

44. Medical Missionary Society, *Report of Medical Missionary Society in China for the Year 1868* (Canton, China: The Medical Missionary Society, 1869).

45. Wong, *History of Chinese Medicine*, 149.

46. Medical Missionary Society, *Report of the Medical Missionary Society in China for the Year 1866* (Canton, China: The Medical Missionary Society, 1867), 9.

47. Cadbury, *At the Point of a Lancet*, 123.

48. Medical Missionary Society, *Report of the Medical Missionary Society in China for the Year 1866* (Canton, China: The Medical Missionary Society, 1867), 9.

49. Wong, *History of Chinese Medicine*, 148.

50. Jia Yuehan (John Kerr), *Weisheng yaozhi* (Essential to hygiene) (Yangcheng boji yiju, 1875).

51. Tso To-Ming, "Sketches of Dr. Kerr," *First Report of the Refuge for the Insane* vol. 38, 18-22, Presbyterian Church Board of Foreign Missions, *China Letters, 1837-1900*, microfilm, Presbyterian Historical Society, Philadelphia, Pennsylvania.

52. J. Oscar Thompson, "To Editor of the Chinese Medical Journal," *China Medial Journal* 26, 3 (May 1912), 208.

53. W.W. Peter, *Broadcasting Health in China* (Shanghai: Presbyterian Mission Press, 1926), 66.

54. Wong, *History of Chinese Medicine*, 249.

55. *Dianshizhai huabao* (Dianshi studio illustrated news) (Guangzhou: Guangdong renmin chubanshe, 1983), 32.

56. Xian Weisun, *Shuyi liuxingshi* (History of the plague) (Guangzhou: the Health and Disease Control Station of Guangdong Province, 1989), 203.

57. Harriet Noyes, *A Light in the Land of Sinim—Forty-Five Years in the True Light Seminar, 1872-1917* (New York: Fleming Revell, 1919), 117-20.

58. R. H. Graves, *Forty Years in China or China in Transition* (Baltimore: Woodward, 1895. Reprint, Scholarly Resource at Wilmington, Delaware, 1972), 234-35.

59. Mary Niles, "Plague in Canton," *China Medical Missionary Journal* 8 (1894): 116-19.

60. John Kerr, "The Bubonic Plague," *China Medical Missionary Journal* 13, 4 (December 1894): 178-80.

61. Mary Niles, "Plague in Canton," *China Medical Missionary Journal* 8 (1894): 116-19.

62. Even after 1898, when the American consul in Canton, Paul Simond, published his classic paper hypothesizing that the rat flea was the missing link in the chain of plague transmission, many Western authorities initially refused to accept it. See Fabian Hirst, *The Conquest of Plague: A Study of the Evolution of Epidemiology* (Oxford: Clarendon Press, 1953), 152-63.

63. John Kerr, "The Bubonic Plague," *China Medical Missionary Journal* 13, 4 (Dec. 1894): 178-80.

64. Seymour to Uhl, June 6, 1894, reel 12, no. 270, Microfilm File Number M 101, Dispatches from Consuls at Canton, 1790-1906, U.S. Department of States, National Archives, Washington, D.C.

65. Mary H. Fulton to Doctor Boone, May 8, 1894, *China Medical Missionary Journal* 8 (1894): 142-43.

66. Elizabeth Sinn, *Power and Charity: The Early History of the Tung Wah Hospital* (Hong Kong: Oxford University Press, 1989), 159; Inspectorate General of Chinese Imperial Customs, *Customs Medical Reports* (Shanghai: Statistical Department of the Inspectorate General of Customs, 1894), no. 48: 20; and "The Plague at Canton," *North China Herald*, May 18, 1894, 774-75.

67. Mary Niles, "Plague in Canton," *China Medical Missionary Journal* 8 (1894): 116-19.

68. It was difficult to hire anyone to assist American doctors. A woman, on whom Dr. Niles had performed an ovariotomy in the early 1894, was employed to attend to the female patients, and a man, a sanitary worker in the hospital, helped take care of male patients but was attacked by the disease and gave up later. "Plague News," *Shen bao*, June 14, 1894.

69. Since a Western woman was attacked by mob in Canton, the Westerners working at the Customs had to take shelters in Westerners' settlement so as not to be attacked. Seymour to Uhl, June 27, 1894, reel 12, no. 272, Microfilm File Number M 101, Dispatches from Consuls at Canton, 1790-1906, U.S. Department of States, National Archives, Washington, D.C.

70. Harriet Noyes, *A Light in the Land of Sinim—Forty-Five Years in the True Light Seminar, 1872-1917* (New York: Fleming Revell, 1919), 118.

71. "Plague News," *Shen bao*, July 3, 1894; "Stop Rumors," Ibid., July 4, 1894; and "Bandits Wanted," Ibid., July 9, 1894.

72. Elizabeth Sinn, *Power and Charity: The Early History of the Tung Wah Hospital* (Hong Kong: Oxford University Press, 1989), 174-76.

73. Liang Longzhang, *Bianzheng qiuzhen* (Seeking the truth) (Guangzhou: Weixin yinwu ju, 1905), 6.

74. "The Southern Plague," *The North China Herald*, June 15, 1894, 946.

75. John Stoddard, *China*, (Chicago: Belford, Middlebrook & Company, 1897), 90.

76. "Cantonese News," *Shen bao*, June 1, 1901.

77. "Guangdong Province," *China Daily*, April 12, 1904.

78. "Yangchen quanchu yapian gonghui guitiao," (Regulations on quitting smoking opium in Canton) *Wanguo congbao* (Global news) 380 (1876).

79. Cadbury, *At the Point of a Lancet*, 126.

80. J. M. Swan, "Opium Poisoning Treated with Atropia-Sulphate," *China Medical Missionary Journal* 3, 2 (June 1889): 143-44.

81. John Kerr, "The Opium Habit," *China Medical Missionary Journal* 3, 2 (June 1889): 143-44.

82. J. G. Kerr, "Introductory—Medical, Missionaries in relation to the Medical Profession," *China Medical Missionary Journal* 6, 3 (1890): 87-99.

83. They were B.C. Atterbury, M.D., American Presbyterian Mission in Beijing; Archdeacon Arthur E. Moule, Church Missionary Society in Shanghai; Henry Whitney, M.D., American Board of Commissioners for Foreign Missions in Kweiyang; the Rev. Samuel Clarke, China Inland Mission in Kweiyang; the Rev. Arthur Shorrock, English Baptist Mission in Taiyuan; and the Rev. Griffith John, London Mission Society in Hankow. See "Missionary Conference," *North China Herald* 16 (May 1890): 602-4.

84. J. G. Kerr and Grainger Hargreaves, "The Opium Question: Report of the Committee on the Opium Traffic," *Chinese Recorder* 22 (August 1891): 371-73.

85. Edward Rhoads, *China's Republican Revolution: The Case of Kwangtung, 1895-1913* (Cambridge, Mass.: Harvard University Press, 1975), 94-6, 124-5, 253, 264.

86. Dr. J. Oscar Thomson to Dr. A. J. Brown, December 10, 1921, File 22, Box 1, Record Group 82, Presbyterian Church in the U.S.A. Board of Foreign Missions. Secretaries Files: China Missions, 1891-1955, Presbyterian Historical Society, Philadelphia, Pennsylvania.

87. "Regulations of the Opium Addict Treatment," *SunYisen boshi yixueyuan yilan* (Information on the Sun Yat-sen Medical College)(Guangzhou, 1935), 148.

88. For an account of the anti-foot binding crusade, see Margaret Burton, *Notable Women of Modern China* (New York, 1912), 131-32; Lu Meiyi, *Zhongguo Funu yundong*, 1840-1921 (China's women movement, 1840-1921) (Zhengzhou: Henan remin chubanshe, 1990); Liu Jucai, *Zhongguo jindai fu nu yundong shi* (History of the modern Chinese women movement) (Beijing: Zhongguo Funu chubanshe, 1989); and Howard S Levy, *Chinese Footbinding: The History of a Curious Erotic Custom* (New York, 1996).

89. John G Kerr, "Small Feet," *Chinese Recorder and Missionary Journal* 6 (June 1870): 22-33.

90. M. Johnstone, "Footbinding," *Woman's Work in the Far East* (Shanghai: Presbyterian Mission Press, 1892), 166-67.

91. Archibald Little, *In the Land of the Blue Gown* 1902 [1908] A photo of the foot that is in the United Sates is shown in Beverley Jackson's *Splendid Slippers* (Berkeley, California: Ten Speed Press, 1997), 135-36.

92. Harriet Noyes, *A Light in the Land of Sinim-Forty-Five Years in the True Light Seminar, 1872-1917* (New York: Fleming Revell, 1919), 157-58.

93. Archibald Little, "Tour in Behalf of the Anti-Foot-binding Society," *The Chinese Recorder* 31 (1900): 258-61.

94. Kang Tongbi, "Qingmo de buchanzu hui" (The Anti-Footbinding Society of the late Qing), *Zhongguo funü* (Chinese women) (May 1957), 12; Lo Jung-pang, ed., *K'ang You-wei: A Biography and a Symposium* (Tucson: University of Arizona, 1967), 38-39.

95. The association finally came to an end without any significant achievements due to the opposition of the strong conservative forces in the district. See Virginia Chui Chao, "The Anti-Footbinding Movement in China, 1850-1912," (M.A. Thesis, Columbia University, 1966), 52.

96. Zheng Guanying, *Sheng shi weiyan* (Taipei: Xue sheng shu ju, 1965 [1892]), 266.

97. In his essay, "Jiechanzu hui xu," (Discussion of the anti-footbinding society), Liang Qichao denoted the cruelty of imposing on ingenuous women the bodily damage produced by fastening the feet. Liang Qichao, *Liang Qichao quanji* (Works of Liang Qichao) (Beijing: Beijing chubanshe, 1999), 80. See also Liang Qichao, "Jiechanzu hui xu" (Discussion of the anti-footbinding society), *Shiwubao* 16 (December 1, 1896), 12a-12b; reprinted in Liang Qichao, *Yinbingshi wenji* (Collected writings from the ice-drinker's studio), vol. 1 (Beijing; Zhonghua shuju, 1989): 120-22.

98. Lin Yutang, Chinese-American writer, translator, and editor, was educated in China and at Harvard University. See Howard S. Levy, *Chinese Footbinding: The History of a Curious Erotic Custom* (New York, 1996), 311.

99. Lo Jung-pang, ed., *K'ang Yu-wei: A Biography and a Symposium* (Tucson: University of Arizona, 1967), 38-39.

100. The Cantonese reformers were able to bring the footbinding issue into public debate and into the reform movement because more Chinese recognized the concept of modern hygienic and China was in a national crisis, defeated in the Sino-Japanese War of 1894-95. They considered the issue of women's footbinding not only the matter of women's health and but the subject of national survival. See Liu Jucai, *Zhongguo jindai fu nu yundong shi* (History of the modern Chinese women movement) (Beijing: Zhongguo Funu chubanshe, 1989), 136.

101. Kang Youwei, "Qing jin funü chanzu zou" (Memorial requesting a ban on the binding of women's feet), dated June 1898, in *Wuxu bianfa* (the 1898 Reform Movement), ed. Zhongguo shixuehui (Chinese historical association) (Shanghai: Shenzhou guoguangshe, 1953), vol. 2, 242-44.

102. Kang Youwei, "Qingjin funu chanzu jie,"in Kang Youwei, *Kang Youwei wenxuan* (Selected works of Kang Youwei) (Shanghai: Shanghai yuandong chubanshe, 1997), 396.

103. Linag Qichiao, *Liang Qichao jia shu* (Liang Qichao's home letters) (Beijing: Zhongguo wenlian chubanshe, 2000), 11.

104. Virginia Chui Chao, "The Anti-Footbinding Movement in China (1850-1912)," (M.A. Thesis, Columbia University, 1966), 115.

105. For the best study of the history of leprosy in China, see Angela Ki Che Leung, *Leprosy in China: A History* (New York: Columbia University Press, 2009).

106. English missionary Wellesley C. Bailey founded in 1874 the Mission to Lepers, an international organization to establish leper asylums in the world.

107. *Medical Times and Gazette* 2 (June 2, 1860): 558-59.

108. John Henry Gray, *Walks in the City of Canton* (Hong Kong: De Souza, 1875): 688-90.
109. James Cantlie, *Report the Conditions under which Leprosy Occurs in China, Indo-China, Malaya, the Archipelago and Oceania* (London: Macmillan, 1897), 65.
110. J. G. Kerr, "Benevolent Institutions of Canton," *China Review* 3 (1874-1975): 108-14.
111. James Cantlie, *Report the Conditions under which Leprosy Occurs in China, Indo-China, Malaya, the Archipelago and Oceania* (London: Macmillan, 1897): 57-65.
112. *History of the South China Mission of the American Presbyterian Church, 1845-1920* (Shanghai: The Presbyterian Mission Press, 1927), 121.
113. R. D. Thomas, *A Trip on the West River* (Canton, China: Baptist Publication Society, 1903): 5-6.
114. *History of the South China Mission of the American Presbyterian Church, 1845-1920*, 121-22.
115. Adolf Razag, *Leprosy in South China: Its Present Condition and Treatment with Special Suggestions* (Canton, 1907), 12.
116. James Cantlie, *Report the Conditions under which Leprosy Occurs in China, Indo-China, Malaya, the Archipelago and Oceania* (London: Macmillan, 1897), 57-65.
117. Adolf Razag, *Leprosy in South China: Its Present Condition and Treatment with Special Suggestions*, 27.
118. Wm. W. Cadbury, "New Methods in the Treatment of Leprosy," *China Medical Journal* 34, 5 (September 1920): 479-81.
119. *Yangchen wanbao* (Guangzho evening daily) June 25, 2008, B5.
120. John E. Kuhne, "The Leper Asylum at Tungkun," *China Medical Missionary Journal* 21, 1 (1907). See also G. Olpp, "The Rhenish Mission Hospital, Tungkun," *China Medical Journal* 23, 3 (1909).
121. James E. Lee, "China and Leprosy," *Chinese Recorder* 57 (May 1926): 856-61.
122. See http://www.csscipaper.com/chinahistory/xdsdt/50420.html.
123. The financial obligations of the Shilong Leprosarium, which had accommodation for 600 lepers, came under the Department of Health of the Canton municipal government, too. The Xiaotan Leprosarium, which had been subsidized since 1921 by the municipal Department of Health for some years, had a capacity of 300 lepers at that time. See "Work Report of the Department of Health of Guangzhou in 1926," *Shizheng gongbao*, 579, 244 (1926): 71-77.
124. "On Anti-Leper Campaign in Canton," *Mafeng jikan* (Leper Quarterly) 7(1933): 3.
125. "Proposal for Government Funding for Support of Leprosariums and Overseas Study of Lepers," *Mafeng jikan* (Leper Quarterly) 10 (1935): 1.
126. Frank Oldt, "Purity Campaign, Canton," *China Medial Journal* 37, 9 (September 1923): 776-82.
127. John Kirk, "Conference Address of Present of CMMA," ibid. 39, 3 (March, 1925): 227-40.
128. "Canton Hospital, Canton," *China Medical Journal* 9, 10 (October 1926), 954.

129. "Reports of C.M.M. A. Biennial Conference, 1925," *China Medial Journal* 39, 2 (February 1925): 151-68.
130. Cadbury and Jones, *Point of a Lancet*, 247, 260-61.
131. *Guangdong jiating weisheng cujinhui gongzou nianbao* (Annual report of the Association of Family Health Promotion of Guangdong) (1933), 4; *Guangdong jiating weisheng cujinhui gongzou nianbao* (Annual report of the Association of Family Health Promotion of Guangdong) (July 1934-June 1935), 17-28.
132. Zhu Qinglan. *Guangdong tongzhi Gao* (The first draft of Guangdong history), vol. 3 (Reprint, Beijing: Zhonghua quan guo tu shu guan wen xian suo wei fu zhi zhong xin, 2001): 1110-3.
133. "General Report of the Department of the Public Health of the Canton Hospital," *Guangzhou weisheng* 1 (October 1935): 155-57.
134. Xiong Yuezhi, *Xi xue dong jian yu wan qing she hui* (The dissemination of Western learning and late Qing society) (Shanghai: Shanghai renmin chubanshe, 1994), 490.
135. *Guangzhou shizhi: Weisheng zhi* (Annals of Guangzhou: Annals of health) (Guangzhou: Guangzhou yiyaozhi weiyuanhui, 1997).
136. Ch'ien Tuan-sheng, *The Government and Politics of China, 1921-1949* (Stanford: Stanford University Press, 1970), 67.
137. "Order of Guangdong Governor Li Yaohan," *Guangdong Gongbao* (Guangdong Bulletin), March 11, 1918.
138. Hu Xuanmin, *Construction of China's Public Health* (Shanghai: East Asia Library, 1928), 5.
139.

Prevention and Health Service	$159,315
Hospital Service	$172,321
Total Expenditure of Municipality	$2,880,000

   See Wong, *History of Chinese Medicine*, 493-94.
140. "Work Report of the Bureau of Public Health in July," *Guangzhou minguo ribao* (Guangzhou Republican Daily), August 17, 1927.
141. Detailed Ordinance of Enforcement of Pubic Health Police by the Bureau of Public Health of Canton, October 29, 1925, Group Number Temporary 2, File Number 2703, Guangzhou Municipal Archives, Guangzhou, China. See also "Announcement of Establishment of Public Health Police Squad," *Guangzhou minguo ribao*, October 30, 1925, 10.
142. Wu Liande, "Zhongguo Gonggong weisheng zhi jingfei wenti" (The expenditure issue of public health in China), *Zhonghua yixue zazhi* (Chinese Medical Journal) 15, 4 (1929): 351-54.
143. *Liangguang jinxinhui yiyuan sanshi zoulien tekan* (The special issue of the thirtieth anniversary of the Two Guang Baptist Hospital) (Guangzhou: Liangguang jinsinhui yiyuan, 1947), 4. See also *Guangzhou Weisheng* 1(October 1935): 83-92.
144. Li Ting'an, "A Public Health Report on Canton, Canton," *China Medical Journal* XI, 4 (August 1925): 324-75.
145. Ibid.
146. Li Zonghuang, *Mofan zhi Guangzhoushi* (The model city of Guangzhou) (Shanghai: Shanwu, 1929),136-37; *Guangzhou shizheng zhangcheng ligui*

huibian (Collection of regulations and rules of Guangzhou municipal government (Guangzhou Municipal Government, Guangzhou, 1924); and "Work Report of the Bureau of Public Health of Guangzhou in 1926," *Shizheng gongbao*, 579, 244 (1926): 71-77.

147. *Guangzhou shizheng gongbao* (Guangzhou government bulletin), Zizheng 2131, 41, Guangzhou Municipal Archive, Guangzhou, China; *Guangzhou shizheng zhangcheng ligui huibian* (A collection of regulations and rules of Guangzhou municipal government) (Guangzhou Municipal Government, Guangzhou, 1924); *Guangzhou shizheng gongbao* (Guangzhou government bulletin), Zizheng 571-69, 54, Guangzhou Municipal Archives, Guangzhou, China.

148. In 1935, Huang Yanpei was elected as member the Central Control Committee of the Chinese Nationalist Party, and became the interim chair of the Yunnan Province in the 1940s. See Huang Yanpei, *Yisui zhi Guangzhou* (One-year old of the city of Guangzhou) (Guangzhou: Shanwu, 1922), 60-61.

149. Appointed by Sun Yat-sen in January 1924 as the delegate to the National Congress of the Chinese Nationalist Party, Li was elected as an alternate member of the Central Executive of the Chinese Nationalist Party.

150. Li Zonghuang, *Xin Guangdong guancha ji* (Observation of new Guangdong)(Shanghai: Shanwu, 1922), 38-40.

151. *Neizheng nianjian* (Yearbook of internal administration) (Shanghai: Shangwu yinshuguan, 1935), (G)45-(G)47.

152. *Difang weisheng xingzheng chuqi shishi fangan* (Plan for the implementation of local health administration in the early stage) Nanjing: Weisheng bu, 1929.

153. *Guangzhou shizheng zhangcheng ligui huibian* (Collection of regulations and rules of Guangzhou municipal government (Guangzhou Municipal Government, 1924).

154. "Discovery of Bubonic Disease in Canton," *Guangzhou minguo ribao* (Guangzhou republican daily), May 12, 1924; "Quiet in Shopping Centers and Crowed in Clinics after Discovery of Bubonic Disease," ibid., May 16, 1924; Editorial, Ibid., May 19, 1924; and "One Case of Disease discovered by the Bureau of Public Health," ibid., July 21, 1924.

155. "Work Report of the Bureau of Public Health of Guangzhou in 1926," *Shizheng gongbao* 579, no. 244 (1926): 71-77.

156. Ibid.

157. "Easy Method to Prevent and Treat Cholera," *Yuehua bao*, July 14, 1932, 5; "Superstitious Activities during the Cholera Epidemic," ibid., June 25, 1932, 1.

158. "Public Health," *Guangzhou nianjian* (Guangzhou year book), vol. 13 (Guangzhou, 1935), 5-7.

159. "Recent Investigation of Cholera in this City," *Yuehua bao*, June 26, 1932, 5; "Medial Bolus Made and Contributed by Commander-in-Chief Chen," ibid., June 28, 1932, 6; *Guangzhou shizhi: Weishen zhi*, vol. 15 (Guangzhou: Guangzhou Local History Committee, 1997), 330; and *Guangdong shengzhi: Weishen zhi* (Guangzhou: Guangdong renmin chubanshe, 2003), 167.

160. *Guangzhou shizheng zhangcheng ligui huibian* (Collection of regulations and rules of Guangzhou municipal government) (Guangzhou Municipal

Government, 1924); *Shimin yaolan* (Essentials for citizens) (Guangzhou: The Bureau of Public Security of Guangdong Province, 1934); and Li Ting'an, "A Public Health Report on Canton," *National Medical Journal of China* 39, 4 (April 1925): 324-25.

161. Li Chunrong, "The Essential Issue of Meat Inspection," *Guangzhuo weisheng* 1 (October 1935), 25-29.

162. John Stoddard, *China*, (Chicago: Belford, Middlebrook & Company, 1897), 88.

163. Edward Bing-Shuey Lee, *Modern Canton* (Shanghai: The Mercury Press, 1936), 60-61.

164. *Neizheng nianjian* (Yearbook of internal administration) (Shanghai: Shangwu yinshuguan, 1935), (G)42-(G)45.

Conclusion

The medical missionary movement in the nineteenth and twentieth centuries played a role in the progress of modern Sino-Western relations. Canton was the first city in Qing China to come into contact with the outside world. The American medical missionary movement of 1835-1935 in south China was one of the important movements to influence the country. It had an impact not only on medical and hygiene modernization, but also on modern women's rights movements, and modern philanthropic campaigns in China generally and in Canton particularly.

Modernization and Social Reform

American medical missionaries went to China to advance Christianity by converting the Chinese. Believing that their task was to cure souls as well as heal bodies, their medical work directly served their evangelistic purpose. The focus of medical missionary work began to shift away from the individual toward social regeneration soon after American doctors started practicing medicine in China. They believed that their task in China was to create a Christian society. In addition to Christian converts, medical missionaries believed that the key to China's regeneration was spiritual salvation through Christianity. They tried to rejuvenate Chinese civilization along Christian principles without changing completely the foundations of Chinese society. They moved away from a determined focus on individual conversion to a broad program designed to meet the material, as well as spiritual, needs of the Chinese. They asserted that their humanitarian efforts to improve the welfare of the Cantonese through education and medication would be sufficient to revitalize Cantonese society. American doctors thus made efforts to improve the welfare of the Cantonese through introduction of medical, public health, educational, and charitable institutions. They contributed to the modern transformation of Canton, which had effects on China.

Medical Modernization

Americans who established Western medicine in Canton were the founders of medical missions in China. The establishment of Canton Hospital, an institution for the care of the sick and the first modern hospital in China, was the decisive step in the spread of medical missions. When the Canton Hospital opened its doors and operated productively, it gave impetus to the spread of missionary hospitals in China. American medical missionaries also initiated the dispensary movement to promote modern medical work in south China. They were the pioneers of the modern rural public health movement and continued playing a role in promoting rural medical programs in south China in the twentieth century.

American doctors in Canton played a role in promoting modern medical education in China. They instituted China's first modern medical college, trained China's first doctors of Western medicine, and first translated Western medical textbooks into Chinese. The establishment of the South China Medical School resulted in the creation of several medical schools in Canton, turning Canton into one of the modern medical education centers in China. The graduates of the medical schools in Canton contributed to the spread of Western medicine when practicing medicine throughout China. A form of hospitalization for patients, a delivery of medical care right to the patients' homes, a supply of curative services in hospitals and clinics, and a system of medical education began to appear in Canton where medical modernization was becoming more systematic and regular.

American doctors in Canton first introduced specific therapies connected with eye treatment and surgery, tumor surgery, lithotomies, and ether chloroform as well as modern medical management measures in China, taking the lead in the development of surgery and modern medical technology in China. American doctors brought in and advanced modern women's medicine in Canton as well. They introduced scientific knowledge about female anatomy and physiology and modern conceptions of women's bodies, instructed Chinese women in social hygiene, and changed their traditional medical ideas. American doctors and Chinese women doctors helped save many women's lives and healed many women and children with modern treatments, introduced modern delivery of babies, and improved conditions and the care of women's health and child welfare in China, particularly in Canton.

American medical missionaries in Canton founded the Medical Missionary Society, the first of its kind in the world, which played a part in the founding of a Chinese national medical association in China. They first published medical journals in China, which helped popularize Western medicine in China. Western medicine and surgery were gradually, but incontestably, moving forward between 1835 and 1935 in China generally, and in Canton particularly. American medical missionaries were some of the pioneers of the modern medicine in Canton and played a part in China's medical transformation.

Hygienic Modernization

Modern hygiene is part of Western medicine. American medical missionaries in Canton started and promoted modern hygienic work with their medical knowledge and experiences. American medical missionaries condemned the Cantonese's wicked unhealthy habits and Canton's unsanitary environment. They encouraged the Cantonese to develop hygienic customs and to improve unsanitary environments, opened the Department of Health at the Canton Hospital, conducted research on contagious diseases, introduced the concepts of civil sanitation and public health as measures to prevent diseases, popularized hygiene education in the cities and the countryside, adopted scientific measures (quarantine, sterilization, and others) to fight epidemic diseases, and provided treatment with preventive medicine to patients with contagious diseases. The Canton Hospital deserved the honor of hosting the first genuinely Chinese institute for cowpox manufacture, and founded China's first organized leprosy clinic to provide scientific treatment of lepers.

The formation of modern hospitals helped the Cantonese to witness Western approaches to hygiene and learn of modern preventive measures to some extent. Many Cantonese began to change their personal hygienic customs, an essential prerequisite for public sanitation. Inspired by Western medicine and preventive measures, and impressed by modern hospitals to some degree, the Cantonese reformers, elites, medical alumni, and foreign-trained physicians began to pay attention to the issue of hygiene. They advocated modern hygiene to improve Chinese health and urged the Chinese to adopt hygienic habits, create clean environments, and adopt a Western-style system of hygiene.

The enlightened Cantonese elite eventually moved to institute Western-style hygienic measures and a modern sanitary system. In 1901, Canton began to publish sanitary regulations, the first local government to enforce sanitary authority in China. In 1906, the Office of Health under the Department of Police of Guangdong was created in Canton, the earliest provincial public health administration in China. In 1920, China's first municipal administration of health was formed in Canton. Canton was the first city in China to separate dietetic hygiene from environmental sanitation. Canton started environmental sanitary work in the 1920s, a time of impressive investment by the Canton municipality in environmental quality in water supply, waste disposal, well-paved clean streets, ventilated and roomier dwellings, and other improvements, which not only helped establish a better, cleaner environment in Canton, but also helped control and reduce the spread of contagious diseases. Canton, one of the cleanest cities in China, served as a model to be emulated by other cities and became one of the cradles of the modern hygienic movement in late Qing dynasty and early Republic China.

Canton efficiently took scientific preventive measures to stop the spread of cholera in 1932, an imperative step and a major accomplishment in hygiene modernization. Canton continued subsequently to be the most enthusiastic place in the modern hygiene movement in the Republic of China. The Cantonese undertook institutional and social change, which medical and hygiene modernization required. Western medicine and American doctors helped transform Canton into a modern hygienic city, although the Cantonese played a crucial role in this transformation.

Modern Women's Rights Movement

American doctors challenged Confucianism's bias against women when removing obstacles to treatment of Chinese women in public places. From the beginning, the Canton Hospital provided treatment to Cantonese women, who became the first Chinese women attended by foreigners in China. American doctors' attention to women at their hospital defied the traditional practice that women could not been treated by male doctors outside the women's quarters and broke the social taboo on Chinese women. For the first time in Chinese history, Chinese women were able to receive foreign medical attention and treatments in public places.

American doctors equipped Chinese women with modern medicine to make their way in a still very male world. They gave their students useful tools, with which they could begin to break away from the old, subordinate role of women in China. American medical missionaries' determination and encouragement helped change many lower-class women's lives and elevate their social status when they practiced medicine after graduation from medical college. American doctors in Canton played a significant role in the feminization of doctors and nurses as a profession in Canton, and medical education allowed Chinese women to participate in modernization by joining the labor force, thus challenging traditional Chinese notions of female passivity and seclusion.

American doctors opened higher education for women, and Chinese women for the first time could go to colleges, an imperative education reform in China. Influenced by the South China Medical School and the Hackett College, the Canton Christian College became the first college in China to admit women students. The Cantonese bravely led in this remarkable direction and conducted the most progressive, coeducational experiments, marking the beginning of coeducation in colleges in China.

American doctors asserted the ideas of women's rights while teaching their students, although their attention remained focused steadfastly on the much more traditional task of arming women to serve the cause of established Christianity. Most female medical students certainly could not have graduated without at least absorbing, in some way, some of these ideas. The Cantonese women doctors, China's first women professionals, not only carried out medical and health work, but also played an important part in modern women's rights movement in China. Advocating women's rights to have political, economic, social, educational, and medical equality with men, Cantonese women doctors contributed to an awareness of women's rights among women and helped promote women's status. They opened new hospitals and dispensaries for women and children, started professional schools for women to learn skills to make a living, taught women the ideology of women's rights, and encouraged other women, like themselves, to play an active role in their communities and the societies. Cantonese women medical doctors not only fought for the elevation of the status of Chinese women, but also participated in the revolutionary movement to overthrow the Manchu regime during the 1911 Revolution movement. It was not surprising that Cantonese women were the first in China to participate in the provincial and local assemblies, and a Cantonese woman was the first in China to serve in the national government after the new Republic was founded.

The modern women's movement in China started with the reform movement in the 1890s. Western medicine in general, and women's medical education in particular, helped, to some degree, to turn Canton into one of the birthplaces of the modern women's movement in China, although many factors were responsible for this transformation.

Modern Philanthropic Movement

Modern missionary hospitals created in the nineteenth century served as medical centers as well as philanthropic and religious institutions in Europe and the United States. When American medical missionaries arrived in China, they founded the Canton Hospital and other dispensaries. The Canton Hospital, the first modern medical charitable institution in China, together with other missionaries' dispensaries and clinics in south China, provided free medical services to many poor Chinese because American medical missionaries believed that medicine and health should be for all, not just the privileged few.

When American medical missionaries in Canton espoused a philosophy, which increasingly defined their task as revitalizing Chinese society, their actions were extended to a humanitarian concern for improving the welfare of the Cantonese, expanding their focus from medical work to welfare work, such as the establishment of the girls' school, the school for the blind, the leper asylum, and the refuge for the mentally ill. The establishment of the Mingxin School for the Blind in 1889, the first one of such kind in south China, and the Kerr's Refuge for the Insane in 1899, the first mental hospital in China, extended American doctors' charitable service from the sick to the blind and to the mentally ill.

American doctors advocated Christian benevolence and encouraged the Chinese to found modern charitable institutions along Christian lines.

Influenced by American doctors' Christian charitable philosophy and impressed by the Canton Hospital to some extent, the enlightened Cantonese elites' social conscience was reinforced. They began to develop modern charitable thought and launched a modern philanthropic movement in Canton in the late nineteenth century. Charitable giving was becoming a new trend in Canton, and the Chinese donations became one of the important sources of finance of the Canton Hospital. Beginning in 1871, the modern charitable institution, Shantang, appeared in Canton. Those Chinese-style benevolent societies, not kin-clan oriented, administered by both professionals and merchants with modern management skills, provided free services to the poor and the needy on a year-round basis. Most of those societies performed medical functions of providing free treatments to the proor with Chinese medicine or Western medicine. Thus the Cantonese elite combined a traditional Chinese benevolent institution with Western hospitals to create a new form of charitable institution, incorporating the characteristics of both Chinese and Western benevolent institutions.

American doctors' new charitable institutions and Americans' medical and health charitable work in Canton in some way contributed to a new philanthropic movement in Canton at the beginning of the twentieth century. More and more Cantonese contributed funds to the philanthropic institutions, societies, and organizations. More Chinese hospitals and dispensaries increasingly provided more free medical and hygienic care to the poor and the needy. A new form of medical philanthropic institution appeared: the Fangbian Hospital became the largest medical charitable institute in south China.

American medical missionaries influenced not only the Cantonese elite, but also the Canton officials in the modern charitable movement. The Mingxin School for the Blind was so successful that the Cantonese government began to send blind children to the School with government financial support. Kerr's Refuge for Insane functioned so well that the Canton municipality began to send mental patients to the hospital with government payments and finally took it over. By that time, Cantonese officials had considered the charitable institutions as important in maintaining social order in society and realized that the government needed to be involved in charitable enterprises and build up a welfare system in Canton. Therefore, in the 1930s, medical and health charitable work in Canton was conducted by both government and private organizations.

American doctors' philanthropic ideology and activities were one of the forces that inspired the Cantonese to found this new form of philanthropic institution, although many forces motivated the Cantonese elite and officials to launch a modern charitable movement in Canton. Both American doctors and the Cantonese played a part in the modern charitable movement in Canton, which had effects on Chinese society at the beginning of the twentieth centuries when more mental hospitals and schools for the blind were founded in China.

Campaigns against Footbinding and Opium

Reform of traditional, wicked behaviors and practices was the first step toward modernization. Social reform was to abolish malevolent habits and dismantle the social construction that safeguarded the old routine. American medical missionaries in Canton were not a driving force of social change deliberately, but they wanted to remodel Chinese society along Christian concepts without transforming its basis. They thus participated in the campaigns to eliminate the malicious customs of the Chinese in an attempt to promote social change in China.

American doctors' efforts took the form of eradicating such evils as opium smoking and footbinding because opium weakened human health and footbinding hurt the human body. Acting as a moving force in the campaign to put an end to the binding of women's feet, American doctors were the first to condemn footbinding in Canton from the hygiene viewpoint so as to help improve Chinese women's health. They not only treated the women patients whose bound feet had created a severe threat to their health, but also persuaded the Cantonese to eliminate this social evil. Inspired by modern hygienic concepts and American doctors to some extent, the Cantonese progressive reformers were the first in China to launch the anti-footbinding movement in Canton, a campaign for women's freedom and a social reform against the traditional evil in Chinese society.

American doctors in Canton were also active in the crusade against opium smoking. They were not content to deal with the opium question merely by attempting to cure those addicts with Western medicine and scientific measures, but also made an effort to prevent the formation of the habit by removing the temptation and popularizing the consideration of opium as a sin. They strongly condemned the evils of opium from the perspective of health. Together with other medical missionaries, American medical doctors determinedly opposed opium and organized campaigns in China to call for the stop of opium traffic. Their efforts had an influence in the anti-opium campaign in China in general and in Canton in particular.

In summary, when transplanting medical institutions and introducing Western medicine into China, American medical missionaries played a role in Canton not only in medical and hygienic modernization, but also in modern women's rights, modern philanthropic campaigns, and social reforms. They were small in number, but their influence on Chinese society was disproportionate to their number. American medical missionaries were not agents of modernization and reform intentionally, but when pushing for a larger role for revitalizing Cantonese society, they brought significant changes, which was praiseworthy but not their purpose.

More importantly, the long-term impact of American models of medical work is still in place, and American medical missionaries' influence continues in China. The medical and charitable institutions established by American medical missionaries, such as the Canton Hospitals, Sun Yet-sen Medical University, the David Gregg Hospital, Kerr's Refuge for the Insane, the School for the Blind, and others, remain in Canton and south China. Their names have been changed, but these institutions are adopting both Western and Chinese measures to improve Chinese health, medical education, and welfare. They are the leading medical and charitable institutions in Canton or in China today.

Western Medicine and the Cantonese

Canton's prevailing humid climate with the intense heat, semitropical in nature, resulted in wide prevalence of dreaded epidemic diseases. The Cantonese were in need of efficient medications to combat frequent epidemics and were enthusiastic to adopt modern hygiene against the different kinds of epidemic diseases in Guangdong Province.

Western medicine came to Canton earlier than other cities in China. When it was introduced into Canton, many Cantonese came to missionary hospitals to seek medical advice to relieve their physical suffering. Western medicine and surgery were gradually becoming popular with the Cantonese because the supremacy of Western medicine over the old Chinese practice was amply demonstrated, and because Western medicine potentially contributed to improving the physical constitution of the people. Cantonese patients satisfied themselves of Western medicine's efficacy, and their skepticism of and antagonism to Western medicine slowly faded away. The successful treatments helped many Cantonese turn to Western medicine. Their desire for physical relief led them to appreciate the superiority of the knowledge and skills of American doctors. The Cantonese thus were the first Chinese in China to appreciate Western medicine and modern hygienic measures. Western medicine extended more widely than other Western learning in south China, being the most popular Western learning in Canton in the nineteenth century.

Western Medicine and the Cradle of Reform and Revolution

Western medicine had an impact on Cantonese society. First, the miracle of Western medicine, combining science with technology, changed many Cantonese attitudes toward Western culture because of its exceptionally effective medication: internal medicine helped cure the disease in the patients' bodies and surgery helped remove disease-stricken parts. From Western medicine, the Cantonese did see the efficiency of Western technology, such as the microscope, scalpel, and other equipment; the advantages of the Western system, such as modern hospital management, modern medical education; and so on. Thus, American medical colleges and hospitals were becoming agencies for overthrowing superstition, removing prejudice, and enlightening the minds of many Cantonese, who were so often the subjects of quacks and frauds. The charitable characteristics of Western hospitals and dispensaries also helped the Cantonese learn about the virtue of humanity, the core of Western culture. American medical missions had an impact on Cantonese common people because of their medical work rather than their missionary work, which had won them few converts, although Americans still tried to change the Chinese attitude toward Westerners through their hospitals so that they would be able to teach the Chinese Christianity. The Canton Hospital and other missionary hospitals and dispensaries in south China facilitated, to some degree, good relations between American medical missionaries and the Chinese in general and the patients in particular.

Second, Western medicine had an influence on the officials in Canton in the nineteenth century when their illnesses were successfully cured by American doctors at the Canton Hospital. Western medicine was one of the forces, if not the sole one, that encouraged the Qing officials in Canton to take a positive attitude towards the Canton Hospital. The officials first recognized and then protected it. They finally adopted more liberal policies towards other Western institutions in China, such as toleration of Christianity. Western medicine, to some extent, inspired high-ranking officials in Canton to take a different attitude towards Westerners in general and Americans in particular and, in part, helped make them become more tolerant and open-minded.

Third, Western medicine had an effect on Cantonese progressive reformers. Three renowned progressive Cantonese reformers, for example, Kang Youwei, Liang Qichao, Zheng Guanying, were in poor health and adopted Western medicine to regain their health. The common people and government officials identified the shortcomings of Chinese medicine and the competence and effectiveness of Western medication, but the Cantonese progressive reformers realized not just the advantages Western medicine offered over the native medicine in individual therapy, but also the importance of Western medicine to Chinese society and the nation at large. In the face of this "dying man" of the Chinese nation, the well-known Cantonese reformers advocated the slogan, "To Rescue China with Western Medicine." They voiced their views that Western medicine and *guojia yixue* (state medicine) were essential for the strength of the nation. They urged medical reform and improvement of Chinese medicine so as to strengthen the race and, through it, the nation. Therefore, reform of Chinese medicine constituted a part of their reform programs. The reform movement of 1898, which included reform of Chinese medicine, failed, but the Cantonese reformers' efforts were not in vain. Thereafter, the Qing government began to adopt new policies to protect and support missionary hospitals and to set up Western hospitals in China, and subsequently the new Republic of China formally legalized the performance of autopsies and dissections under the new Chinese laws.

More importantly, Western medicine was one of the forces to inspire the enlightened Cantonese reformers to cry for social and political reform. Cantonese reformers identified scientific ways and rational thinking in Western medicine. They encouraged the Chinese to apply Western medical principles to Chinese society: the law of suiting the remedy to the Chinese case. They urged the Chinese to learn the virtue of Western culture and to eliminate the evils of the Chinese traditional customs and cultures, especially those social diseases resulting in Chinese sickness. They asserted that the Chinese health problem was not only a medical or hygienic issue, but also a problem of poverty, ignorance, superstition, and many other social issues. They argued that modern medicine could cure disease, but could not cure social problems. As a result, they argued that reform was one of the most effective means for removing the sources of disease in China, and that without social reform or political reform, China's problems could not be solved. It was not surprising that Canton was the starting point of the political and social reform movement in late Qing China.

Finally, American doctors not only trained China's first physicians of Western medicine, but also generated modern China's earliest reformers and revolutionaries. American doctors criticized the backwardness of Chinese society, condemned the evil customs and manners of the Chinese, and advocated the transformation of China into a modern state under Christian influence. They came to China with not only medical arts, but also with Western values and culture. It is not clear how the Cantonese students received progressive ideas or adopted the new Western concepts from their American teachers, along with their training in Western medicine. It was clear, however, that the Canton Hospital and the Hackett College were missionary medical institutions where it was hard for the Qing government to ban progressive and radical ideas. Thus the missionary hospitals and colleges provided a new public sphere to the Cantonese. With this advantage, the medical students had the opportunity and freedom to discuss their ideas of reform and revolution. Their disappointment with China's current conditions and their new thoughts were nurtured at the missionary medical institutions where their experiences laid down the foundation of their reform and revolutionary thinking. While practicing medicine, the medical alumni gradually realized that Western medicine alone could not cure the ills of Chinese society, and that only social and political reform would rescue the Chinese nation. They thus became engaged in the reform and revolutionary movements with an agenda to modernize China's traditional society. Some of them, such as Sun Yat-sen, Kang Guangren, and Zheng Shiliang, took the lead in the reform and revolutionary movement.

In short, Western medicine became one of the many agencies, if not the sole one, for removing the Cantonese' prejudice, enlightening their minds, and changing their attitude toward Western culture. Western medicine turned into one of the many factors in the formation of the Cantonese reformers' reform ideology. Western medicine, to some extent, helped inspire the prominent Cantonese reformers to take the lead in the social and political reform movement to stimulate modern transformation of China. The Cantonese medical alumni and elite, like the progressive reformers, advocated social and political reforms because those reforms were more crucial than their medical practice for the good of the Chinese. Western medicine was one of the many forces that helped make Canton become the cradle of reform and revolution in modern China, although many other factors were responsible.

Western Medicine and Anti-Western Nationalism

Ironically, Western medicine was one of the sources of the rise of Chinese nationalism in Canton. At the beginning of the twentieth century, China was still under the oppression of imperialism. It was natural that Chinese intellectuals first developed Chinese nationalism and then tried to awaken national consciousness among the Chinese people. The Cantonese medical elite were concerned about educational sovereignty in general, and medical educational sovereignty in particular.

The Cantonese medical students' national consciousness was reinforced at the beginning of the twentieth century. They realized that Western medicine, an important tool in nation-building, was extraordinarily critical, not only to individual health, but also to the Chinese nation, and that if China's modern medical institutions were monopolized by foreigners, Chinese lives would be in the hands of other countries. The medical students and alumni also believed that Chinese-controlled modern medical education and services would be a victory in China's fight to master modern medicine, and in regaining sovereign rights lost in the unequal treaties of the nineteenth century. To express their awareness and concern about the destiny of the nation, they launched a campaign to regain modern medical education rights in Canton.

The Guanghua Medical School was a product of Chinese nationalism. Liang Peiji, John Kerr's student, and other elite Cantonese practitioners of Western medicine asserted that China had to control its own medical education institutions. Therefore, they established in 1908 China's first Chinese-style medical school run entirely by Chinese, where Chinese taught medicine in the Cantonese dialect.

The shift of administration of the private Gongyi Medical College to the Cantonese government was a good example in point of Chinese nationalism. Promoted by both the Nationalists and the Communists, the medical students in Canton launched an anti-imperialism and anti-religion campaign in the

1920s in order to develop Chinese-controlled modern medical education and services. The private Gongyi Medical College experienced this kind of agitation in 1925. The medical students strongly condemned the College for attempting to let American financiers and bankers control the medical college by securing Rockefeller Foundation donations during the financial crisis in Gongyi. They denounced cultural imperialism at Gongyi because American medical missionaries were teaching at and administering the college. They appealed to the government to take over Gongyi. Under the pressure of the Gongyi students, the Cantonese government finally took control of the college in 1929.

Hackett was another case in point. Hackett's alumnae participated in the anti-U.S. campaign in 1905 and its students took part in the anti-Britain movement in the 1920s. Hackett's students and faculty members advocated the restoration of medical rights to the Chinese in 1926. The rise of nationalism in Hackett was so powerful that the administrative authority of the Hackett College had to be transferred from missionaries to Chinese Christians in 1930.

For the purpose of nation-building, the Cantonese medical elite had taken over all medical educational institutions in Canton by 1935. Medical students and professionals in Canton helped promote Chinese nationalism. Many reasons explained the rise of strong anti-West nationalism among the Chinese medical elite at the beginning of the twentieth century, such as Western powers' China policies, the Communists' propaganda, and the Nationalists' mass mobilization strategy, but Western medicine was one of them.

Technological Transmitters in Modern Globalization

Modern globalization implies the breaking of social and technological barriers across the world toward the creation of a one-world network of increasing connection, interdependency, and homogeneity. The medical missionary movement in Canton was a campaign in globalizing modernity that altered Western countries as well as traditional China in the nineteenth and twentieth centuries.

In contrast to the American businessmen who came first before them, American medical missionaries to China were strong-minded enough to break through the cultural stumbling blocks and the various restrictions imposed by the Chinese government, which had segregated the Chinese from Westerners for a long time. From the start, American medical missionaries tried to use one of the most efficient tactics—the founding of hospitals and dispensaries—to promote Christianity in China. With such an approach, American medical missionaries, endowed with a means of social interaction with the Chinese, did break social barriers between the Chinese and American doctors. From the commencement of the work at the hospitals and dispensaries in Canton as well as in south China, American medical missionaries put emphasis on not only the healing of the body but also on the teaching of Christianity, and they worked as diligently for the latter as they did for the former.

The Chinese, however, were more interested in the missions' medical work than their religious work. Many Chinese had a high regard for Western hospitals, but only a few of them were converted to Christianity. For this reason as well others, medical missionaries realized that it was crucial to first heal the wounds of the bodies of the Chinese before treating "infections" of their spirit—medical work first and religious work second. The formation of the Medical Missionary Society in 1838 indicated that American medical missionaries had already adjusted themselves to Chinese society when implanting a Western institution into China. They had to put the medical work before the religious work because most Cantonese were more interested in Americans' medical arts and technology than their sermons at the hospital. Since then, the Canton Hospital, as well as other missionary hospitals in China in the following decades, became mainly a medical center rather than a religious center, although it was performing those two functions.

American medical missions were successful in breaking technological barriers, bringing the benefits of Western medical knowledge to the Chinese. To adjust themselves to Cantonese society, American doctors were interested in Sino-Western medical integration and were motivated to study Chinese medicine at the Canton Hospital. They also tried to adopt some Chinese remedial methods in the treatment of patients so as to make Western medicine more efficient. They translated medical textbooks into Chinese and used the Cantonese dialect in teaching, an important approach to remove the technological barriers and promote medical technology in China.

The Chinese responded to, other than acquiescing in, Americans' call for medical modernization during that time. American medical missionary movement in Canton was a process of the Cantonese to "localize" Western knowledge and technology. Western medicine was culturally reinterpreted as it moved from its original cultural location to Canton when the Cantonese tried to understand and to modify Western technology with Chinese tradition, although medical modernization in Canton was in large part the systematic assimilation of Western medical models and practices. The Cantonese doctors trained at the Canton Hospital combined both Chinese and Western medications together to produce a new form of medication to facilitate the introduction of Western medicine, effectively fulfilling the cultural and social needs of the Chinese people. The enlightened Cantonese elite and the physicians of Chinese medicine took Western preventive measures and medications to battle contagious diseases while continuing to use Chinese traditional ways and methods. The combination of Sino-Western preventive measures and medications was efficient and practical to some degree in the anti-epidemic campaigns. The Cantonese physicians of both

Chinese tradition and Western medicine reinterpreted, modified, and adopted, vaccination, which made it acceptable by many Cantonese officials and commoners. The Cantonese taught Western medicine in Cantonese at medical institutions, translated Western medical texts into Chinese, published medical and hygienic journals in Chinese, and established their own medical associations.

The involvement of Canton and the Cantonese in medical modernization of China was a process of interaction and integration between American doctors and the Chinese and was a complicated development of the Cantonese to combine Western technology with Chinese tradition. Western medicine became the first crucial step in modernization of Cantonese society, and American medical missionaries in Canton acted as the transmitters in China of the globalization of modern medical technology.

Glossary

Aiguo nüxuexiao	爱国女学校
Aiyu	爱育
Anya bao	安雅报
Bagu	八股
Baoguo hui	保国会
Baoguohui yanshuoci	保国会演说辞
Baosheng	保生
Baoyu shanhui	保育善会
Beihai	北海
Beiji yanfang	备急验方
Bidesheng yaofang	必得胜药房
bing	病
Bingli cuoyao	病理撮要
bo	播
Boji	博济
Bowen bao	博闻报
Buguozu hui	不裹足会
Cen Chunxuan	岑春宣
Chen Ruihua	陈瑞华
Chen Apeng	陈阿鹏
Chen Baitan	陈伯坛
Chen bao	晨报
Chen Dingtai	陈定泰
Chen Huipu	陈惠普
Chen Jiongming	陈炯明
Chen Jitang	陈济棠
Chen Lunhun	陈沦魂
Chen Mengnan	陈梦南
Chen Nianzu	陈念祖
Chen Shuren	陈树人
Chen Weiliang	陈伟良
Chen Xiangjing	陈相靜
Chen Xiqi	陈锡祺

Chen Yanfen 陈衍芬
Chen Yinci 陈引驰
Chen Zhen'ge 陈珍阁
Choban yiwu shimo 筹办夷务始末
Chongzhen 崇正
Chouji bian 筹济编
Chouyi yanjin yapian zhangcheng jie 筹议严禁鸦片章程折
Chu Qinglan 朱庆澜
zhuan 传
chuanran 传染
chubanshe 出版社
Cuiheng 翠亨
Daliang 大良
Daoguang chao 道光朝
Daoguang 道光
Daqing dezong (Guangxu) huangdi shilu 大清德宗（光绪）皇帝实录
Datong shu 大同书
datong 大同
dazhong 大众
Deng Yusheng 邓雨生
Dianshi 电视
Dianshizhai huabao 点石斋画报
Difang weisheng xingzheng chuqi 地方卫生行政初期实施方案
   shishi fang'an
Ding Wenjiang 丁文江
Diqiu renshi ji 地球人事记
Dongguan 东莞
Dongshan 东山
Dongwu bijiaoJiepou tu 动物比较解剖图
Dong xi yang kao mei yue tong ji zhuan 东西洋考每月统记传
Du xixue shu fa, 读西学书法
duizheng xiayao 对症下药
erke 儿科
Fan Zhongyan 范仲淹
Fangbian yuekan 方便月刊
Fangbian 方便
Fangcun (Fong Tsuen) 芳村
Feng Ziyou 冯自由
Foshan 佛山
Humen 虎门
Fuqiang shi yu weisheng lun 富强始于卫生论
Fushenggongbao lun chuangjian yiyuan shu 复盛宫保论创建医院书
Fumin 福民

Fuzhou	福州
Gao Xinrong	高欣荣
Gaoyao	高要
Geming yishi	革命逸史
Gezhi huibian	格致汇编
Gongyi nuxue	公益女学
Gu Songquan	顾松泉
Guagndong shi bao	广东时报
Guangzhou jinbainien jiaoyu shiliao	广州近百年教育史料
Guan Kaixi	关凯熙,
Guan Xianhe	关相和
Guang Yadu (Kwan Ato)	关亚杜
Guangan xiyaofang	广安西药房
Guangdong minzheng gongbao	广东民政公报
Guangdong sheng zhi: minzhengzhi	广东省志：民政志
Guangdong wenshi ziliao	广东文史资料
Guanghua biye Tongxuehui tekan	光华毕业同学会特刊
Guanghua weisheng bao	光华卫生报
Guanghua yishi hui tekan	光华医师会特刊
Guanghua yishi weisheng zazhi	光华医事卫生杂志
Guanghua	光华
Guangsan	广三
Guangzhou shizheng gongbao	广州市政公报
Guangzhou shizhi	广州市志
Guangzhou wenshi ziliao	广卅文史资料
Guangzhou zhinan	广卅指南
Guiping	桂平
guji	古籍
Guo Fenglu	郭风律
Guo Youcheng	郭友诚
Hainan	海南
Han Rixiu	韩日修
Hanlin	翰林
He Ronhui	何永辉
He Litian	何利田
He Qiwei	何其伟
He Zijing	何子敬
Hongzhong yiyao	宏中医药
Hu Xuanming	胡宣明
Hu Yisheng	胡毅生
Huabao	画报
Huadi	花地
Huamin	化民

Huang Entong	黄恩彤
Huang Kuan (Wong Fun)	黄宽
Huang Mei	黄梅
Huang Xuezhen	黄雪贞
Huangpu	黄埔
Huaxue chujie	化学初阶
Huaxue weisheng lun	化学卫生论
Huayang zangfutuxiang hezuan	华洋脏腑图象合纂
Huayang zangxiang yuezuan	华洋脏象约纂
Huiai	惠爱
Huiji (Wai-Tsai)	惠济
Huiming ju	惠民局
Huixing shanyuan	惠行善院
Huizhou	惠州
Humen	虎门
Huoluan yanfang	霍乱验方
Huxi shiyi yiyuan	沪西时疫医院
ji	急
ji	集
Jia Yuehan	嘉约翰
Jiang Yihua	姜义华
Jianhua yiji yuan	健华颐疾园
Jiechanzu hui	戒缠足会
Jiefang hua bao	解放画报
jiefang	解放
Jiepou shiti guize	解剖尸体规则
Jilong (Kee-lung)	基隆
Jin Baoshan	金宝善
Jindai zhongguo shiliao congkan	近代中国史料丛刊
Jindaishi ziliao	近代史资料
jingshenbing	精神病
Jingzhong ribao	警钟日报
Jinkui yaolue qianzhu	金匮要略浅注
Jinlifan	金利藩
jinshi	进士
Jiushi jieyao	救时揭要
juren	举人
Juzhu weisheng lun	居住卫生论
Kang Guangren	康广仁
Kang Nanhai zibian nianpu	康南海自编年谱
Kang Youwei	康有为
Kang Youwei quanji	康有为全集
Kang Youwei wenxuan	康有为文选

Kang Youwei zhenglun shangji	康有为证论：上集
Kesou wan	咳嗽丸
Kong Peiran	孔沛然
Jiangmen	江门
Kunwei	坤维
Guan Yadu	关亚杜
leshan	乐善
Li Bida	李必达
Li Duo	黎铎
Li Fengzhen	李风珍
Li Fulin	李福林
Li Hanzhang	李瀚章
Li Jiehong	黎解鸿
Li Jiliang	李济良
Li Shufen	李树芬
Li Ting'an	李廷安
Li Xisuo	李喜所
Li Yaohan	李耀汉
Li Zonghuang	李宗黄
Liang Ganchu	梁乾初
Liang Huanzhen	梁焕真
Liang Peiji	梁培基
Liang Qichao chuan	梁启超传
Liang Qichao dushu shengya	梁启超读书生涯
Liang Qichao nianpu changbian	梁启超年谱长编
Liang Qichao	梁启超
Liang Qichao jia shu	梁启超家书
Liang Shenyu	梁慎余
Liang Xiaochu	梁晓初
Liang Xiguang	梁钖光
Liang Yiwen	梁毅文
liangguang	两广
Liangguang Jinxinhui	两广浸信会
Liangrengong xiansheng nianpuchangbian	梁任公先生年谱长编
liangyue	两粤
Lianzhou (Lien Chow)	连州
Liu Jiwen	刘纪文
Liu Deye	刘德业
Liu Jucai	刘巨才
Liu Suzhi	刘叔治
Liu Weijun	刘维均
Liu Wu	刘务
Liu Xinci	刘心慈

Liu Zhenlin	刘桢麟
Liu Zhiqin	刘志琴
Liu Zihuai	刘子怀
Lixing quefa de qimeng	理性缺乏的启蒙
Lu Haodong	陆皓东
Lu Jinghui	卢镜辉
Lu Meiyi	吕美颐
Lu Xingyuan	卢兴原
Lun Neizi	论内痔
Luo Kaitai	罗开泰
Luo Xiuyun	罗秀云
Mafeng jikan	麻风季刊
miaoshou huichun	妙手回春
Mei Yalian	梅亚怜
Mei Yagui	梅亚桂
Minli bao	民立报
mingxin	明心
Minsheng ribao	民生日报
Nanshitou	南石头
Nanfu	南福
nannu shoushou buqin	男女授受不亲
Nantong	南通
Neizheng nianjian	内政年鉴
neizhi	内痔
Ni Xipeng	倪锡鹏
Nianjian	年鉴
Ningbo	宁波
Nongxue hui	农学会
nubei	奴婢
nujiao	女教
Nuzi hongshizi hui zhi kejing	女子红十字会之可敬
Nuzi shougong chuanxi suo	女子手工传习所
Nuzi xingxue baoxian hui	女子兴学保险会
pai	排
Pan Peiru	潘佩如
Pan Shicheng	潘仕成
Pan Yunhe	潘允和
Panyu	番禺
Peng Lianxi	彭莲喜
Peng Hui	彭回
pian	篇
Puyu tang	普育堂
Qi Dadeng	齐大登

Qi Shihe	齐思和
Qiangxue hui	强学会
Qigongbao shuzeng	耆宫保书赠
Qingdao	青岛
qingjin funu chanzu	请禁妇女缠足
Qingyi bao	清议报
Qishier hang shang bao	七十二行商报
Qiying	耆英
Qizheng lueshu	奇症略述
Quanxue pian	劝学篇
Quanyue she hui shi lu	全粤社会实录
Quanyue shehui shi lu chu bian	全粤社会实录初编
Renji	仁济
renlei gongli	人类公理
Renmin zhou kan	人民周刊
Renti zuzhi lanyao	人体组织揽要
Riben shumu zhi	日本书目志
Rouji	柔济
Sanlian	三联
Sanshui	三水
Shamian	沙面
shanju	善举
Shantou	汕头
shangwu	商务
Shaoguan	韶关
Shen Yunlong	沈云龙
Shen bao	申报
Sheng Xuanhuai	盛宣怀
sheng	省
Shengshi weiyan	盛世危言
Shengyu guangxun	圣谕广训
shengyuan	生员
Shi Jianru	史坚如
Shi Meiqing	施梅卿
Shi Meixing	施梅兴
Shiban buchanzu hui jianming zhangcheng	试办不缠足会简明章程
shifan	师范
Shili gongfa quanshu	实理公法全书
Shilong	石龙
Shiwu bao	时务报
Shaotan	稍潭
Shiyi ju	施医局
Shizheng zhangcheng ligui huibian	市政章程例规汇编

shizhi	市志
Shunde	顺德
Shuyi liuxingshi	鼠疫流行史
Sipailou	四牌楼
Su Daoming	苏道明
Suishi xunfeng	穗石熏风
Sun Ke	孙科
Sun Yixian boshi yixueyuan yilan	孙逸仙博士医学院一览
Sun Zhongshan nianpu changbian	孙中山年谱长编
Sun Zhongshan quanji	孙中山全集
Sun Zhongshan xuanji	孙中山选集
suo	所
Taian	泰安
Taichan juyao	胎产举要
taixi	泰西
Tan Yunchang	谭元昌
Tan Zhushan	谭竹山
Tang Zhijun	汤志钧
Tang Shiyi	唐拾义
Tang Shiyi yaochang jianshi	唐拾义药厂简史
Tao Shanming	陶善敏
Tianjin	天津
Tianzu hui	天足会
Tiecheng	铁成
Difu	堤富
Tongde dajie	同德大街
Tongmeng hui	同盟会
tongren	同仁
Tongwen guan	同文馆
Wang Dexin	王德馨
Wang Jingwei	汪精卫
Wang Kangnian	汪康年
Wang Kangnian shiyyou shuzha	汪康年师友书札
Wang Kentang	王肯堂
Wang Qingren	王清任
Wang Xincai	王心裁
Wang Yiliang	王怡良
Wanguo gongbao	万国公报
Wangxia	望厦
Wanmu caotang	万木草堂
Weisheng baihua bao	卫生白话报
Weisheng yaozhi	卫生要旨
Wen Tianmou	温天谋

wenji	文集
wenlian	文联
wenyi	文艺
Wu Shaorong	伍绍荣
Wu Tingfang	伍庭芳
Wuchang	武昌
Wuzhou	梧州
wuxu bianfa	戊戌变法
Xi'nan	西南
Xia Dongyuan	夏东元
Xia Qiaoyun	夏巧云
Xia Xiaohong	夏晓红
Xiagu zhonghun: Zheng Shiliang chuan	侠骨忠魂—郑士良传
Xiamen	厦门
Xian Weisun	冼维逊
xiangbao	香包
Xiaochuan wan	哮喘丸
xiaodu	消毒
Xiaolan	小榄
Xie Aiqiong	谢爱琼
Xie Zhantai	谢缵泰
Xinan	西南
Xinbao	新报
Xindoulan	新豆栏
Xinhai geming jianshinianjianshi lun xuanji	辛亥革命前十年间时论选集
Xinhui	新会
Xinmin congbao	新民丛报
Xinxue yuebao	新学月报
Xinyi yiyuan	信义医院
Xixue	思雪
Xixue shumu biao	西学书目表
Xiyi xinbao	西医新报
xiyi	西医
Xu Gangliang	许刚良
Xu Ganlai	徐甘来
Xu Guangjin	徐广缙
Xu Qin	徐勤
xuan	选
Xushi zuzhi (Xin lun)	须氏组织(新论)
Yadong cong bao	亚东丛报
Yanbu	盐步
Yangcheng quanchu yapian gonghui guitiao	羊城劝除鸦片公会规条

Yangcheng wanbao	羊城晚报
Yangcheng boji yiju	羊城博济医局
Yangjiang (Yeung Kong)	阳江
Ye Chendeng	叶臣登
Ye Fangpu	叶芳圃
Ye Peichu	叶培初
yidao	医道
Yigang zongshu	医纲总枢
yijiu ninwu nian fanmei aiguo yundong	一九〇五年反美爱国运动
Yili lueshu	医理略术
Yilin gaicuo	医林改错
Yin Duanmo	尹端模
Yinbingshi heji	饮冰室合集
Yishizhiguangzhou	一岁之广州
Yitan Chuanzhen	医谈传真
Yixue bao	医学报
Yixue shanhui	医学善会
Yixue shanhui xu	医学善会序
Yixue weisheng bao	医学卫生报
Yixuepian	医学篇
Yiyan	易言
You Yutang	尤裕堂
Youtong weisheng lun	幼童卫生论
Yu Meide	于美德
yuandong	远东
Yuehua	越华
Yuezhong buchanzu hui	粤中不缠足会
Yushan	禺山
Yuxian nuxue	育贤女学
Yuying yuan	育婴院
Zanyu xueshe	赞育学社
Zanyu yuekan	赞育月刊
Zhang He	张贺
Zhang Shusheng	张树声
Zhang Xinji	张新基
Zhang Jian	张謇
Zhang Yunwen	张允文
Zhang Zhidong	张之洞
Zhang Zhujun	张竹君
zhanshi difang	战时地方
Zhaoqing	肇庆
Zheng Guanying	郑观应
Zheng Guanying zhuan	郑观应传

Zheng Hao	郑豪
Zheng Shiliang	郑士良
Zheng Yuxiu	郑毓秀
Zheng Zaoru	郑藻如
Zhengguang guangrong jianshi	真光光荣简史
Zhengguang	真光
Zhengsha	增沙
Zhixin bao	知新报
Zhong Rongguang	鍾荣光
Zhongdou yaojue	种痘要诀
Zhongguo funü yundong	中国妇女运动
Zhongguo jindai funü yundong shi	中国近代妇女运动史
Zhongguo jindai shi ziliao	中国近代史资料
Zhongguo jindai xueji shiliao	中国近代学制史料
Zhongguo nüzi yaojiu canzheng de xianshen	中国女子要求参政的先声
Zhongguo nüzi yixue jiaoyu	中国女子医学教育
Zhongguo xinnüjie	中国新女界
Zhonghua shuju	中华书局
Zhonghua yixue zazhi	中华医学杂志
Zhongshan	中山
Zhongwai weisheng yaozhi	中外卫生要旨
Zhongxi Dayaofang	中西大药房
Zhou Guangmin	周贯民
Zhou Huomin	周活民
Zhou Jingting	周镜廷
Zhou Shuanglan	周双兰
Zhu Qinglan (Chue Hing Lan)	朱庆澜
Zhu Zhixin	朱执信
zilaishui	自来水

Bibliography

Archival Collections

Guangdong Provincial Archives, Guangzhou, China. Mingxin School Archives, Folder 430, Catalogue 1, Record Group 92.

____. Mary Niles Papers, Folder 4, Record Group 92.

____. Letters of South China Mission (Presbyterian Church in the United States), Folder 4, Record Group 92.

____. Records of the Board of Trustee of the Ming Sum School, Folder 1, Record Group 17.

____. Hackett Medical College Documents, Folder 42, Record Group 65.

____. Material Relating to the Hospital for the Instance, Folder 73, Record Group 65.

____. Materials Relating to Weiai Hospital, 1926-1927, Folder 33, Record Group 65.

Guangzhou Municipal Archives, Guangzhou, China. Records of the Board of Trustee of the Ming Sum School for Blind, 1918-1945, Folder 1.

____. Department of Health Documents, Folder 2703, Group Number Temporary 2.

____. A Brief History of the Hackett Women College, November 29, 1934, Folder 43, Group Number 18.

____. History of Fangbian Hospital, 1934, Folder 8, Record Group 18.

____. The Plan to Clean Every Big City in Guangdong Province, 1913, Folder 503, Record Group 7.

____. The Work Reports of the Department of Health of Guangzhou, 1921-1926.

____. *Guangzhou shizheng gongbao* (Guangzhou government bulletin), 1921-1935.

Hong Kong Baptist University Library, Hong Kong. Presbyterian Church Board of Foreign Missions, Missions Correspondence and Reports (1833-1911).

Presbyterian Historical Society, Philadelphia, Pennsylvania. Presbyterian Church in the U.S.A. Board of Foreign Missions. Secretaries Files: China Missions, 1891-1955, Record Group 82. Canton Christian College—Correspondence and Reports, 1906-1917, Folder 5, Box 1.

____. South China Mission—Canton, True Light Seminary Correspondence, 1906-17, Folder 5, Box 1.

____. Canton—Correspondence re Medical situation, 1909-1925, Folder 18, Box 1.

____. Canton—Ming Sum School, 1909-1947, Folder 19, Box 1.

____. Canton—True Light Seminary-Correspondence, 1912-22, Folder 9, Box 4.

____. Canton—Hackett Medical College, 1912-1946, Folder 4, Box 5.

____. Canton—Hackett Medical College, 1925-1930, Folder 21, Box 28.

____. Canton Hospital, 1916-1923, Folder 22, Box 11.

____. Canton Hospital, 1924-1942, Folder 8, Box 27.

____. Kwangtung—Yeuang Kong—Correspondence and Report, 1912-1920, Folder 7, Box 5.

____. Karcher, Mrs. J. F. "Dear Friends" letter, Canton, November 18-December 22, 1936, Folder 17, Box 53.

Presbyterian Historical Society, Philadelphia, Pennsylvania. Presbyterian Church in the U.S.A. Board of Foreign Missions-China Mission Secretaries' Files, 1893-1957, Record Group 129. Notes on A Historical, Sketch of the American Presbyterian Mission Hainan China, 1899.

United States. Department of State. Dispatches from Consuls at Canton, 1790-1906. (Microfilm.)

____. Records of the United States Department of State Relating to the Internal Affairs of China, 1910-1929.

Yale Divinity School Library, Yale University. United Board for Christian Higher Education in Asia, Record Group 11: Lingnan University (Canton Christian College).

____. The Trustees of Lingnan University, Record Group 14.

Books and Periodicals

A Brief Sketch of the History of Kung Yee. Hong Kong: Victoria Printing Press, 1925.

"A Form of Prayer to the God of Heaven with Preface, by Qiying, Governor of the Two Kwang Provinces." Translated by Sixensis. The North China Herald, April 12, 1851, 146.

A Guide to the City and Suburbs of Canton. Kelly & Walshi, 1904.

A Report of the Mission Hospital in the Western Suburbs of Canton under the Care of Dr. Hobson, 1853-1854. Canton, 1855.

"A Short History of the Private Guanghua Medical College." Guangzhou wenshi ziliao 26 (1982): 139-154.

"Abstract from Chinese Report of the Kwangtung Kung Yee Medical College and Hospital, 1914-1915." China Medical Missionary Journal 30, 6 (1916).

"Absurd Chinese Notions: Remarkable Ignorance of Medicine and Surgery in China." The New York Times, April 2, 1890.

Alexander, Mary. Seedtime and Harvest in the South China Mission of the Southern Baptist Convention, 1845-1933. Richmond, Virginia: Foreign Mission Board Southern Baptist Convention, 1934.

Allyn, Harriet M. "The Hackett Medical College: The Healing of His Seamless Dress by Chinese Beds of Pain." The Presbyterian Magazine (April, 1922): 218.

____. "Is a Woman's Medical College Worth While in China?" Post Jubilee News 5 January 1921.

Anderson, Mary. A Cycle in the Celestial Kingdom. Mobile, Alabama: Press of Heiter-Starke, 1943.

Anderson, Rufus. *History of the Missions of the American Board of Commissioners for Foreign Missions to the Oriental Churches.* 2 vols. Boston, 1872.

Anderson, Warwick. "Introduction: Postcolonial Technoscience." *Social Studies of Science* 32, 5 (2002): 648-50.

"Announcement of Establishment of Public Health Police Squad." *Guangzhou minguo ribao,* October 30, 1925, 10.

"Annual Meeting of the Canton Medical Missionary Society." *Canton Gazette,* January 23, 1924.

Annual Report of the David Gregg Hospital for Women and Children, Hackett Medical College for Women, Turner Training School for Nurses, Yau Tsai School of Pharmacy. Canton: Shameen Printing Press, 1931.

Annual Report of the Presbyterian Board of Foreign Missions. New York: The Board of Foreign Missions, Presbyterian Church in the U.S.A., 1854.

Annual Report of the Presbyterian Board of Foreign Missions. New York: The Board of Foreign Missions, Presbyterian Church in the U.S.A., 1884.

Annual Report of the Presbyterian Board of Foreign Missions. New York: The Board of Foreign Missions, Presbyterian Church in the U.S.A., 1889.

Annual Report of the Presbyterian Board of Foreign Missions. New York: The Board of Foreign Missions, Presbyterian Church in the U.S.A., 1890.

Annual Report of the Presbyterian Board of Foreign Missions. New York: The Board of Foreign Missions, Presbyterian Church in the U.S.A., 1891.

Annual Report of the Presbyterian Board of Foreign Missions. New York: The Board of Foreign Missions, Presbyterian Church in the U.S.A., 1894.

Annual Report of the Presbyterian Board of Foreign Missions. New York: The Board of Foreign Missions, Presbyterian Church in the U.S.A., 1895.

Annual Report of the Presbyterian Board of Foreign Missions. New York: The Board of Foreign Missions, Presbyterian Church in the U.S.A., 1902.

Annual Report of the Presbyterian Board of Foreign Missions. New York: The Board of Foreign Missions, Presbyterian Church in the U.S.A., 1903.

Annual Report of the Presbyterian Board of Foreign Missions. New York: The Board of Foreign Missions, Presbyterian Church in the U.S.A., 1904.

Annual Report of the Presbyterian Board of Foreign Missions. New York: The Board of Foreign Missions, Presbyterian Church in the U.S.A., 1905.

Annual Report of the Presbyterian Board of Foreign Missions. New York: The Board of Foreign Missions, Presbyterian Church in the U.S.A., 1909.

Apter, D. M. *The Politics of Modernization.* Chicago: University of Chicago, 1965.

Arnold, David. *Colonizing the Body: State Medicine and Epidemic Disease in 19th-Century India.* Berkeley: University of California Press, 1993.

Ayers, William. *Chang Chih-tung and Educational Reform in China.* Cambridge, MA: Harvard University Press, 1971.

Ballantyne, Lereine. *Dr. Jessie MacBean and the Work at Hackett Medical College, Canton, China.* Toronto, Canada: Women's Missionary Society of the Presbyterian Church in Canada, 1934.

Balme, Harold. *China and Modern Medicine: A study in Medical Missionary Development.* London: London Missionary Society, 1921.

"Bandits Wanted." *Shen bao* (Shanghai daily), July 9, 1894.

Barnet, Suzanne Wilson, and John King Fairbank, eds. *Christianity in China: Early Protestant Missionary Writings.* Cambridge, MA, 1985.

Bays, Daniel H. *China Enters the Twentieth Century: Chang Chih-tung and the Issues of a New Age, 1895-1909*. Ann Arbor: University of Michigan Press, 1978.

Bays, Daniel H. ed. *Christianity in China: From the Eighteen Century to the Present*. Stanford, CA, 1996.

Beahan, Charlotte L. "In the Public Eye: Women in Early Twentieth Century China." In *Women in China: Current Directions in Historical Scholarship*, ed. Richard W. Guisso and Stanley Johannesen. New York: Philo Press, 1981.

Benedict, Carol. *Bubonic Plague in Nineteenth-Century China*. Stanford: Stanford University Press, 1996.

Bergere, Marie-Claire. *Sun Yat-sen*. Stanford, California: Stanford University Press, 1994.

Bermann, Gregorio. "Mental Health in China." In *Psychiatry in the Communist World*, ed. A. Kiev. New York: Science House, 1968.

"Biography of Miss Zhang Zhujun." *Dagong bao* (Unselfishness daily), October 19, 1902.

"Biography of Miss Zhang Zhujun, Part 2." *Dagong bao* (Unselfishness daily), October 21, 1902.

Bliss, Edward Jr. *Beyond the Stone Arches: An American Missionary Doctor in China, 1892-1932*. New York: John Wiley, 2001.

"Book Review: Manual of Nursing." *China Medical Missionary Journal* XX, 2 (March 1906), 86.

Boone, Henry William. "Medical Mission Work at Shanghai." *China Medical Missionary Journal* XV (1901), 24-5.

Bowers, John Z., and Elizabeth F. Purcell. eds. *Medicine and Society in China*. New York: Josiah Macy, Jr., Foundation, 1974.

Bowers, John. *Science and Medicine in Twentieth-Century China*. Ann Arbor: The University of Michigan Press, 1988.

Braibanti, R., and J. Spengler. *Tradition, Values, and Socio-economic Development*. Durham, NC: Duke University Press, 1961.

Brand, Jeanne. *Doctors and the State*. Baltimore, Md.: John Hopkins University Press, 1965.

Bridgman, E. C. "Canton Dispensary." *Chinese Repository* 2 (October 1833), 276.

Bridgman, Eliza, and J. Gillett, ed. *The Pioneer of American Missions in China: The Life and Labors of Elijah Coleman Bridgman*. New York: Anson D. F. Randolph, 1864.

Brown, G. Thompson. *Earthen Vessels and Transcendent Power: American Presbyterians in China, 1837-1952*. Maryknoll, N.Y.: Orbis Books, 1997.

Broyelle, Claudie. *Women's liberation in China*. Atlantic Highlands, NJ: Humanities Press International, Incorporated, 1977.

Buck, Peter. *American Science and Modern China*. Cambridge: Cambridge University Press, 1980.

Bulletin of the David Gregg Hospital for Women and Children, Hackett Medical College for Women, Julia Turner School of Nursing. Canton, 1929.

Burton, Margaret. *Notable Women of Modern China*. New York, 1912.

Cadbury, W. W. *At the Point of a Lancet: One Hundred Years of the Canton Hospital, 1835-1935*. Shanghai: Kelly & Walsh, 1935.

____. *Lingnam Hospital for the Care of College Workmen and Neighboring Villages.* Canton: Knipp Memorial Press, 1925.

Cadbury, William Warder. "Mission Hospital and Medical Educational Work in Canton." *China Medical Journal* (October 1933): 1-2.

Cadbury, Wm. W. "New Methods in the Treatment of Leprosy." *China Medical Journal* (1920): 479-81.

Cadbury, William Warder. "The 1918 Pandemic of Influenza in Canton." *China Medical Journal* 34, 1 (January 1920): 1-17.

Callery, J. M. and Melchior Yvan. *History of the Insurrections in China with Notices of the Christianity, Creed, and Proclamations of the Insurgents.* New York: Harper and Brothers, 1853.

Cantlie, James. *Report the Conditions under which Leprosy Occurs in China, Indo-China, Malaya, the Archipelago and Oceania.* London: Macmillan, 1897.

Cantlie, James, and Jones, C. Sheridan, *Sun Yat-sen and the Awakening of China.* London: Jarrold and Sons, 1912.

"Canton Christians Opposing British Gunboat Policy." *Renmin zhou kan* (People's weekly) 25 (1926).

Canton Hospital. *Annual Report of the Canton Hospital for the Year 1914.* Canton: Too Leung Printing Press, 1915.

____. *Annual Report of the Canton Hospital for the Year 1916.* Canton: Too Leung Printing Press, 1917.

____. *Annual Report of the Canton Hospital for the Year 1917.* Canton: Too Leung Printing Press, 1918.

____. *Annual Report of the Canton Hospital for the Year 1918.* Canton: Too Leung Printing Press, 1919.

____. *Annual Report of the Canton Hospital for the Year 1920.* Canton: Too Leung Printing Press, 1921.

____. *Annual Report of the Canton Hospital for the Year 1922.* Canton: Too Leung Printing Press, 1923.

____. *Annual Report for the 99th Year of the Sun Yat-sen Memorial of the Canton Hospital.* Canton: Too Leung Printing Press, 1934.

____. *Annual Report for the 104th year of Canton Hospital, 1938-1939.* Canton: the Canton Hospital, 1939.

____. *Annual Report for the 106th year of Canton Hospital, 1940-1941.* Canton: Canton Hospital, 1941.

"Canton Hospital." *The Canton Gazette*, October 8, 1924, 6.

"Canton Hospital, Canton." *The China Medical Journal* 9 (1926): 954.

"Canton Hospital: Celebration of the Eightieth Anniversary." *The Hong Kong Daily Press*, December 21, 1916.

"Canton Hospital: Its Work in 1919." *South China Morning Post*, July 31, 1920, 8.

"Cantonese News," *Shen bao* (Shanghai daily), June 1, 1901.

Cao Zengyou. *Jidu jiao yu ming qing ji zhongguo she hui: zhong xi wen hua de tiao shi yu chong zhuang* (The Protestant movement in China between the Ming and Qing dynasties: the Sino-Western Cultural exchanges). Beijing: Zuojia chubanshe, 2006.

"Case of Tumors, and other Morbid Growths." *Chinese Repository* 19 (1850): 271-72.

Ch'ien Tuan-sheng. *The Government and Politics of China, 1921-1949.* Stanford: Stanford University Press, 1970.

Chan, Ming K. "A Turning Point in the Modern Chinese Revolution: The Historical Significance of the Canton Decade, 1917-27." In *Remapping China: Fissures in Historical Terrain,* eds. Gail Hershatter, Emily Honig, and others. Stanford: Stanford University Press, 1996.

Chang Hao. *Liang Ch'i-ch'ao and Intellectual Transition in China, 1898-1907.* Cambridge, MA: Harvard University Press, 1971.

Chang Hsin-pao. *Commissioner Lin and the Opium War.* Cambridge, Massachusetts: Harvard University Press, 1964.

Chang Po-chen. *Nanhai Kang xiansheng Zhuan* (Biography of Mr. Kang of Nanhai). Beijing, 1932.

Chao, Virginia Chui. "The Anti-Footbinding Movement in China (1850-1912)." M.A. Thesis, Columbia University, 1966.

"Charity Donations." *Guangzhou minguo ribao* (Guangzhou republic daily), May 13, 1928, 2.

Chen bao (Morning daily) (Beijing).

Chen, Janet Yi-chun. "Guilty of indigence: the Urban Poor in China, 1900-1949." Ph.D. Dissertation, Yale University, 2005.

Chen Weiliang, ed. *Liang Qichao wenji* (Liang Qichao's works). Beijing: Yanshan chubanshe, 1997.

Chen Xiqi, ed. *Sun Zhongshan nianpu changbian* (A chronicle record of Sun Yat-sen's life) Beijing: Zhonghua shuju, 1991.

Chestnut, Eleanor. "Medical Work in Lien-Chow, Kwangtung." *China Medical Missionary Journal* 14, no. 2 (1900): 123.

Cheung Yuet-wah. *Missionary Medicine in China: A study of Two Canadian Protestant Missions in China before 1937.* Lanham, Md.: University Press of America, 1988.

Ch'ien Tuan-sheng. *The Government and Politics of China, 1921-1949.* Stanford: Stanford University Press, 1970.

China Medical Missionary Journal. vols. 1-50, 1887-1936. Published vol. 21 – vol. 45 as *China Medical Journal* and vol. 46-50 as *Chinese Medical Journal.* Beijing, Shanghai, etc.

China Review. Hong Kong, 1877-1900.

China Year Book, 1935, 1936. Tianjin and Shanghai: Tianjin Press, 1936.

China Year Book, 1913. London: H. T. Montague Bell & H. B. W. Woodhead, 1913.

Chinese Recorder, vols. 1-20, 1868-1887. Fuzhou, 1868-1872; Shanghai, 1874-1887.

Chinese Repository. vols. 1-2. Ed. E. C. Bridgman and S. Wells Williams. Macao and Canton, monthly, 1832-1851.

Chinese Year Book, 1929-1930.

Choa, G. H. *"Heal the Sick" was Their Motto: The Protestant Medical Missionaries in China.* Hong Kong: Chinese University Press, 1990.

Chow, Rey. *Woman and Chinese Modernity: The Politics of Reading between West and East.* Theory and History of Literature, vol. 75. Minneapolis, MN: University of Minnesota Press, 1991.

Christian Observer (Philadelphia), 1839-1852.

Chu Hsi-ju, and Daniel G. Lai. "Distribution of Modern-Trained Physicians in China." *Chinese Medical Journal* 49 (1935): 544-46.

Cohen, Warren. *American Response to China: A History of Sino-American Relations.* New York: Columbia University Press, 1989.

"Cold Milk Banned at Ice Cream Houses." *Guangzhou minguo ribao* (Guangzhou Republican daily), September 25, 1927.

Colledge, Thomas R. *The Medical Missionary Society in China.* Philadelphia, 1838.

Corbett, Charles Hodge. *Lingnan University.* New York: The Trustees of Lingnan University, 1963.

Couling, Samuel. *Encyclopedia Sinica.* Shanghai, 1917.

Craftree, Loren W. "Andrew P. Happer and Presbyterian Mission in China, 1844-1891." *Journal of Presbyterian History,* vol. 62, no. 1.

Croizier, Ralph. *Traditional Medicine in Modern China: Science, Nationalism, and the Tensions of Cultural Changes.* Cambridge: Harvard University Press, 1968.

Curtin, Philip D. *Disease and Empire: the Health of European Troops in the Conquest of Africa.* New York: Cambridge University Press, 1998.

Dagong bao (Unselfishness daily), 1901-1910.

Danton, George H. *The Culture Contacts of the United States and China, 1784-1844.* New York, 1931.

Daqing dezong (Guangxu) huangdi shilu (The record of Emperor Guangxu of Great Qing) vol. 6. Taipei: Huawen shuju, 1960.

Deng Chanxian. "General Report of the Second Municipal Hospital for Insane," *Guangzhuo weisheng* (Guangzhou health) 1 (October 1935): 107-10.

Deng Yusheng. *Quanyue shehui shilu* (A record of the Guangdong society). Guangzhou: Guangdong xuewu gongsuo, 1910.

Diamant, Neil. "China's Great Confinement? Missionaries, Municipal Elites and Police in the Establishment of Chinese Mental Hospitals." *Republican China* 19 (1) 3-50.

Dianshizhai huabao (Dianshi studio illustrated news) Guangzhou: Guangdong renmin chubanshe, 1983.

Dictionary of American Biography. New York, 1928-1936.

Difang weisheng xingzheng chuqi shishi fangan (A plan for the implementation of local health administration in the early stage). Nanjing: Weishengbu, 1929.

"Different Aspects of the Epidemic." *Yuehua bao* (Yuehua daily), July 15, 1932, 1.

Dikötter, Frank. *The Discourse of Race in Modern China.* Stanford, Calif.: Stanford University Press, 1992.

Ding Wenjiang. *Liangrengong xiansheng nianpuchangbian chugao* (First draft of a chronological biography of Liang Qichao). Taipei: Shijie, 1959.

Ding Wenjiang. *Liang Qichao nianpu changbian* (Chronicled biography of Liang Qichao) Shanghai: Shanghai renmin chubanshe, 1983.

"Discovery of Bubonic Disease in Canton." *Guangzhou minguo ribao* (Guangzhou Republican Daily), May 12, 1924.

"Disturbance of Employment of Women Telephone Operators." *Guangzhou minguo ribao* (Guangzhou Republican daily), May 11, 1924.

"Diyici guonei geming zhangzheng shiqi de Guangdong funu yundong" (The women's movement in Guangdong during the first revolutionary civil war). In *Guangdong dangshi ziliao* (Source materials on party history in Guangdong), vol. 8. Guangzhou, 1986.

Dongfang zazhi (Asian journal), 1904-1905.

Dong xi yang kao mei yue tong ji zhuan (Eastern western monthly magazine, 1833-1838). Canton, 1833-1838. Reprint, Beijing: Zhonghua shuju, 1997.

Downing, C. T. *The Stranger in China*. vol. 2. Philadelphia: Lea & Blanchard, 1838.

Drucker, Alison R. "The Role of the Y.W.C.A. in the Development of the Chinese Women's Movement, 1890-1927." *Social Serve Review* 53 (Dec. 1979): 420-28.

Duffy, John. "History of Public Health and Sanitation in the West since 1700." In *The Cambridge World History of Human Disease*, ed. Kenneth Kiple. Cambridge, Eng.: Cambridge University Press, 1993.

"Easy Method to Prevent and Treat Cholera." *Yuehua bao* (Yuehua daily), July 14, 1932.

Editorial. "Chinese Women, to Demand Social Status!" *Shanghai minguo ribao* (Shanghai Republican daily), February 18, 1921.

Elman, Benjamin. *A Cultural History of Civil Examinations in Late Imperial China*. London: University of California Press, 2002.

____. *On their Own Terms: Science in China, 1550-1900*. Cambridge: Harvard University Press, 2005.

"Epidemic at Canton." *The Chinese Repository* 19 (1850): 288-343.

"Establishment of Schools for Blind and Deaf." *Shen bao* (Shanghai daily), Feb. 25, 1905.

Evans, David James. *Obstetrics: A Manual for Students and Practitioners*. New York: Lea, 1900.

Fairbank, John King, ed. *The Missionary Enterprise in China and America*. Harvard University Press, 1974.

Fan, Hong. *Footbinding, Feminism, and Freedom: The Liberation of Women's Bodies in Modern China*. Ilford, Essex: Frank Cass Publishers, 1997.

"Fangbian Hospital in West Canton." *Fangbian yuekan* (Fangbian monthly journal) 2 (1936).

"Fangbian Hospital's Entertainment Park." *Guangzhou minguo ribao* (Guangzhou Republic Daily), December 9, 1925.

Fee, Elizabeth and Dorothy Porter. "Public Health, Preventive Medicine and Professionalization: England and America in the Nineteenth Century." In *Medicine in Society: Historical Essays*, ed. Andrew Wear. Cambridge, England: Cambridge University Press, 1992.

Feng Ziyou. "Nü yishi Zhang Zhujun" (Female doctor Zhang Zhujun). In *Geming yishi* (Unofficial history of the revolution), ed. Feng Ziyou. Vol. 2. Taibei: Taiwan shangwu yinshuguan, 1965.

Feng Ziyou. *Geming yishi* (Unofficial history of the revolution). 3 vols. Shanghai: The Commercial Press, 1981.

Feuerwerker, Albert. *China's Early Industrialization: Sheng Hsuan-huai (1844-1916) and Mandarin Enterprise*. Cambridge, Mass.: Harvard University Press, 1958.

First Annual Report of the American Presbyterian Mission in the Island of Hainan, China for the Year 1893. Nodoa: Hainan Mission Press, 1894.

Flynt, Wayne, and Gerald W. Berkley. *Taking Christianity to China: Alabama Missionaries in the Middle Kingdom, 1850-1950*. Tuscaloosa: University of Alabama Press, 1997.

"From the Scholars and Merchants of the Entire Province of Kwangtung." *Chinese Repository* XVI (April 1847): 196.

Fullerton, Anna. *Nursing in Abdominal Surgery and Diseases of Women.* Philadelphia: P. Blakiston, 1891.

Fulton, Mary H. "Hackett Medical College for Women, Canton." *The China Medical Missionary Journal* XXIII, 5 (1909): 324-29.

Fulton, Mary H. *"Inasmuch": Extracts from Letters, Journals, Papers, Etc.* West Medford, Mass.: The Central Committee of the United Study of Foreign Missions, n.d.

Fulton, Mary H. to Doctor Boone, May 8, 1894, *The China Medical Missionary Journal* 8 (1894): 142-43.

Church at Home and Abroad (monthly). 24 vols. 1887-1898.

Gaynor, Lucy A. "A Nurses Association." *China Medical Journal* XXIII, 2 (March 1909): 118-20.

"General Letter." *Missionary Herald* XXXVI (March 1840): 82.

"General Report of the Department of the Public Health of the Canton Hospital." *Guangzhou weisheng* (Guangzhou health) 1 (October 1935): 155-57.

Gienow-Hecht, Jessica. "Cultural Transfer." In *Explaining the History of American Foreign Relations*, 2nd ed, ed. Michael J. Hogan and Thomas J. Paterson. New York, 2004.

Gilmartin, Christina. *Engendering China: Women, Culture, and the State.* Cambridge: Harvard University Press, 1994.

Goulet, Denis. *The Uncertain Promise: Value Conflicts in Technology Transfer.* New York: IDOC, 1977.

Graham, Gael. *Gender, Culture, and Christianity: American Protestant Mission Schools in China, 1880-1930.* New York: Peter Lang, 1995.

Graves, R. H. *Forty Years in China or China in Transition.* Baltimore: Woodward, 1895. Reprint, Scholarly Resource at Wilmington, Delaware, 1972.

_____."Some Personal Reminiscences of Thirty Years' Mission Work." *Chinese Recorder* XVII (November 1886): 421-35.

Gray, John Henry. *Walks in the City of Canton.* Hong Kong: De Souza, 1875.

Guangda yike zhou nian ji nian hao (The special issue of the first anniversary of the Medical School of Guangdong University). Guangzhou, Guangdong yike da xue yi xue yuan, 1926.

Guangdong gongyi xiaoyuan di ba, jiu zhou nian bu gao (Report on the eighth and ninth anniversary of Gongyi medical school). Guangzhou: Guangdong gongyi, 1918.

Guangdong gongyi xiaoyuan di shi yi, er zhou nian bu gao (Report on the eleventh and twelfth anniversary of Gongyi medical school). Guangzhou: Guangdong gongyi, 1924.

Guangdong gongyi yixue zhuanmen xuexiao, guoli guangdong daxue yike, zhongshan daxue yixueyuan biyeshen mingce, 1909-1955 (The graduate register of Guangdong medical school, medical department of national Guangdong university, and medical college of Zhongshan University). Guangzhou, 1962.

Guangdong jiating weisheng cujinhui gongzou nianbao (Annual report of the Association of Family Health Promotion of Guangdong). Guangzhou, 1933.

Guangdong jiating weisheng cujinhui gongzou nianbao (Annual report of the Association of Family Health Promotion of Guangdong). Guangzhou, July 1934-June 1935.

Guangdong minzheng gongbao (Guangdong civil government bulletin). Guangzhou: Guangdong minzhenju, 1929.

"Guangdong Province." *China Daily,* April 12, 1904.

Guangdong shengzhi: minzhen zhi (Annals of Guangdong Province: annals of civil administration). Guangzhou, Guangdong renmin chubanshe, 1993.

Guangdong shengzhi: weishen zhi (Annals of Guangdong Province: annals of the health administration). Guangzhou: Guangdong renmin chubanshe, 2003.

Guagndong shi bao (Guagndong news daily) 1911.

Guangdong wenshi ziliao (History and literature of Guangdong). Guangzhou: Guagndong sheng wenshi ziliao weiyuan hui. 34 vols., 1958-1991.

Guanghua biye tongxuehui tekan (Special issue of Guanghua medial alumni). Guangzhou, 1935.

Guanghua weisheng bao (Guanghua health journal). Guangzhou, 1918-1919.

Guanghua yishi hui tekan (Special issue of the Guanghua Medical School). Guangzhou, 1929.

Guanghua yishi weisheng zazhi (Guagnhua medical and health journal).

Guangzhou jibainien jiaoyu shiliao (Sources of education in Guangzhou in the past 100 years). Guangzhou: Wenshi ziliao weiyun hui, 1983.

Guangzhou shi dierrenmin yiyuan shi (The History of the Second Guangzhou Municipal Hospital, 1899-1999). Guangzhou: Guangzhou shi dierrenmin yiyuan yuanshi weiyuan hui 1999.

Guangzhou shi diyirenmin yiyuan shi (The History of the First Guangzhou Municipal Hospital, 1899-1999). Guangzhou: Guangzhou shi diyirenmin yiyuan yuanshi weiyuan hui 1999.

Guangzhou shi jingshen binyuan shi, 1899-1998 (The History of the Guangzhou Municipal Mental Hospital, 1899-1998). Guangzhou: Guangzhoushi jingshenbing yiyuan yuanshi weiyuan hui 1998.

Guangzhou shizheng zhangcheng ligui huibian (Collection of Regulations and Rules of Guangzhou Municipal Government). Guangzhou: Guangzhoushi zhengfu, 1924.

Guangzhou shizhi: Minzheng zhi (Annuals of Guangzhou: Annals of civil administration). vol. 10. Guangzhou: Guangzhou shizhi weiyuan hui, 2000.

Guangzhou shizhi: weishen zhi (Annuals of Guangzhou: Annals of health). Guangzhou: Guangzhou difang shi weihuan hui, 1997.

Guangzhou weisheng (Journal of Guangzhou health). Guangzhou, 1935.

Guangzhou wenshi ziliao (History and literature of Guangzhou). Guangzhou: Guangzhoushi wenshi ziliao weiyuan hui. 43 vols., 1961-1991.

Guangzhou zhinan (Guide to Canton). Shanghai: Shanghai xinhua shuju, 1919.

Guangzhou zhinan (Guide to Canton). Guangzhou: Guangzhoushi zhengfu, 1934.

Guangzhoushi ge yiyuan yange (History of the hospitals in Canton). Guangzhou, 1934.

Gulick, Edward V. *Peter Parker and the Opening of* China. Cambridge, Mass.: Harvard University Press, 1973.

"Hackett Medical College, Canton." *China Medical Journal* XLI, 7 (July 1927): 667-68.

"Hackett Medical College and Affiliated Institution." *China Medical Journal* XLIV (September 1930): 961-62.

"Hackett Medical College." *China Medial Missionary Journal* XV, 3 (July 1901): 243-44.

"Hackett Medical College: The Opening Ceremony." *The China Mail*, June 26, 1913.

Harding, Gardner L. *Present-Day China: A Narrative of a Nation's Advance.* New York, 1916.

He Xiaolian. *Xi yi dong jian yu wen hua tiao shi* (Introduction of Western medicine to China and cultural accommodation). Shanghai: Shanghai guji chubanshe, 2006.

Heinrich, Larissa N. *The Afterlife of Images: Translating the Pathological Body between China and the West.* Durham: Duke University Press, 2008.

Henry, B.C. "Strategic Importance of Lien Chow." *The Church at Home and Abroad* 6 (September 1889): 244.

Hershatter, Gail. *Women in China's Long Twentieth Century.* Berkeley: University of California Press, 2007.

Hirst, Fabian. *The Conquest of Plague: A Study of the Evolution of Epidemiology.* Oxford: Clarendon Press, 1953.

History of the South China Mission of the American Presbyterian Church, 1845-1920. Shanghai: The Presbyterian Mission Press, 1927.

Ho, Virgil K. Y. *Understanding Canton: Rethinking Popular Culture in the Republican Period.* New York: Oxford University Press, 2005.

Hofmann, J. Allen. "A Short Historical Sketch of Hackett Medical College and Affiliated Institutions." *The China Medical Journal* 8 (1926): 776-79.

Holden, R. *Yale in China: The Mainland 1901-1951.* New Haven, Conn.: Yale in China Association, 1964.

Hsiao, Kung-chuan. *A Modern China and a New World: K'ang Yu-wei, Reformer and Utopian, 1858-1927.* Seattle: University of Washington Press, 1975.

Hsueh, Chun-tu. *Hunag Hsing and the Chinese Revolution.* Stanford University Press, 1961.

Hu Xuanmin, *Construction of China's Public Health.* Shanghai: East Asia Library, 1928.

Huang, Philip C. *Liang Ch'i-ch'ao and Modern Chinese Liberalism.* Seattle: University of Washington Press, 1972.

Huang Zifang. "Zhongguo weisheng zhouyi" (On sanitation of China). *Zhonghua yixue zazhi* 13, no. 5 (1927): 339.

Huang Yanpei, *Yisui zhi Guangzhou* (One-year old of the city of Guangzhou). Guangzhou: Shanwu, 1922.

Huang Zhongye. "Tang Shiyi yaochang jianshi" (History of Tang Shiyi's Medical Factory). *Guangdong wenshi ziliao* (History and literature of Guangdong) 20 (1980): 95-104.

Huayan Zangxiang Yuezuan (The drawings of viscera of the Chinese and Europeans), Foshan, 1893.

Hunt, Michael. *The Making of a Special Relationship: The United States and China to 1914.* New York: Columbia University Press, 1983.

Hunter, Jane. *The Gospel of Gentility: American Women Missionaries in Turn-of-the-Century China.* New Haven: Yale University Press, 1984.

Hunter, W. *The "Fan Kwae" at Canto, Before Treaty Days 1825-1844.* London: Kean Paul, Trench, 1855.

"Impact of Epidemic on Business." *Yuehua bao* (Yuehua daily), June 21, 1932.

"Inserting Water into Meat." *Guangzhou Minguo ribao* (Guangzhou Republican Daily), September 19, 1925.

Inspectorate General of Chinese Imperial Customs, *Customs Medical Reports.* Shanghai: Statistical Department of the Inspectorate General of Customs, 1894.

Jackson, Beverley. *Splendid Slippers.* Berkeley, California: Ten Speed Press, 1997.

Jeanne Brand, *Doctors and the State.* Baltimore, Md.: John Hopkins University Press, 1965.

Jefferys, W. Hamilton, and James L. Mazwell. *The Disease of China.* Philadelphia: P. Blakiston's Son, 1910.

Jia Yuehan (John Kerr). *Huaxue chujie* (Elementary chemistry), 4 volumes, Yangcheng boji yiju, 1870.

____. "Lun neizhi" (On internal piles). *Wanguo gongbao* (Global news), March 5, 1881.

____. *Qizheng lunshu* (On special illness). Guangzhou: Yangcheng boji yiju 1886.

____. *Weisheng yaozhi* (Essentials of hygiene) Guangzhou: Yangcheng boji yiju, 1875. Reprint, 1884.

Jiang Yihua. *Lixing quefa de qimeng* (The Irrational enlightenment). Shanghai: Sanlian chubanshe, 2000.

Jin Baoshan. *Zhanshi defang weisheng xingzheng gaiyao* (Local health administration during the war). Chongqing: Zhongyang xunlian tuan dang zheng xunlian ban, 1940.

Jingzhong ribao (Alarm bell daily). Shanghai, 1904-1905. Taiwan, reprint, 1968.

"John G. Kerr Hospital for the Insane, Canton." *The China Medical Journal,* 41(1927): 164-68.

John G. Kerr Hospital for the Insane, Report for the Years 1907-1908. Canton: China Baptist Publication Society, 1909.

John G. Kerr Hospital for the Insane, Report for the Years 1916-1917. Canton: Wai Hing Printing, 1918.

John G. Kerr Hospital for the Insane, Reports for the Years 1918-1921. Canton: Wai Hing Printing, 1921.

Johnston, James F. *Chemistry of Common Life.* New York: D. Appleton and Company, 1853.

Johnstone, M. "Footbinding." In *Woman's Work in the Far East.* Shanghai: Presbyterian Mission Press, 1892.

Judge, Joan. *The Precious Raft of History: The Past, the West, and the Woman Question in China.* Stanford, California: Stanford University Press, 2008.

Kang Guangren. "Sino-British Alliance against Japan." *Zhixin bao* (China reformer) 45 (1898): 44-46.

Kang Tongbi. "Qingmo de buchanzu hui." (The Anti-footbinding society of the late Qing) *Zhongguo funü* (Chinese women), May 1957.

Kang Youwei. *Datong shu* (Great Harmony). 1902. Reprint, Beijing: Beijing guji chubanshe, 1956.

____. *Datong shu* (Great Harmony). 1902. Reprint, Zhengzhou: Zhongzhou guji chubanshe, 1998.

____. *Datong shu* (Great Harmony). Shanghai: Zhonghua shuju, 1935.

____. "Kannanhai zibian nianpu" (A self-compiled chronological biography of Kang Youwei). In *Wuxu bianfa* (The reform movement of 1898), ed. Jian Bozhang. Vol. 4. Shanghai: Shengzhou guoguang she. 1953.

____. *Kangnanhai zibian nianpu* (A self-compiled chronological biography of Kang Youwei). Beijing: Zhonghua shuju, 1992.

____. "Kang Nanhai nianpu." In *Wuxu bianfa* (The 1898 reform movement). Shanghai: Shanghai renmin chubanshe, 1972.

____. *Kang Youwei quanji* (Works of Kang Youwei), ed. Jiang Yihua. Vol. 3. Shanghai: Guji chubanshe, 1992.

____. *Kang Youwei quanji* (Works of Kang Youwei). Ed. Jiang Yihua. vol. 1. Shanghai: Guji chubanshe, 1987.

____. "On Parliament Government's Hands off Public Customs." In *Jindai zhongguoshiliao congkan* (Historical materials of modern China), ed. Shen Yulong. Vol. 38. Taiwan: The Wenhai Press, 1988.

____. "Qingjin funu chanzu jie." In *Wuxu bianfa* (The reform movement of 1898), ed. Jian Bozhang, 2: 243. Shanghai: Shanghai renmin chuban she, 1961.

____. "Qingjin funu chanzu jie." In Kang Youwei, *Kang Youwei wenxuan* (Selected works of Kang Youwei). Shanghai: Shanghai yuandong chubanshe, 1997.

____. "Riben shumu zhi" (Japanese Bibliography). In *Kang Youwei quanji*. (Works of Kang Youwei), ed. Jiang Yihua. Vol. 3, Shanghai: Guji chubanshe, 1992.

____. "Wuxu Chougao." In *Jindai Zhongguo shilao chongkan* (Collected primary sources in modern Chinese history), ed. Shen Yunlong. Taipei: Wenhai chubanshe 1966.

Kao, John J. *Three Millennia of Chinese Psychiatry*. New York: The Institute for Advanced Research in Asian General topic of insanity in traditional Chinese medicine, 1979.

Kaya, Ibrahim. "Modernity, Openness, Interpretation: A Perspective on Multiple Maternities." *Social Science Information* 43, 1 (2004): 49-50.

Kazuko, Ono. *Chinese Women in a Century of Revolution, 1850-1950*. Stanford, CA: Stanford University Press, 1989.

Kerr, J. G. "A Chinese Benevolent Association." *The China Medical Missionary Journal* 3, no. 4 (1889): 152-55.

____. *Medical Missions: At Home and Abroad*. San Francisco: A. L. Bancroft, 1878.

____. "Introductory—Medical, Missionaries in relation to the Medical Profession." *The China Medical Missionary Journal* 6, 3 (1890): 87-99.

____. "Visical Calculus in Canton Province, China, Including the Report of a Personal Experience in 1894 Operations." *The China Medical Missionary Journal* 8 (1894): 104-16.

____. "The Native Benevolent Institutions of Canton." *China Review* 2 (Sept./Oct. 1873), 88-95.

____. "Benevolent Institutions of Canton." *China Review* 3 (1874-1875): 108-114.

____. "Training Medical Students." *China Medical Missionary Journal* 3, 2 (1889): 135-40.

Kerr, J. G., and Grainger Hargreaver. "The Opium Question: Report of the Committee on the opium Traffic." *Chinese Recorder* 22 (August, 1891), 371-72.

Kerr, John. "Chinese Materia Medica." *China Medical Missionary Journal* 1, 2 (June 1887): 79-80.

____. "Opening of the Hong Kong College of Medicine for Chinese." *China Medical Missionary Journal* 1, 4 (December 1887): 169.

____. "The Bubonic Plague." *China Medical Missionary Journal* 3 (1894): 178-80.

____. "The Sanitary Condition of Canton." *China Medical Missionary Journal*, 2, no. 3 (September 1888): 134-35.

____. "Cleanliness." *China Medical Missionary Journal* 11, 3 (September 1888): 156-57.

____. "Preservation of Health A Duty." *China Medical Missionary Journal* 5, no. 1 (March, 1891): 1-2.

____. *"Report of the Medical Missionary Society in China for the Year 1860,"* *Report of the Medical Society's Hospital at Canton for the Year 1860.* Canton, Friend of China Press, 1861.

____. "Canton Mental Hospital." *Chinese Medical Missionary Journal* 12, 4 (1898).

____. "Report of the Medical Society's Hospital at Canton for the Year 1860." In Medical Missionary Society, *Report of the Medical Missionary Society in China for the Year 1860.* Canton, Friend of China Press, 1861.

____. "The Opium Habit." *China Medical Missionary Journal* 3, 2 (June 1889): 143-44.

Kerr, John G. "Small Feet." *Chinese Recorder and Missionary Journal,* June (1870), 22-33.

Kerr, John Glasgow. "History of Medical Missionary Society's Hospital, Canton." *China Medical Missionary Journal* 10, no.1 and no. 3 (1896): 55-7, 95-8.

____. "Is It an Advance?" *China Medical Missionary Journal* 3, 2 (1889): 66-67.

____. "Medical Missions." *Records of the General Conference of the Protestant Missionaries of China Held at Shanghai, May 10-24, 1877.* Shanghai, Presbyterian Mission press, 1878.

____. "Training Medical Students." *China Medical Missionary Journal* IV (1890): 137.

____. "Self-Support in Mission Hospitals." *China Medical Missionary Journal* 9, 3 (1895): 136.

"Killed by Cold Milk." *Guangzhou minguo ribao* (Guangzhou Republican daily), July 22, 1927.

Kirk, John. "Canton Branch," *The China Medical Journal* 23, 3 (March 1909): 202.

____. "Conference Address of Present of CMMA." *China Medical Journal* 39, 3 (March, 1925): 227-40.

Kobayashi, T. "Chang Chu-chün for Women's Rights." *Journal of the Oriental Society of Australia* II (1976): 62-80.

Koo, T. Z. "Educational Conditions and Student Life in China Today." In T. T. Lew, *China Today through Chinese Eyes.* London: Student Christian Movement, 1926.

Kuhne, John E. "The Leper Asylum at Tungkun." *China Medical Missionary Journal* 21, 1 (1907).

Kuisel, Richard F. *Seducing the French: The Dilemma of Americanization.* Berkeley, CA, 1993.

"Kung Yi Hospital and Medical school." *China Medical Journal* 39, 9 (September 1925), 853.

Kwok, Pui-Lan. "Chinese Women and Protestant Christianity at the Turn of the Twentieth Century." In *Christianity in China from the Eighteenth Century to the Present*, ed. Daniel H. Bays. Stanford: Stanford University Press, 1996.

Latourette, Kenneth S. *The Chinese: Their History and Culture*. New York: The Macmillan, 1929.

Lazich, Michael C. *E. C. Bridgman (1801-1861): America's First Missionary to China*. Lewiston: The Edwin Mellen Press, 2000.

Lee, Edward Bing-Shuey. *Modern Canton*. Shanghai: The Mercury Press, 1936.

Lee, James E. "China and Leprosy." *Chinese Recorder* 57 (1926): 856-61.

Lee T'ao. "Some Statistics on Medical Schools in China for the Year 1933-1934." *Chinese Medical Journal* 49 (1935): 894-902.

Lennox, William G. "The Distribution of Medical School Graduates in China." *Chinese Medical Journal* 46 (1932): 406.

Lerner, Barron H. "The University of Pennsylvania in China: Medical Missionary Work, 1905-1914." BA Thesis, University of Pennsylvania, 1982.

"Letter from Doctor Parker, August 1, 1844." *Missionary Herald* XLI (February, 1845): 53.

Leung, Angela Ki Che. *Leprosy in China: A History*. New York: Columbia University Press, 2009.

Levenson, Joseph R. *Liang Ch'i-ch'ao and the Mind of Modern China*, 2d ed. Berkeley: University of California Press, 1970.

Levy, Howard S. *Chinese Footbinding: The History of a Curious Erotic Custom*. New York, 1996.

Lew, T. T. *China Today through Chinese Eyes*. London: Student Christian Movement, 1926.

Li Chunrong. "The Essential Issue of Meat Inspection." *Guangzhuo weisheng* 1 (October 1935), 25-29.

Li Duo. "History of Guangdong Gongyi Medical College and its Hospital." *Guangzhou wenshi ziliao* (History and literature of Guangzhou) 21 (1980): 169-174.

Li, Jingwei, and Yan Liang bian. *Xi xue dong jian yu zhongguo jin dai yi xue si chao* (Introduction of Western learning and modern medical ideology in China). Wuhan: Hubei ke xue ji shu chubanshe, 1990.

Li Tingan. "A Public Health Report on Canton." *National Medical Journal of China* 11 (1925): 324-75.

Li Xisu, *Liangqichao zhuan* (Biography of Liang Qichao). Beijing: Renmin chubanshe, 1993.

Li Yuning, and Zhang Yufa, eds. *Jindai zhongguo nuquan yundong shiliao 1842-1911* (Documents on the women's rights movement in modern China, 1842-1911). 2 vols. Taipei, 1975.

Li Zonghuang. *Xin Guangdong guancha ji* (Observation of new Guangdong). Shanghai: Shanwu, 1922.

Li Zonghuang. *Mofan zhi Guangzhoushi* (The model city of Guangzhou). Shanghai: Shanwu, 1929.

Lian, Xi. *The Conversion of Missionaries: Liberalism in American Protestant Missions in China*. University Park: Pennsylvania State University Press, 1997.

Liang Longzhang. *Bianzheng qiuzhen* (Seeking the truth). Guangzhou: Weixin yinwu ju, 1905.
Liang Peiji. "To Organize Public Lectures on Medicine to Enforce Cleanness Policy." *Yixue weisheng bao* (Medical and hygienic daily) 7 (1909): 55.
Liang Qichao. "Baoguohui yanshuoci"(Speech on safeguard of Congress). *Zhixin bao* (China reformer journal) 55 (April 1898): 718-19.
____. "Baoguohui yanshuoci"(Speech on safeguard of Congress). In *Yinbingshi heji* (Writings from the ice-drinker's studio) 1 (1898): 27-29. Reprint, Beijing: Zhonghua shuju, 1989.
____. "Bianfa tongyi--lun nü xue." In *Yinbingshi heji* (Writings from the ice-drinker's studio) 1 (1896): 37-43. Reprint, Beijing: Zhonghua shuju, 1989.
____. "Biography of Six Martyrs." In Chen Yinci, *Liang Qichao's Academic Works* (Shanghai: East China Normal Press, 1998), 449.
____. "Diqiu renshi ji."(The record of human beings and the events). *Qingyi bao* (China discussion), vol. 41.
____. "Du xixueshu fa" (On reading books of Western learning). In Liang Qichao, *Yinbingshi heji* (Writings from the ice-drinker's studio). Beijing: Beijing daxue chubanshe, 2005, 1159-1170.
____. "Jiechanzu hui xu" (Discussion of the Anti-Footbinding Society) *Shiwubao* 16 (December 1, 1896): 12a-12b.
____. "Jiechanzu hui xu." (Discussion of the Anti-Footbinding Society) in Liang Qichao, *Yinbingshi wenji* 1 (1896): 120-22. Reprint, Beijing: Zhonghua shuju, 1989.
____. "Kang Guangren zhuan" (Biography of Kang Guangren). *Qingyi bao* (China discussion journal) 6 (Feb. 1899).
____. "Kang Guangren zhuan" (Biography of Kang Guangren). In *Yinbingshi heji* (Liang Qichao's works). Beijing: Zhonghua shu ju, 1989.
____. "Kang Guangren zhuan" (Biography of Kang Guangren). In *Liang Qichao wenji* (Liang Qichao's works), ed. Chen Weiliang. Beijing: Yanshan chubanshe, 1997.
____. "Kang Guangren zhuan" (Biography of Kang Guangren). In *Liang Qichao wenxuan* (Liang Qichao's selected works), ed. Xia Shaohong. Vol. 1. Beijing: Zhongguo guangbodianshi chubanshe, 1992.
____. *Kang Youwei zhuan* (Biography of Kang Youwei). Beijing: Tuan jie chubanshe, 2004.
____. "Kang Youwei zhuan" (Biography of Kang Youwei). In *Liang Qichao wenji* (Liang Qichao's works), ed. Chen Weiliang. Beijing: Yanshan chubanshe, 1997.
____. *Liang Qichao jiashu* (Liang Qichao's home letters). Beijing: Zhongguo wenlian chubanshe, 2000.
____. *Liang Qichao quanji* (Works of Liang Qichao). Beijing: Beijing chubanshe, 1999.
____. "Lun guohui"(On Parliament). In Liang Qichao, *Yinbingshi wenji* (Works of Liang Qichao). Vol. 3. Beijing; Zhonghua shuju, 1989.
____. "Shibian buchanzu hui jianming zhangcheng."(Concise rules of the experimental Anti-Footbinding Society). *Shiwubao* 25 (April 11, 1897).
____. "Shibian buchanzu hui jianming zhangcheng"(Concise rules of the experimental Anti-Footbinding Society). In Liang Qichao, *Yinbingshi heji* 1 (1897): 20-23. Reprint, Beijing: Zhonghua shuju, 1989.

____. "Xixue shumubiao"(A list of Western books). In Liang Qichao, *Yinbingshi heji* (Writings from the ice-drinker's studio). Beijing: Beijing daxue chubanshe, 2005.

____. *Yinbingshi heji* (Writings from the ice-drinker's studio). Vols. 1-3. Beijing: Zhonghua shuju, 1989.

____. *Yinbingshi wenji* (Collected writings from the ice-drinker's studio). Shanghai, 1916.

____. "Yixue shanhui xu" (The Discussion of the medical philanthropy society), *Shiwubao* 38 (August 11, 1897).

____. "Yixue shanhui xu." In *Wuxu bianfa* (the 1898 reform). *Zhongguo jindai shi ziliaocongkan*. Vol. 4. Shanghai: Shanghai renmin chubanshe, 1961.

____. "Yixue shanhui xu." In Liang Qichao, *Yinbingshi heji* (Writings from the ice-drinker's studio). Vol. 1 (1897): 68-72. Reprint, Beijing: Zhonghua Shuju, 1989.

Liang Yiwen. "Recollections of Xiage Medical College for Women," *Guangzhou wenshi ziliao* (History and literature of Guangzhou) 35 (1986): 147-151.

Liangguang jinhui yiyuan sanshi zoulien tekan (The special issue of the thirtieth year anniversary of two guang baptist hospital. Guangzhou: Liangguang jinxinhui yiyuan, 1947.

Lin Zexu. *Lin Zexu quanji* (Lin Zexu's works). Vol. 7. Fuzhou: Haixia wenyi, 2002.

"Ling Nam Hospital, Canton," *Chinese Medical Journal* 4 (1926).

Little, Archibald. *In the Land of the Blue Gown*. New York: Appleton, 1909.

Liu Jucai. *Zhongguo jindai fu nu yundong shi* (History of Modern Chinese women movement) Beijing: Zhongguo funu chubanshe, 1989.

Liu Xinchi. *Zhengguang guangron jianshi* (A brief history of true light seminar). Hong Kong, Heyintang chubanshe, 1972.

Liu Zhiqin, ed. *Jindai Zhongguo shehui wenhua bianqianlu* (History of modern social and cultural changes in China). Vol. 3. Hangzhou: Zhejiang chubanshe, 1998.

Lo Hsianglin. *Sun Yat Sen's University Days*. Taipei: The Commercial Press, 1954.

Lo Jung-pang, ed. *K'ang You-wei: A Biography and a Symposium*. Tucson: University of Arizona Press, 1967.

Lodwick, Kathleen L. *Crusades against Opium: Protestant Missionaries in China, 1874-1917*. Lexington: University Press of Kentucky, 1996.

Lorber, Judith. *Women Physicians: Careers, Status, and Power*. New York: Tavistock, 1984.

Lu Meiyi. *Zhongguo Funu yundong, 1840-1921* (China's Women Movement, 1840-1921). Zhengzhou: Henan Remin chubanshe, 1990.

Lu Yu. "Guangzhou's Fangbian Hospital." *Guangdong wenshi ziliao* (History and literature of Guangdong) 8 (1963): 139-150.

Lucas, AnElissa. *Chinese Medical Modernization: Comparative Police Continuities, 1930-1980s*. New York: Praeger, 1982.

Lutz, Jessie Gregory, ed. *Pioneer Chinese Christian Women: Gender, Christianity, and Social Mobility*. Bethlehem: Lehigh University Press, 2010.

Ma Junwu. "Zhang Zhujun zhuan." *Xinmin congbao* (Renovation of the people journal) 7 (May 1902).

Macpherson, Kerrie. *A Wilderness of Marshes: The Origins of Public Health in Shanghai, 1843-1893.* Oxford University Press, 1987.

Man-Cheong, Iona. *The Class of 1761: Examinations, the State and Elites in Eighteenth-Century China.* Stanford: Stanford University Press, 2004.

"Mary W. Niles." *Chinese Recorder* 64, 3 (March 1933), 176.

McCandliss, Carolyn. *Of No Small Account: the Life of John Glasgow Kerr.* The Washang Press, 1996.

McCartney, J. Lincoln. "Neuropsychiatry in China; A Preliminary Observation." *China Medical Journal* XL, 7 (July 1926): 617-26.

"Medial Bolus Made and Contributed by Commander-in-Chief Chen." *Yuehua bao,* June 28, 1932.

"Medical Missionary Society: Regulations and Resolutions, Adopted at a Public Meeting Held at Canton on the 21st of February, 1838." *Chinese Repository* VII (March, 1838).

Medical Missionary Society. *The Medical Missionary Society in China: Address, With Minutes of Proceedings.* Canton, 1838.

____. *The Hospital Reports of the Medical Missionary Society in China for the Year 1839.* China: the Office of the Chinese Repository, 1840.

____. *Report of the Medical Missionary Society in China: The Fourteenth Report of the Ophthalmic Hospital, Canton.* Canton: The Chinese Repository, 1848.

____. *Report of the Medical Missionary Society in China for the Year 1860.* Canton, Friend of China Press, 1861.

____. *Report of the Medical Missionary Society in China for the Year 1861.* Canton: Tung-Hing Office, 1862.

____. *Report of the Medical Missionary Society in China for the Year 1866.* Canton, China: The Medical Missionary Society, 1867.

____. *Report of the Medical Mission Society in China for the Year 1868.* Canton: The Medical Missionary Society, 1869.

____. *Report of the Medical Missionary Society in China for the Year 1871.* Canton, China: The Medical Missionary Society, 1872.

____. *Report of the Medical Missionary Society in China for the Year 1880.* Canton, China: The Medical Missionary Society, 1881.

Medical Times and Gazette, 1860.

Minden, Karen. *Bamboo Stone: the Evolution of a Chinese Medical Elite.* Toronto: University of Toronto Press, 1994.

Ming Sum School for the Blind, 50th Anniversary Report, 1889-1939. Hong Kong: Standard Press, 1939.

Minli bao (People's daily), 1910-1915.

Minsheng ribao (People's living daily), 1912-1913.

Minutes of the Annual Meeting of the Medical Missionary Society in China. Macao: N. P. 1857.

"Missions in China." *The Church at Home and Abroad* 15 (February 1894): 113.

"Missionary Conference." *North China Herald* 16 (May 1890): 602-3.

Missionary Herald, ed. American Board of Commissioners for Foreign Missions, Boston, monthly, 1821-1951.

Missionary Review of the World, February 1935.

Moldow, Gloria. *Women Doctors in Gilded-Age Washington: Race, Gender, and Professionalization.* University of Illinois Press, 1987.

Nanhai Xianzhi (A gazetteer of Nanhai county). 17 vols. 1691-1911.
National Medical Journal, 1925-1929.
Neizheng nianjian (Yearbook of internal administration). Shanghai: Shangwu yinshuguan, 1935.
Ng, Vivien W. *Madness in Late Imperial China: From Illness to Deviance.* University of Oklahoma Press, 1990.
Niles, Mary W. "Native Midwifery in Canton." *China Medical Missionary Journal* 4, no. 2 (1890): 52.
Niles, Mary. "Plague in Canton." *China Medical Missionary Journal* 8, no (June 1894): 116-19.
North China Herald. Shanghai, weekly, 1850-1867.
Notable American Women 1607-1950: A Biographical Dictionary, vol. 1 (A-F). Cambridge, Mass.: The Belknap Press of Harvard University Press, 1971.
Noyes, Harriet. *A Light in the Land of Sinim-Forty-Five Years in the True Light Seminar, 1872-1917.* New York: Fleming Revell, 1919.
____. "Fifty Years in the Foreign Field." *The Continent,* May 13, 1920.
"Officials Sent by the Health Department to inspect Man-made Ice," *Guangzhou Minguo ribao* (Guangzhou Republican Daily), September 23, 1925.
Oldt, Frank. "Purity Campaign, Canton." *China Medial Journal,* 1923, 776.
Oldt, F. "Scientific Medicine in Kwangtung." *Chinese Medical Journal* 48 (1934): 663-71.
Olpp, G. "The Rhenish Mission Hospital, Tungkun." *China Medical Missionary Journal* 23, no. 3 (1909).
"On Anti-Leper Campaign in Canton." *Mafeng jikan* (Leper Quarterly) 7(1933): 3.
"On Fangbian Fund Raising." *Guangzhou minguo ribao* (Guangzhou Republic Daily) February 3, 1926.
"On Tongren Dispensary in 1877." *Sheng bao* (Shanghai daily), December 22, 1877.
"One Case of Disease discovered by the Bureau of Public Health." *Guangzhou minguo ribao* (Guangzhou Republican Daily), July 21, 1924.
"Order of Guangdong Governor Li Yaohan." In *Guangdong Gongbao* (Guangdong Bulletin). March 11, 1918.
Pang Suk Man. "To Save Life and Spread the True Light: the Hackett Medical College for Women in China (1899-1936)." MA Thesis, Hong Kong Baptist University, 1998.
Pan Zhuo'an. "Sili Guangdong Guanghua yixue yuan shilue" (The outline of the history the private Guangdong Guanghua Medical College). *Guangzhou wenshi ziliao* (History and literature of Guangzhou) 26 (1982): 139-155.
Papers Relative to Hospitals in China. Boston: J. R. Butts, 1841.
Parker, Peter. "Eleventh Report of the Ophthalmic Hospital at Canton for the Term Commencing 1st January and Ending 17th June, 1840." *Chinese Repository* XIII (May 1844): 240-43.
Parker, P. "First Quarterly Report of Ophthalmic Hospital at Canton." *Chinese Repository* 4 (February 1836): 461-62.
____. "Second Quarterly Report of Ophthalmic Hospital at Canton." *Chinese Repository* 5 (May 1836): 31-33.
____. "Third Quarterly Report of Ophthalmic Hospital at Canton." *Chinese Repository* 5 (August 1836): 187-88.

____. "Fourth Quarterly Report of Ophthalmic Hospital at Canton." *Chinese Repository* 5 (November 1836): 187-88.

____. "Seventh Quarterly Report of Ophthalmic Hospital at Canton." *Chinese Repository* 6 (January 1838): 438-39.

Parker, Peter. *Statements Respecting Hospitals in China. Preceded by a Letter to John Abercrombie.* Glasgow: Maclehose, 1842.

Parker, P, and E. C. Bridgman. "Suggestions for the Formation of A Medical Missionary Society." *Chinese Repository* 5 (December 1836): 369-71.

Parker, Peter. "Thirteenth Report of the Ophthalmic Hospital at Canton, Including the Period from the 1st January, 1844 to the 1st July, 1845" *Chinese Repository* XIV, 10 (October 1845): 452-57.

Parker, Theodore. *Genealogical and Biographical Notes of John Parker of Lexington and His Descendant.* Worcester, Mass.: Press of C. Hamilton, 1893.

Peake, Cyrus H. *Nationalism and Education in Modern China.* New York, 1932.

Pearson, A. "Report submitted to the Board of the National Vaccine Establishment, respecting the introduction of the practice of vaccine inoculation into China, AD 1805," *Chinese Repository* 2 (May 1833), 35-41.

Pearson, Veronica. "The Development of Modern Psychiatric Services in China 1891-1949." *History of Psychiatry* 2 (1991): 133-47.

Peter, W.W. *Broadcasting Health in China.* Shanghai: Presbyterian Mission Press, 1926.

"Plague News." *Shen bao* (Shanghai daily), July 3, 1894.

"Plague News." *Shen bao* (Shanghai daily), June 14, 1894.

Polachek, James. *The Inner Opium War.* Cambridge, MA: Harvard University Press, 1992.

Preston, T. J. "The Chinese Benevolent Institutions in Theory and Practice." *Chinese Recorder and Missionary Journal* 28 (1907): 245-53.

"Proposal for Government Funding for Support of Leprosariums and Overseas Study of Lepers." *Mafeng jikan* (Leper Quarterly) 10 (1935): 1.

"Prospectus of Medical Colleges and Schools." *Chinese Medical Journal* 49 (1935): 998-1034.

"Public Health." *Guangzhou Nianjian* (Guangzhou year book) 13 (1935): 2-5.

Qi Shihe, ed. *Choban yiwu shimo, daoguan chao* (The history of foreign affairs during the reign of Daoguan). 6 vols. Beijing: Zhonghua shuju, 1964.

Qingyi bao (China discussion journal), 1894-1898.

Qishier hang shang bao (Commercial daily of all sorts of occupations), 1913-1926.

"Quiet in Shopping Centers and Crowed in Clinics after Discovery of the Bubonic Disease." *Guangzhou minguo ribao* (Guangzhou republican daily), May 16, 1924.

Graves, R. H. *Forty Years in China or China in Transition.* Baltimore: Woodward, 1895. Reprint, Scholarly Resource at Wilmington, Delaware, 1972.

Ramesh, J., and C. C. Weis, eds. *Mobilizing Technology for World Development.* New York: Praeger, 1979.

Rankin, Mary. *Early Chinese Revolutionaries: Radical Intellectuals in Shang and Chekiang, 1902-1911.* The Cambridge University Press, 1971.

Razag, Adolf. *Leprosy in South China: Its Present Condition and Treatment with Special Suggestions.* Canton, 1907.

"Recent Investigation of Cholera in this City." *Yuehua bao* (Yuehua daily), June 26, 1932.

"Records of the General Conference of the Protestant Missionaries of China. Shanghai, Presbyterian Mission Press, 1878.

Reeves, Caroline Beth. "The Power of Mercy: the Chinese Red Cross Society, 1900-1937." Ph. D. Dissertation, Harvard University, 1998.

"Regulations of the Opium Addict Treatment." In *Sun Yisen boshi yixueyuan yilan* (Information on the Sun Yat-sen Medical College). Guangzhou, 1935.

"Regulations of the Schools for Blind and Deaf," *Shen bao* (Shanghai daily), October 16, 1907.

Renshaw, Michelle Campbell. *Accommodating the Chinese: The American Hospital in China, 1880-1920.* New York: Routledge, 2005.

"Reports of C.M.M. A. Biennial Conference, 1925." *China Medial Journal* 39, 2 February 1925): 151-68.

"Report of the Medical Missionary Society." *Chinese Repository* 12 (April 1843): 190-191.

"Report on Income and Expenses in 1935." *Fangbian yuekan* (Fangbian monthly journal) 1 (1936).

Rhoads, Edward. *China's Republican Revolution: The Case of Kwangtung, 1895-1913.* Cambridge, Mass.: Harvard University Press, 1975.

Ride, L. T. *Sun Yat Sen.* Hong Kong: The Hong Kong Press, 1970.

Robb, Isabel Hampton. *Nursing: Its Principles and Practice for Hospital and Private Use.* Cleveland: E. C. Koeckert, 1906.

Rogaski, Ruth. *Hygienic Modernity: Meanings of Health and Disease in Treaty-Port China.* Berkeley, California: University of California Press, 2004.

Ross, Margaret Taylor. "A Child Welfare Clinic." *China Medical Journal* 41 (1927): 250-54.

Ross, Robert M. "Mental Hygiene." *The China Medical Journal* (January 1926): 8-13.

Rouji Duanna Hushi Xuexiao Zhang cheng, 1934-1935 (The catalog of the Rouji Hospital and Turner Nursing School, 1934-1935). Guangzhou, 1935.

Rubinstein, Murray A. *The Origins of the Anglo-American Missionary Enterprise in China, 1807-1840.* Lanham, Md: Scarecrow Press, 1996.

Schlesinger, Arthur M. Jr."The Missionary Impulse and Theories of Imperialism." In *The Missionary Enterprise in China and America,* ed. John Fairbank.

Selden, C. C. "Work Among the Chinese Insane and Some of its Results." *China Medical Missionary Journal* 19, 1(1905): 2-3.

____. "The John G. Kerr Refuge for the Insane: The Opening of the Insane." *China Medical Journal* 23, 1 (March 1909): 82-91.

____. "A Work for the Insane in China." *The Chinese Recorder,* May 1909, 262.

____. "II. Treatment of the Insane," *China Medical Journal* 23, 4 (July 1909): 221-22.

____. "III. Treatment of the Insane," *China Medical Journal* 23, 6 (November 1909): 374.

____. "The Story of the John G. Kerr Hospital for the Insane." *Chinese Medical Journal* 52 (November 1937): 705-14.

Selden, Charles C. "The Life of John G. Kerr: Forty-three Years Superintendent of the Canton Hospital." *Chinese Medical Journal* 2 (1935): 364-76.

Selden, Chas C. "The Need of More Hospital for Insane in China." *China Medical Journal* 24 (1910): 326.

Shen bao (Shanghai daily), 1877-1901.

Shen Yanshen. "Recollections of Rouji Hospital." *Guangzhou wenshi ziliao* (History and literature of Guangzhou) 45(1993): 144-158.

Shimin Yaolan (Essentials for citizens). Guangzhou: Guangdongsheng gonganju, 1934.

Shiwu bao (Chinese progress journal), Shanghai, 1896-1898.

Shizheng gongbao (Municipal administration bulletin).

Shixue. "Nüzi hongsshizi hui zi kejing." *Minli bao* (People's daily), October, 10, 1911.

Sili Guangdong Guanghua yixue yuan gai kuang (The outline of the private Guangdong Guanghua Medical College history). Canton, Guanghua yixueyuan, 1936.

Sinn, Elizabeth. *Power and Charity: The Early History of the Tung Wah Hospital.* Hong Kong: Oxford University Press, 1989.

Smith, Arthur Henderson. *Chinese Characteristics.* Shanghai: North China Herald and S.C. & C Gazette, 1890.

Spence, Jonathan. *To Change China: Western Advisers in China 1620-1960.* Boston: Little, Brown and Company, 1969.

____. *The Search for Modern China.* New York: W.W. Norton, 1990.

Starr, Paul. *The Social Transformation of American Medicine.* New York: Basic Books, 1982.

Stevens, George B. and W. Fisher Markwick. *The Life, Letters, and Journals of the Rev. and Hon. Peter Parker, M.D., Missionary, Physician, and Diplomatist, the Father of Medical Missions and Founder of the Ophthalmic Hospital in Canton.* Boston: Congregational Sunday School and Publishing Society, 1896.

Stoddard, John. *China.* Chicago: Belford, Middlebrook & Company, 1897.

"Stop Rumors." *Shen bao* (Shanghai daily), July 4, 1894.

"Students of Midwifery School Demanded for Improvement of Treatment." *Guangzhou minguo ribao* (Guangzhou Republican daily), March 27, 1927.

Sun Yat-sen, *Knapped in London.* London: China Society, reprint,1969.

Sun Zhongshan. *Sun Zhongshan quanji* (Works of Sun Yat-sen). Vols. 1-6. Beijing: Zhonghua shuju, 1981-1986.

Sun Zhongshan. *Sun Zhongshan xuanji* (Selected works of Sun Yat-sen). Beijing: Beijing Renmin, 1956.

"Superstitious Activities during the Cholera Epidemic." *Yuehua bao* (Yuehua daily), June 25, 1932.

"Swan." *China Medical Missionary Journal* 34 (1920): 106-107.

Swan, J. M. "Opium Poisoning Treated with Atropia-Sulphate." *China Medical Missionary Journal* 3, 2 (June 1889): 143-44.

Swan, John. "Caesarean Section." *China Medical Journal*, September 1893, 173-77.

Swan, John M. "South China Medical College." *China Medical Journal* 23, 5 (September 1909): 303-306.

Tang Zhijun. *Kang Youwei zhenglun. shangji* (Kang Youwei's political essays, part 1). Beijing: Zhonghua shuju, 1981.

Tao S. M. "Medical Education of Chinese Women." *Chinese Medical Journal* 47 (1933): 1010-28.

Tao Shanming. "Zhongguo zi yixue jiaoyu." *Zhonghua yixue zazhi* (Chinese medical journal) 19, no. 6 (1933): 849-64.

Teresa, Meade, and Mark Walker, eds. *Science, Medicine and Cultural Imperialism.* New York: St. Martin's Press, 1991.

The China Year Book, 1929-30. Kraus reprint, 1969.

The Isle of Palms, Sketches of Hainan: The American Presbyterian Mission. Shanghai: the Commercial Press, 1919. Reprint, the Garland Publishing, 1980.

"The Southern Plague." *The North China Herald*, June 15, 1894.

The Hundred Years History of the Canton Hospital. The Organization Committee of the Sun Yat-sen Medical College, Lingnan University, Canton, 1935.

The Twentieth Annual Report of the Board of Foreign Missions of the Presbyterian Church in the United States of America. New York, 1857.

The Twenty-Fourth Annual Report of the Board of Foreign Missions of the Presbyterian Church in the United States of America. New York, 1861.

Thomas, R. D. *A Trip on the West River.* Canton, China: Baptist Publication Society, 1903.

Thomson, J. C. "Medical Missionaries to China." *China Medial Missionary Journal* 1 (January 1887): 45-49.

____. "Medical Publication in Chinese." *China Medical Missionary Journal* 1, 3 (September 1887), 115.

Thomson, J. Oscar. "A Century of Medical Work in China." *The Missionary Review of the World* 2 (February 1935), 55-59.

____. "The Medical Educational Situation in Canton." *China Medical Journal* 40 (1926): 790-97.

____. "To Editor of the Chinese Medical Journal." *China Medial Journal* 26, 3 (May 1912), 208.

Thompson, Laurence G. ed. *Ta T'ung Shu: The One-World Philosophy of K'ang Yu-we.* London: George Allen & Unwin, 1958.

Todd, O. J. "Co-Operation with the Chinese in Medical Education Work." *China Medical Journal* XXVII (May 1913): 143-47.

Tsin, Michael T. W. *Nation, Governance, and Modernity in China, Canton, 1900-1927.* Stanford, California: Stanford University Press, 1999.

Tucker, Sara. "A Mission for Change in China: The Hackett Women's Medical Center of Canton, China, 1900-1930. In *Women's Work for Women: Missionaries and Social Change in Asia*, ed. Leslie A. Flemming. Boulder: Westview, 1989.

____. "The Canton Hospital and Medicine in Nineteen Century China, 1835-1900." Ph.D. dissertation, Indiana University, 1982.

"Twenty-Eighth Annual Meeting of the Board." *Missionary Herald* (November 1837), 473.

Twenty-Eighth Annual Report of the American Board of Commissioners for Foreign Missions Boston, 1837.

Tyau, Min-Ch'ien T. Z. *China Awakened.* New York: The Macmillan, 1922.

"University Medical School, Canton." *China Medical Missionary Journal* 23, 6 (1909): 406-07.

Vogel, Ezra F. *Canton under Communism: Program and Politics in a Provincial Capital, 1949-1968.* Harvard University Press, 1969.

Vorst, Van. *A Girl from China* (Soumay Tcheng). New York: Frederick A Stokes Company, 1926.

Wagnleiter, Reinhold. *Coca-Colonization and the Cold War: The Cultural Mission of the United States in Austria after the Second World War,* trans., Diana M. Wolf. Chapel Hill, N.C.: University of North Carolina Press, 1994.

"Walks About Canton-Extracts from a Private Journal." *Chinese Repository* 4, no. May (1835): 45.

Waley, Arthur. *The Opium War Through Chinese Eyes.* London, England: George Allen & Unwin, 1958.

Wang Hongjin. "Qingmo Minchu de Guangdong yihui zhengzhi" (Guangdong parliamentary politics at the end of the Qing and beginning of the Republic). In *Guangdong xinhai geming ziliao* (Materials on Guangdong in the 1911 Revolution). Guagndong: Guangdong renmin chubanshe, 1981.

Wang Kangnian shiyou shuzha (Collection of Wang Kannian's letters). Shanghai: Guji chubanshe, 1986.

Wang, Meixiu. *Jidu jiao shi* (The history of the Protestant movement). Nanjing: Jiangsu ren min chubanshe, 2006.

Wang, Qingren. *Yilin gaicuo* (Correction of medical theory).1830. Reprint, Beijing: Zhongguo zhongyi yao chubanshe, 1995.

Wang Xincai. *Liang qichao dushu shengya* (Liang Qichao's reading books). Wuhan: Changjiang wenyi, 1998.

Wang Yilian. *Xiagu zhongyun: Zheng Shiliang chuan* (Biography of Zheng Shiliang). Taipei: Modern China, 1983.

Wang, Ping. *Aching for Beauty: Footbinding in China.* Minneapolis: University of Minnesota Press, 2000.

Wanguo Gongbao (Global news), 1876-1881.

Watts, Sheldon. *Epidemics and History: Disease, Power, and Imperialism.* New Haven and London: Yale University Press, 1997.

Wei Waiyang. *Xuanjiao shiye yu jindai zhongguo* (The missionary enterprises and modern China). Taibei: Yuzhou guang chuban she, 1992.

Weisheng tongji (Health statistics). Chongqing: Neizheng bu, 1938.

Whitney, H. T. "A Quarterly Medical Journal in Chinese." *China Medical Missionary Journal* 2, 2 (June 1888): 59.

Wibur, C. Martin. *The Nationalist Revolution in China, 1923-1928.* Cambridge: Cambridge University Press, 1983.

"Witness in the Epidemic." *Yuehua bao* (Yuehua daily), June 28, 1932.

Wong K. Chimin and Wu Lien-teh. *History of Chinese Medicine: Being a Chronicle of Medical Happenings in China from Ancient Times to the Present Period.* Tientsin: Tientsin Press, 1932.

____. *History of Chinese Medicine.* Shanghai: National Quarantine Service, 1936.

Wong, K. C. "A Short History of Psychiatry and Mental Hygiene in China." *Chinese Medical Journa* 68 (Jan.-Feb. 1950).

"Work Report of the Department of Health of Guangzhou in 1926." *Shizheng gongbao,* 579 (1926): 71-77.

"Work Report of the Department of Health in July." *Guangzhou minguo ribao* (Guangzhou Republican daily), August 17, 1927.

Wu Liande. "Zhongguo Gonggong weisheng zhi jingfei wenti" (The expenditure issue of public health in China), *Zhonghua yixue zazhi* (Chinese Medical Journal) 15, 4 (1929): 351-54.

Wu Lien-teh. "A Hundred Years of the Modern Medicine in China." *China Medical Journal* 50, 2 (February 1936).

Wu limin. *Liang Qichao he ta de er numen* (Liang Qichao and his children). Shanghai: Shanghai renmin chubanshe, 1999.

Wu, Ziming. ed. *Zhongguo jiao hui da xue li shi wen xian yan tao hui lun wen ji* (Essays on historical archives of Christian higher education in China). Hong Kong: Chinese University Press, 1995.

Wuhan shizhi: weishen zhi (Annuals of Wuhan: Annals of health) Wuhan: Wuhan difang shi weiyuan hui, 1993.

Wuhan wenshi ziliao (History and literature of Wuhan). Wuhanshi wenshi ziliao weiyuan hui, vol. 9, 2002.

Wuxu bianfa (the 1898 reform movement). Ed. Jian Bozhang. Shanghai: Shenzhou guoguangshe, 1953.

Wuxu bianfa (the 1898 reform movement). *Zhongguo jindai shi ziliaocongkan.* Vol. 4. Shanghai: Shanghai renmin chubanshe, 1961.

Wylie, A. *Memorials of Protestant Missionaries.* Shanghai: American Presbyterian Mission Press, 1867.

Xiage nu yi xue xiao zhang cheng (The regulations of xiage medical school for women). Guangzhou: Xiage nuyi xue xiao, 1919.

Xiage yike da xue sanshi zhounian jinian lu (The thirtieth anniversary of the Hackett Medical College for Women). Guangzhou: Xiage yike daxue, 1929.

Xian Weisun. *Shuyi liuxingshi* (History of the plague) Guangzhou: the Health and Disease Control Station of Guangdong Province, 1989.

Xinmin congbao (Journal of New Citizen), 1900-1909.

Xinxue yuebao (Monthly journal of new learning), 1897-1898.

Xiong Yuezhi. *Xixue dongjian yu wan qing shehui* (The dissemination of Western learning and late Qing society). Shanghai: Shanghai renmin chubanshe, 1994.

Yadong cong bao (East Asia journal).

"Yangchen quanchu yapian gonghui guitiao" (Regulations on quitting smoking opium in Canton). *Wanguo congbao* (Global news) 380 (1876).

Yangchen wanbao (Guangzhou evening daily).

Yao, Esther Lee. *Chinese Women, Past and Present.* Mesquite, TX: Ide House, 1983.

Ye Nezhen. "Record on Guangzhou's New Drug Industry and Anya Drug Factory." *Guangzhou wenshi ziliao* (History and literature of Guangdong) 30 (Guangzhou): 152-160.

Yie Fangpu. "Biography of Medical Doctor John Kerr." *Yixue weishe bao* (Medical and hygienic daily) 4 (1908): 25-30.

"Yijiu ninwu nian fanmei aiguo yundong" (The 1905 anti-American patriotic campaign). In *Jindaishi ziliao* (Sources of modern history), vol. 1. Beijing, 1954.

Ying, Hu. *Tales of Translation: Composing the New Woman in China, 1899-1918.* Stanford: Stanford University Press, 2000.

Yip, Ka-che. *Health and National Reconstruction in Nationalist China: The Development of Modern Health Services, 1928-1937,* Monograph and Occasional Paper Series. Ann Arbor: Association for Asian Studies, 1995.

Yixue weisheng bao (Journal of Medicine and Hygiene), 1908-1918.

You, Heng. "Alice Carpenter and the Chinese Ming Sum School for the Blind." *Journal of Presbyterian History* 58 (Winter 1990): 259.

Yu Xinzhong. *Qing dai Jiang nan de wen yi yu she hui : yi xiang yi liao she hui shi de yan jiu* (Plague and society in south China during the Qing Dynasty). Beijing: Zhongguo ren min da xue chu ban she, 2003.

____. ed. *Qing yi lai de ji bing, yi liao he wei sheng: yi she hui wen hua shi wei shi jiao de tan suo* (Disease, medicine, and hygiene since the Qing Dynasty: A study from a social and cultural perspective). Beijing: Sheng huo, du shu, xin zhi san lian shu dian, 2009.

Yuehua bao (Yuehua daily), 1926-1932.

Zaccarini, M. Cristina. *The Sino-American Friendship as Tradition and Challenge: Dr. Ailie Gale in China, 1908-1950*. Bethlehem: Lehigh University Press, 2001.

"Zai weisheng Jiangxi hui chengli hui shang de yanshuo." *Jingzhong ribao* (Alarm bell daily), May 24 and 25, 1904.

Zhang Daqing. *Zhongguo jin dai ji bing she hui shi: 1912-1937* (A social history of diseases in modern China). Jinan: Shandong jiao yu chubanshe, 2006.

Zhang Zhidong. *Quan xue pien* (Leaning). Taipei: Wenhai, reprint, 1967.

____. "Buchanzuhui xu." *Zhixin bao* 27 (1897): 8-9.

____. China's *Only Hope: An Appeal by her Greatest Victory, Chang Chih-tung*. Trans. Samuel I. Woodbridge. New York: F. H. Revell, 1900.

____. "Jiechanzu hui zhangcheng xu" (Discussion of the rules of the Anti-Footbinding Society). *Shiwubao* 38 (August 11, 1897).

Zhang Zhujun. "Lun chuzhi nuzi jundui"(On organizing women's army). *Dongfang zazhi* (Asian journal) 8, no. 10 (1912): 6.

____."Announcement of the Women's Association for Security through Learning." *Jingzhong ribao* (Alarm bell daily), April 1904.

____. "Zai weisheng jiangxi hui chengli hui shang de yanshuo" (Speech at the meeting of the establishment of the association of the health study). *Jingzhong ribao* (Alarm bell daily), May 24 and 25, 1904.

____. "Nüzi xinxue baoxian hui xu" (Introduction to women society of learning and security). *Zhongguo xinnüjie* (New Chinese women's world) (Tokyo) 4 (May 1907), in *Xinhai geming jianshinianjianshi lun chunji* (A collection of the essays published ten years before the 1911 Revolution). Vol. 2. Shanghai: Shanlian chubanshe, 1977.

"Zhang Zhujun's Speech, President of the Red Cross Society." *Shen bao* (Shanghai daily), December 27, 1911.

"Zhang Zhujun's Speech, President of the Red Cross Society." *Shen bao* (Shanghai daily), December 30, 1911.

Zheng Entao. *Liangguangjinxinhui yiyuan baogaoshu* (Report on the two guang Baptist hospital). Guangzhou: Liangguangjunhui yiyuan, 1946.

Zheng Guanying. "Nujiao"(Women education). In *Zheng Guanying ji* (The Works of Zheng Guanying). Vol. 1. Shanghai: Shanghai renmin chubanshe, 1982.

Zheng Guanying. *Shengshi weiyan* (Words of warning to an affluent age).1892. Reprint, Taipei: Xueheng shuju, 1965.

Zheng Guanying. "Yidao"(Medical essences). In *Zheng Guanying ji* (The Works of Zheng Guanying). Vol. 1. Shanghai Renmin chubanshe, 1982.

Zheng Guanying. *Zheng Guanying ji* (The Works of Zheng Guanying). Ed. Xia Dongyuan. 2 vols. Shanghai: Shanghai renmin chubanshe, 1982, 1988.

Zheng Guanying. *Zhongwai weisheng yaozhi* (Chinese and foreign essentials to hygiene). 1890, 1895.

Zheng Hong. *Guoyi zhishang: Bainian zhongyi chenfu lu* (Tragedy of Chinese medicine in the past one hundred years of ups and downs). Guangzhou: Guangdong keji chu ban she, 2010.

____. "Wanqing zhongxi yi de weitong yu lunzheng" (Discussion on the Sino-Western medical integration during the late Qing dynasty*). Nanfang dushi bao* (South China city daily), October 21, 2009, B14.

Zheng, Yangwen. *The Social Life of Opium in China: A History of Consumption from the Fifteenth to the Twentieth Century.* Cambridge University Press, 2005.

Zhixin bao (China Reformer journal), 1897-1898.

Zhongguo Guomindang zhongyang tongjichu (Central statistical bureau of the Guomindang), *Minguo ershier nian zhi jianshe* (Reconstruction in 1933). Nanjing: Central Statistical Bureau of the Guomindang, 1934.

Zhongguo jindai xueji shiliao (Sources of the educational system of modern China). Vol. 2. Shanghai: Huadong shifan daxue chubanshe 1989.

"Zhongguo nüzi yaojiu canzheng de xianshen" (The first cry for Chinese women's participation in government). *Jiefan hua bao* (Liberation pictorial journal) 5 (Shanghai, May 1920).

Zhongguo xinnüjie (New Chinese Women's World) (Tokyo) 1907.

Zhongping. "Lun shantung yiyuan yi she xiyi," (On adoption of Western medicine by charitable hospitals). *Zanyu yuekan* 22 (1922): 4

Zhu Qinglan. *Guangdong tongzhi gao* (The first draft of Guangdong history). 5 vols. Reprint, Beijing: Zhonghua quan guo tu shu guan wen xian suo wei fu zhi zhong xin, 2001.

Zi xi cu dong: Malixun mu shi lai Hua er bai zhou nian ji nian (Meeting of East-West culture: celebrating the 200th anniversary of Rev. Robert Morrison's arrival in China). Xianggang: Xianggang Zhongwen daxue chong ji xue yuan zong jiao yu zhongguo shehui yanjiu zhong xin, 2007.

Zou Jincheng. "Zheng shiliang chun lue" (A short biography of Zheng Shiliang). *Guangdong wenshi ziliao* (History and literature of Guangdong) 63 (1986): 127-133.

Index